Outcome Research and the Fut‚ Psychoanalysis

Outcome Research and the Future of Psychoanalysis explores the connection between outcome studies and important and complex questions of clinical practices, research methodologies, epistemology, and sociological consider-ations. Presenting the ideas and voices of leading experts in clinical and extra-clinical research in psychoanalysis, the book provides an overview of the state of the art of outcome research, its results and implications. Furthermore, its contributions discuss the basic premises and ideas of outcome research and in which way the contemporary Zeitgeist might shape the future of psychoanalysis.

Divided into three parts, the book begins by discussing the scientific basis of psychoanalysis and advances in psychoanalytic thinking as well as the state of the art of psychoanalytic outcome research, critically analyzing so-called evidence-based therapies. Part II of the book contains exemplary research projects that are discussed from a clinical perspective, illustrating the dialogue between researchers and clinicians. Lastly, in Part III, several psychoanalysts review the importance of critical thinking and research in psychoanalytical education.

Thought-provoking and expertly written and researched, this book is a useful resource for academics, researchers and postgraduate students in the fields of mental health, psychotherapy, and psychoanalysis.

Marianne Leuzinger-Bohleber was Director in charge of the Sigmund-Freud-Institut (SFI) in Frankfurt a.M., Germany (2001–2016), now senior scientist at SFI and University Medicine Mainz, as well as staff member of the IDeA Center in Frankfurt a.M.

Mark Solms is Chair of Neuropsychology at the University of Cape Town and Groote Schuur Hospital and Chair of the Research Committee of the International Psychoanalytical Association.

Simon E. Arnold is a Research Assistant at the Sigmund-Freud-Institut in Frankfurt a.M., Germany.

Outcome Research and the Future of Psychoanalysis

Clinicians and Researchers in Dialogue

Edited by Marianne Leuzinger-Bohleber,
Mark Solms and Simon E. Arnold

Routledge
Taylor & Francis Group

LONDON AND NEW YORK

First published 2020 by Routledge

2 Park Square, Milton Park, Abingdon, Oxon OX14 4RN
605 Third Avenue, New York, NY 10017

Routledge is an imprint of the Taylor & Francis Group, an informa business

First issued in paperback 2021

British Library Cataloguing-in-Publication Data
A catalogue record for this book is available from the British Library

Library of Congress Cataloging-in-Publication Data
A catalog record has been requested for this book

ISBN: 978-0-367-23666-3 (hbk)
ISBN: 978-1-03-217466-2 (pbk)
DOI: 10.4324/9780429281112

Typeset in Bembo
by Wearset Ltd, Boldon, Tyne and Wear

Contents

Contributors

Carolina Altimir is Professor of Psychology, Universidad de Las Américas, with a PhD from the Universidad Católica de Chile. She is the Deputy Director at the Center for Psychotherapy Research, CIPsi, Santiago de Chile.

Simon E. Arnold, Dipl.-Psych. is research associate at the Sigmund Freud Institut in Frankfurt a.M. He studied psychology, literary studies, art history and philosophy in Konstanz, Paris, and Beer Sheva. His research interests include clinical psychoanalysis and the history of science—especially neurology, forensics and psychiatry—social psychology and critical theory. Currently he works on a study on trauma and psychosocial support for refugees and is part of a research group on the aftermath of the Holocaust on Jewish and non-Jewish Germans. He is member of the *Gesellschaft für psychoanalytische Sozialpsychologie* and writes a column on the quotidianity of myths.

Ulrich Bahrke, is a PD Dr. med. for Psychiatry and Psychotherapy and psychoanalyst (DPV/IPA) at the Sigmund-Freud-Institut in Frankfurt a.M., Germany.

Manfred E. Beutel, Prof. Dr. med., is the Director of the Clinic for Psychosomatic Medicine and Psychotherapy University Medicine Mainz (since 2004), and the Postgraduate Training Program for psychodynamic psychotherapy at the Johannes Gutenberg University Mainz, Germany. He has conducted numerous psychotherapy trials, especially RCTs on the efficacy of psychodynamic psychotherapy (online and offline). He co-edits the series of psychodynamic treatment manuals (Hogrefe, Göttingen).

John F. Clarkin, PhD, is Clinical Professor of Psychology in Psychiatry at the Weill Cornell Medical College, New York City. He serves as the Co-Director of the Personality Disorders Institute (PDI) of the New York Presbyterian Hospital, the university hospital of Cornell and Columbia. Dr. Clarkin is the author of numerous articles and books on psychopathology, differential treatment planning, and personality disorders. He has worked with Dr. Otto Kernberg and the interdisciplinary members of the

PDI since 1980 in a concentrated effort to empirically investigate the symptom patterns, traits, and neurocognitive functioning in patients with borderline personality disorder, and relate these findings to a focused treatment approach. Dr. Clarkin is a past president of the international Society for Psychotherapy Research (SPR). He has served on study groups at the National Institute of Mental Health (NIMH), and is a reviewer for major journals such as the *American Journal of Psychiatry*, *Journal of Personality Disorders*, and *Personality Disorders: Theory, Research and Treatment*.

Esther Dreifuss-Kattan PhD, PhD CB-ATR, was president of the New Center for Psychoanalysis in LA from 2016 to 2018, is a senior faculty member, and chair of the Archival Committee. She holds a PhD in Psychooncology/ Art Therapy and a PhD in Psychoanalysis. Her book published by Routledge in 2016 is called *Art and mourning: The role of creativity in healing trauma and loss*. It addresses the creative mourning work of different, mostly Modernists artists. Her new book *Cancer and Creativity: A Psychoanalytic Guide to Therapeutic Transformation* written in collaboration with seven artists/cancer survivors and was published by Routledge in November 2018. For 16 years she has led an art-psychotherapy-based support group for adult cancer patients and survivors at the Simms/Mann UCLA Center for Integrative Oncology. Her psychoanalytic and psychotherapy practice is in West Los Angeles. Dreifuss-Kattan is also a practicing artist and curator of art exhibitions.

Morris N. Eagle, PhD, is Distinguished Faculty Member, New Center for Psychoanalysis (NCP) and Professor Emeritus, Derner Institute of Advanced Psychological Studies, Adelphi University. He is Former President of the Division of Psychoanalysis, American Psychological Association (APA) and Co-chair (with Linda Goodman) of Research Education Section of the Department of Psychoanalytic Education (American Psychoanalytic Association). He is recipient of the New York Attachment Consortium Award for his contribution to interface between attachment theory and psychoanalysis (2002) and the Sigourney Award (2009). He was awarded for Distinguished Scientific Achievement (Division of Psychoanalysis, APA). He is elected Fellow of Royal Society of Canada and Diplomate in Psychoanalysis for the American Board of Professional Examiners in Psychology and was Erikson Scholar in Residence at the Austen Riggs Center (1993-1994). He is editor of *Psychological Issues*, on the Board of Editors of *Journal of the American Psychoanalytic Association, Psychoanalytic Psychology, Psychoanalysis & Contemporary Thought, American Journal of Psychotherapy*, as well as at the Advisory Board of *Journal of the American Psychoanalytic Association*. He is author and editor of 10 books, about 150 journal articles and chapters in edited books and more than 150 presentations. In addition, he is a private practice in psychoanalytic psychotherapy.

Robert N. Emde, Emeritus Professor of Psychiatry at the University of Colorado, School of Medicine, has a CV that lists over 300 publications in the fields of early socio-emotional development, sleep research, infant mental health, diagnostic classification, early moral development, evaluation of early childhood intervention, psychoanalysis, behavioral genetics, and research education.

Mareike Ernst MSc. Psych. is a research psychologist working at the University Medical Center Mainz (Dept. of Psychosomatic Medicine & Psychotherapy).

Georg Fiedler, Dipl.-Psych., is a research assistant at the University Medical Centre Hamburg-Eppendorf, Germany (1990–2016). He is Secretary of the National Suicide Prevention Program (2002–2015), co-responsible for the BMG project "Suicide Prevention Germany—Current Status and Perspectives." In 2018 he was honored with the Hans Rost Prize of the German Society for Suicide Prevention.

Linda S. Goodman, PhD is a psychoanalyst and clinical psychologist in private practice in Los Angeles, California. She is a senior faculty member of the New Center for Psychoanalysis. As president of the Los Angeles Psychoanalytic Society and Institute she fostered the successful merger of LAPSI and SCPSI and served as inaugural co-president of the New Center for Psychoanalysis. She has chaired or co-chaired the LAPSI & NCP Research Committee collectively over 20 years, now co-chairing it with Morris Eagle, PhD. With Linda Mayes, M.D. and Stuart Hauser, MD, PhD she originated the APsaA Research Poster Session and co-chaired it for 12 years. She currently (with Morris Eagle) co-chairs the Research Education Section of APsaA Department of Psychoanalytic Education, and has developed a yearly panel "Research Education Dialogues" at the National Meeting.

Les Greenberg, PhD. He co-founded emotion-focused therapy (EFT). He is also the director for the Emotion-Focused Therapy Clinic housed at York University. Greenberg co-founded the Society of the Exploration of Psychotherapy Integration (SEPI) and the Society for Constructivism in Psychotherapy (SCP). He is the author of several books, including *Emotion-Focused Couples Therapy: The Dynamics of Emotion, Love and Power* and *Emotion-Focused Therapy for Depression*. Greenberg has been recognized for his contributions to psychology with the Distinguished Contribution to the Profession from the Canadian Psychological Association, and the Distinguished Research Career award from the International Society for Psychotherapy Research.

Simone Hauck, MD, MSc, PhD, is an assistant professor and preceptor of the psychiatry residence program at the Universidade Federal do Rio Grande do Sul (UFRGS/HCPA), Brazil. She is Coordinator of the Psychoanalysis and Psychodynamic Psychotherapy Research Group.

Martin Hautzinger is Professor of Psychology at the Eberhard Karls University Tübingen. Since 1996 he has been Head of the Clinical Psychology and Psychotherapy working group at the Department of Psychology and the local Psychotherapeutic Outpatient Clinic; partly responsible for the behavioral therapy institutes TAVT and TAKT. He has numerous publications, relating in particular to affective disorders and psychotherapy research.

Juan Pablo Jiménez, is a Professor of Psychiatry at Universidad de Chile, Doctor Med. University of Ulm, Germany. He is a Director at the Millennium Institute for Research on Depression and Personality, MIDAP, Santiago de Chile.

Horst Kächele, Prof. Dr. Dr., studied medicine in Marburg, Leeds (England), and Munich (1963–1969) and trained in psychoanalysis at the Ulm Institute of Psychoanalysis (IPA, 1970–1975). He was Chair of Department Psychosomatic Medicine and Psychotherapy at the Faculty of Medicine Ulm University and since 2010 has been a Professor at International Psychoanalytic University Berlin.

Lisa Kallenbach, Dipl.-Psych., was a research associate (2010–2017) at the SFI with a focus on the LAC Study. Since 2014 she has taught at the Frankfurt Psychoanalytical Institute (FPI), and is a Federal candidate spokeswoman for the DPV.

Johannes Kaufhold, Dipl.-Psych., is a psychoanalyst in Frankfurt a.M. In 1993–1999 he was a research associate at the Institute for Psychoanalysis of the Goethe University Frankfurt, an in 2000–2005 was a research assistant at the Department of Psychosomatic Medicine and Psychotherapy of the Goethe University Hospital. Since 2012 he has collaborated in research on the LAC Study.

Richard D. Lane, M.D., PhD, is Professor of Psychiatry, Psychology and Neuroscience at the University of Arizona. A clinical psychiatrist and psychodynamic psychotherapist with a PhD in Experimental Psychology, he was one of the first researchers to perform functional brain imaging studies of emotion in the 1990s and continues studies on emotion, emotional awareness and neurovisceral integration to the present using fMRI. His research on emotion, the brain and heart disease has been funded by a variety of sources including K and several RO1 grants from NIH. He is the author of 180 papers and book chapters. As an educator he served as director of the psychotherapy curriculum for psychiatric residents at the University of Arizona for over two decades and has received seven awards for teaching and mentoring. He was President of the American Psychosomatic Society from 2005-2006, elected member of the American College of Neuropsychopharmacology, Distinguished Life Fellow of the American

Psychiatric Association and elected Honorary Fellow of the American College of Psychoanalysts.

Falk Leichsenring, DSc, is Professor of Psychotherapy Research in the department of Psychosomatics and Psychotherapy at the University of Giessen. He is a psychologist and a training and supervising analyst (DGPT). Falk Leichsenring has carried out several randomized control trials and meta-analyses on the efficacy of psychodynamic therapy. He has developed treatment manuals for anxiety disorders, depressive disorders obsessive-compulsive disorder, post-traumatic stress disorder, and personality disorders. The focus of his research is on the evidence base of psychodynamic therapy. Falk Leichsenring has published numerous articles in research journals, as well as books and book chapters. He was awarded the Heigl-Award for Psychotherapy Research (2005), the Hamburg Prize for Research on Personality Disorders (2006) and the Adolf-Ernst-Meyer-Award (2011) for Psychotherapy Research.

Marianne Leuzinger-Bohleber, Prof. Dr. Phil., Professor emeritus of Psychoanalysis at the University Kassel. She was the Director in charge of the Sigmund-Freud-Institut (SFI) (2001–2016) and a Senior Scientist at the SFI and at the University of Mainz; Teaching Analyst (DPV/IPA); Visiting professor at University College London; Co-Chair for Europe of the Research Board of International Psychoanalytical Association (IPA). She was awarded with the Mary Sigourney Award 2016 and the Haskell Norman Prize for Excellence Awarded in Psychoanalysis 2017. She works on clinical and empirical research in psychoanalysis, adolescence, psycho-analytic Developmental Psychology, Early Prevention.

Reed Maxwell is a licensed clinical psychologist and clinical assistant professor of psychology in psychiatry at University of Kansas Medical Center.

Alexa Negele, Dr. Phil., Dipl.-Psych. She was a research associate at the SFI in Frankfurt a.M. with a focus on the LAC Study. She is a psychoanalyst with her own practice in Frankfurt a.M.

Joshua Pretsky is Associate Clinical Professor of Psychiatry at the David Geffen School of Medicine at UCLA where he is the founding director of the concentration in psychodynamic psychotherapy and immediate past-president of the Psychiatry Clinical Faculty Association. He is a senior faculty member at the New Center for Psychoanalysis where he is a past chair and longstanding member of the research committee. He maintains a full-time private practice of psychiatry and psychotherapy in Los Angeles with a focus on accelerated experiential psychodynamic psychotherapy and holistic psychiatry.

Clara Raznoszczyk Schejtman, PhD, is a Permanent Professor, Director of Research and Community programs, Faculty of Psychology University de Buenos Aires. Training analyst Argentine Psychoanalytic Association, IPA.

Jonathan Shedler, PhD is known internationally as an author, consultant, and master clinician and teacher. His article "The efficacy of psychodynamic psychotherapy" won worldwide acclaim for establishing psychoanalytic therapy as an evidence-based treatment. He is a leading expert on personality styles and disorders and their treatment. Dr. Shedler leads professional workshops nationally and internationally and consults to clinicians, organizations, and U.S. and international government agencies.

Mark Solms is Professor of Neuropsychology at the University of Cape Town, South Africa, President of the South African Psychoanalytical Association, Director of the Science Department of the American Psychoanalytic Association, Co-chair of the International Neuropsychoanalysis Society and Chair of the Research Committee of the International Psychoanalytical Association. He was awarded with the Mary Sigourney Award in 2011.

Julia F. Sowislo earned her PhD in Psychology from the University of Basel, Switzerland. She is also a Swiss-state licensed psychotherapist (psychodynamic psychotherapy). Currently, she functions as a Visiting Researcher with the Personality Disorder Institute (Weill Cornell Medical College, New York) founded through the Swiss National Science Foundation. Her main current research interest lies in empirically studying the relation of different aspects of self-esteem to object–relation models of personality.

Harriet Wolfe, M.D., is President-elect of the IPA, Clinical Professor of Psychiatry at the University of California San Francisco School of Medicine, and Training and Supervising Analyst at the San Francisco Center for Psychoanalysis. Her scholarly interests include organizational processes, clinical application of neuroscientific research, female development and therapeutic action. She teaches analysts-in-training, psychiatric residents and junior faculty psychodynamic understandings of severely ill patients and the value of listening to listening in the clinical setting. She has a private practice of psychoanalysis, psychoanalytic psychotherapy, and couples and family therapy in San Francisco.

Introduction

Outcome research and the future of psychoanalysis

Marianne Leuzinger-Bohleber and Simon E. Arnold

A basic question

Can outcome research save the future of psychoanalysis? This question—the original title of a Sandler Research Conference, held in Los Angeles at the Children's Hospital in early May 2018 (local host: Bradley Peterson, MD) and a recurrent theme throughout our volume—refers to the view of some clinical colleagues, scholars in the field of psychotherapy research and health policy-makers. For them, the future of psychoanalysis in times of evidence-based medicine depends on proving the outcome of treatments for different patient groups. In fact, it implies that psychoanalysis would have no future without competing in this race and that it is a matter of pure survival. Such prophecies of doom are not new: speaking of the future, we will take a moment and look back on the history of psychoanalysis, and some tendencies in psychoanalytical research, before giving an overview of the contributions to the volume, you are about to read.

But let's take one step at a time and remember the backstory of this volume: in the 1990s an international psychoanalytic research conference was brought to life by Annemarie and Joseph Sandler, with the support of Arnold Cooper, Robert Wallerstein, Peter Fonagy, and many more, as a productive answer to a changing Zeitgeist in the realm of science. It has—together with the Research Training Program of the International Psychoanalytic Association (IPA) in London that was founded five years later—contributed essentially to embedding psychoanalysis in a new way in the world of science and in the general public.

Therefore the Sandler Conferences are closely connected to the topic of this volume: the founders of the conference have been convinced that empirical research, and particularly outcome research, would prove to be essential for the future of psychoanalysis. However, as we will discuss in this introduction, not all psychoanalysts are sharing their view. Empirical outcome research was controversial in the psychoanalytical community at that time—and it still is today. Thus one central aim of the Sandler Conferences was and still is the dialogue between researchers and clinicians. Joseph and Annemarie Sandler, both experts in the so-called conceptual research in psychoanalysis,

were two of the most successful bridge-builders between the world of
psychoanalytic researchers on the one hand, who often are engrossed in the
academic discourse and the clinicians on the other hand, working in their
private offices and having their professional exchange almost exclusively in
their psychoanalytical institutions.

The potential danger of splitting between researchers and clinicians has
interesting historical roots. In the following sections, we are developing some
thoughts on these splits. However, of course the historical remarks must
remain very fragmentary within the frame of this introduction.[1] We must
confine ourselves to a few thoughts on this complex topic that are of interest
to this volume. We will focus on some developments in Germany[2] (and in
particular in Frankfurt a.M.) to highlight in an exemplary way some problematic ruptures and polarizations between clinicians and (empirical) researchers,
especially in outcome research, due to the traumatic history of psychoanalysis
in the twentieth century.[3]

Clinical and extraclinical research in psychoanalysis—some historical remarks

The beginnings ...

George Makari (2008) impressively traces back the origins of psychoanalysis
to the beginning of the twentieth century and shows its entrenchment in
European cultural and intellectual history. He argues that Freud succeeded in
integrating various trends of biology, physiology, psychophysics, and psychology
at the time. For instance, the controversies surrounding a new understanding
of psychopathology around Charcot at the world-famous Salpêtrière Hospital
in France, as well as the scientific study of human sexuality by Krafft-Ebing,
Ehrenfels, Weinberger, Moll, Hirschfeld, and others into his theories of
psychosexual development, the unconscious and the psychodynamics of
mental disorders (see Makari, 2008, p. 120). Moreover, in this scientific orientation Freud was strongly influenced by Darwinism, which saw man as an
organism driven by needs that he tries to satisfy under specific environmental
conditions. Therefore, Freud defined "*Triebe*" (drives) at the border between
the somatic and the psychic. He understood psychological qualities, the
developmental stages of sexuality and the ego functions as the product of a
long evolutionary history in which man continuously adapted to inner and
outer realities (cf. also Jones et al., 1960; Gay, 1988; Zaretsky, 2004, pp. 473ff.;
Whitebook, 2010).

One of the great achievements of Freud in discovering psychoanalysis is,
undisputedly, that he kept up with the natural sciences of his time, but also
integrated so-called humanities and cultural sciences. Freud, as a young man,
was very interested in philosophy and other humanities before he turned to the
natural sciences with a remarkably violent emotional reaction. In the laboratory

at the Physiological Institute of Ernst Brücke, he got to know a strictly positivistic understanding of science that attracted him throughout his life. Nevertheless, Freud later turned away from the neurology of his time, because he recognized its limits in understanding the psyche. With the *Interpretation of Dreams* (1900), he defined psychoanalysis as *pure psychology*. However, he continued to see himself as a physician who observed complex clinical phenomena like a natural scientist. According to Joel Whitebook (2010), his desire for a precise "empirical" examination of hypotheses and theories protected Freud from his own inclination to wild speculation. As a "philosophical physician" he was thus able to establish a new "specific science of the unconscious"—psychoanalysis.

Makari (2008) as well as Zaretsky (2004) give detailed accounts how, even in the early days of psychoanalysis, Freud and his followers tried to find a way between, on the one hand, an open, innovative discussion, with constant questioning so-called "truths"—as they characterized a scientific discourse—and, on the other hand, the search for a common identity, the specific characteristics of "psychoanalysis."

According to Makari (2008), this effort of psychoanalysis has been a key to its success. Freud followed a gut feeling and stuck to his understanding of psychoanalysis in times of great conflicts—both content-related and institutional. He resisted integrating psychoanalysis either into the world of medicine or into that of philosophy and the humanities and therefore retained its autonomy as a scientific discipline. In 1909 Freud considered integrating psychoanalysis into the medical organization *Internationaler Verein für medizinische Psychologie und Psychotherapie* of August Forel or even into the *Orden für Ethik und Kultur*. Fortunately, he decided during the Sylvester night 1910, to found his own organization, the International Psychoanalytical Association (IPA, see Falzeder, 2010). With this decision, the independence of psychoanalysis as a scientific discipline with its own research methodology and institution was protected. Afterward, Freud always emphasized that psychoanalysis did not deserve to be "swallowed up" by medicine. Instead he said, "as a 'deep-psychology', a theory of the mental unconscious, it can become indispensable to all the sciences which are concerned with the evolution of human civilization and its major institutions such as art, religion and the social order" (Freud, 1926, p. 248).

However, as Michael Schröter (2019) argues for the years 1918 to 1932, the Viennese group around Freud was characterized by a continuing openness towards the academic world, psychiatry, and other sciences.

> Unlike Berlin (or Germany in general), in Vienna there were major overlaps between the representatives of academic psychiatry and psychoanalysis. This was largely due to the chair-holder Julius Wagner-Lauregg, who despite his personal resentment of psychoanalysis gave his academic staff the freedom to engage in research on it.
>
> (Schröter, 2019, p. 290, translation MLB)

Schröter (2019) discusses three exponents of this concatenation: Otto Plötzl,[4] Paul Schilder, and Heinz Hartmann. All of them played a central part outside their therapeutic offices in working on empirical confirmation of psychoanalytic theory and encouraging further development. Other well-known psychoanalysts such as Helene Deutsch, Hermann Nunberg, and Erwin Stengel had positions in psychiatry or at medical departments of the Viennese University. Felix Deutsch was a doctor of internal medicine, Josef Karl Freidjung worked with children and adolescents, and Charlotte and Karl Bühler were famous professors in Psychology. Hans Kelsen was a full professor of state and administrative law and August Aichhorn and Lili Roubiczek (Peller) were devoted to education and social work. All of them were either psychoanalysts themselves or interested in the interdisciplinary dialogue with psychoanalysis, at that time the new, challenging science of the unconscious.

As an example, Schröter (2019) depicts the Association for Applied Psychopathology and Psychology, founded in 1920, as a forum for lively and unusual discussions. Their aim was to promote the study and application of psychopathological and scientific knowledge to practical and social life, to cultural research and history. Erwin Stansky, Professor at the Neurological Psychiatric University Clinic, was in charge of the discussion and organized a series of lectures by psychoanalysts (Bernfeld, Ferenczi, Aichhorn, and Schilder) and non-psychoanalysts (Allers, Kelsen, and Stransky, etc.). Afterward he was very proud and described the events as the first serious academic discussion, at least in the German-speaking world, in which clinicians and psychoanalysts participated. Stransky formulated a wish: "May both—but especially psychoanalysts—descend from their towers! Intolerance and science are incompatible" (Stransky & Dattner, 1922, p. 1, quoted after Schröter, 2019, p. 282, translation MLB).

Within the framework of this introduction, we can only mention that problems of empirical research in psychoanalysis were raised already during these early controversial discussions that are still relevant today. For example, Heinz Hartmann gave a lecture on *Empirism in Psychoanalysis*. His talk was followed by fierce controversies on the scientific understanding of psychoanalysis and tensions in the dialogue with the academic-scientific community (e.g., Hartmann, Pappenheim, & Stranksky, 1931). According to Schröter (2019, pp. 284ff.), after some years it became apparent that there was no common ground on which the older generation of psychoanalytical practitioners impressed by their therapeutic experiences (and faithfully bound to Freud) could meet with methodically trained and methodically demanding academics and scientists. However, it is historically interesting that in Vienna many psychoanalysts and other researchers endeavored to create a common ground with the non-psychoanalytical scientific world and—despite all the difficulties just mentioned—to not simply ignore academic and cultural discourses. In contrast, according to Schröter (2019), there were hardly any crossing borders in Berlin. The psychoanalytical community in Berlin concentrated much more on internal education or theory development—and the "internal differentiation" of psychoanalysis (Binnendifferenzierung), as Schröter calls it.⁵

The traumatic history of psychoanalysis and some of its epistemological and methodological consequences

The divergent developments in Vienna as well as in Berlin were brought to a tragic end by the rise of National Socialism and anti-Semitism in the early 1930s: many psychoanalysts were persecuted and murdered in the concentration camps, a few emigrated and others, especially the non-Jewish Germans, "adapted" to Nazi-Germany. The many traumatic events due to National Socialism and the Shoah, the following of Nazism of German psychoanalysts as well as the death of Sigmund Freud—all this had a decisive influence on the development of psychoanalysis and led, for example, to the fact that to this day hardly any coherent history of psychoanalysis as a movement and a science exists in the various countries (e.g., Young-Bruehl & Schwartz, 2011).

Bohleber (2019) proceeds from this thesis and examines in his Abraham lecture how the aforementioned traumatizations of psychoanalysis have affected the development of theory in German Psychoanalysis:

> The exploration of their history in the decades after 1945 was long overshadowed and under the spell of the confrontation with their involvement in the Nazi regime. [...] For a long time German psychoanalysis was dominated by a certain narrative with which it described its development after 1945 as a path leading from liberation from the relics of the Göring-Institut and especially from synoptic psychotherapy to the "rebirth" of "Sigmund Freud's unadulterated psychoanalysis". At the same time, however, the idea of a completely new beginning resulted in amnesia of the historical reality of the ideas of that time. Some achievements of depth-psychological psychotherapy (*Tiefenpsychologie*) and psychoanalysis, which had emerged from a fruitful dialogue with philosophical, phenomenological and anthropological thinking, were forgotten. [...] [T]he rupture with the theoretical and therapeutic approaches of that time was not only a liberation, but also a loss of seminal insights. Psychoanalysis here experienced a second rupture in the 1980s. Its causes also have to do with the long shadow of the Nazi past.
>
> (Bohleber, 2019, p. 1, unpublished manuscript)

Such ruptures and discontinuities can also be observed in relation to the attitude of clinicians to empirical research in psychoanalysis, especially to outcome research as will be discussed shortly in the next sections.

Some remarks on the development of psychoanalytic (outcome) research in Germany after 1945

Understandably, in Germany these ruptures—or distortions—in the theory developments, in the clinical treatment technique, as well as in the attitudes towards empirical research after 1945 proved to be particularly serious. It took decades before a critical and self-critical reflection of the history of psychoanalysis in Germany during National Socialism became possible.

After the war, the psychoanalysts who had remained in Germany or immediately came back were primarily concerned with existential questions of survival, their professional establishment, but also with the confrontation with crimes during the Nazi-era. Alexander Mitscherlich, one of the leading figures of German psychoanalysis in the 1950s and 60s, is a good example for these developments after 1945. He was one of the observers of the Nürnberg Doctors' Trial and their involvement in National Socialism. His book *Doctors of Infamy* (1949, but in Germany under the title *Medizin ohne Menschlichkeit* not before 1960), which he published together with Fred Mielke, made him well known internationally but at the same time a persona non grata in the world of German academic medicine. He was regarded as fouling his own nest and never received a full professorship at one of the medical faculties in Germany. However, as Bohleber (2019) pointed out, the ruptures in the scientific career of Mitscherlich also led to ruptures in his own scientific thinking, his theory formation and his attitude towards various forms of empirical research. For example, his first book *Freiheit und Unfreiheit in der Krankheit* (Freedom and Unfreedom in Illness, 1948) was strongly influenced by anthropological positions. Until 1955 he tried to develop a synopsis of anthropology and psychoanalysis, which also meant that he felt more connected to philosophy and the humanities than to pure natural science. He had read Freud intensively during the war and expressed his gratitude to Freud in his first work with the words: "whose deep view also helped the darkness of the past years to wander through ..." Bohleber (2019) pronounces:

> But Mitscherlich understands Freud in the years after the war through the glasses of his own anthropological-existentialistic therapy concept. This changed after his research stay in the USA in 1951, during which he became acquainted with American ego psychology. [...] At first he criticizes ego psychologists from his own concept of anthropological therapy and considers them too conformist to the American way of life. But more and more he adopted their positions in the following years. In 1956 Mitscherlich's version of a natural scientific first-person psychology was widely received, and at the same time he was on his way to his own version of first-person psychology, which he further developed over the

next few years. Mitscherlich increasingly distanced himself from his original synoptic view of psychotherapy at that time.[6]

(Bohleber, loc. cit. p. 14)

With regard to empirical research, it is interesting to note that identification
with an ego-psychological understanding of psychoanalysis as a (natural)
science, also meant being open to empirical research at least for some of the
psychoanalysts who worked in psychiatry, Helmut Thomä, for example.[7] In
contrast, many psychoanalysts at the Sigmund-Freud-Institut (SFI) in Frankfurt
am Main—founded with the support of Max Horkheimer and closely connected with the *Institut für Sozialforschung*—were keen on following the sharp
critique of positivism in Critical Theory. Mitscherlich was a close friend of
Jürgen Habermas and, as a charismatic personality, shaped the heyday of psychoanalysis in the following decades. However, personally he has never dealt
extensively with distancing the positivistic understanding of ego-psychology
with which he was identified deeply. A few more remarks on these
contradictions.

Alexander Mitscherlich: charismatic personality and "one-man-army" in the heyday of psychoanalysis[8]

As Plänkers (2010) points out, it is interesting that the SFI owes its existence
not primarily to the universities (and certainly not to empirical research!), but
to politics. In particular, the good relations of Mitscherlich with the Hessian
prime minister Georg-August Zinn and the ministerial councilor Helene von
Bila, as well as the longstanding comrades-in-arms, Max Horkheimer and
Theodor W. Adorno at the *Institut für Sozialforschung* made it possible. On a
lecture celebrating Freud's 100th birthday, which Mitscherlich organized
together with the *Institut für Sozialforschung* in the summer of 1956, prime
minister Zinn announced the establishment of a professorship for psychoanalysis at Frankfurt University. Mitscherlich saw himself close to his goal of
finally being able to represent the subject of psychoanalysis as a full professor
at a German university, but he was disappointed again: the medical faculty of
the University of Frankfurt refused to appoint him as professor. Nevertheless,
he did not give up the fight: he tirelessly tried to use the good contacts with
the Hessian Ministry and the *Institut für Sozialforschung* to establish a psychoanalytical training and research institute despite all the resistance and with
much political and rhetorical skill. Again, after almost unimaginable obstacles
and intrigues, the time had finally come on April 27, 1960: Alexander
Mitscherlich ceremoniously opened an institute and training center for psychoanalysis and psychosomatic medicine in Frankfurt, which in 1964
received the name *Sigmund-Freud-Institut* (SFI). The SFI developed into an
inspiring center of psychoanalysis, also thanks to the many foreign guests who
came to Frankfurt often and with pleasure. Most of them were close friends

of the Mitscherlich couple, such as Piet Kuiper and Jeanne Lampl-de Groot from Amsterdam, Otto von Mehring from Pitsburg, Willi Hoffer, Michael Balint and Paula Heimann from London, Heinz Kohut and many others from the U.S. Alexander Mitscherlich also advocated the German translations of many important publications, one more reason why psychoanalysis met with enormous public and professional interest in the 1960s and experienced the greatest bloom in its history in Germany.

In recent decades it has become strangely quiet around Mitscherlich. This extensive forgetting of the charismatic personality, Alexander Mitscherlich, especially among younger generations, can only be understood in connection with the enormous societal changes in the last five decades—changes that naturally also affect psychoanalysis. For many psychoanalysts, thinking about these transformations is associated with grief work, because today we no longer live in a "heyday." In psychoanalysis, but also in the world of contemporary globalized sciences, the times of a "one-man army," as Erikson once characterized him, seem to belong to the past. New fields of tension have emerged in which psychoanalysis must assert itself and unfold as a "specific science of the unconscious" without losing its critical potential. In this context, it is also a question of a changed significance of empirical research in psychoanalysis and, in particular, of outcome research.

Alexander Mitscherlich can be seen as a prototype of an advocate of a "new psychoanalytical ethic." He passionately committed himself to shed light on the unconscious effects of National Socialism on the German postwar period. The SFI owes its existence to this commitment, which was perceived publicly and politically closely with psychoanalysis as an indispensable force of enlightenment. It was indeed the combination of a precise, "scientific" observation of complex phenomena with current sociological and philosophical theory that contributed to the attractiveness of psychoanalysis at that time—even among politicians. To our knowledge, not a single empirical psychoanalytic therapy study was carried out at the SFI in the first decades: in contrast to the research group led by Thomä and Kächele at the University of Ulm, where already in the 1970s national and international empirical studies from the field of psychoanalytic therapy research were conducted.[9] But within the German Psychoanalytic Association (DPV), empirical research in the 1980s and 1990s were met with great skepticism (see also Bohleber, 2019). At the time, many German psychoanalysts felt a polarization between the critical "Mitscherlich tradition" at the SFI or in Giessen (represented by H.E. Richter) and the research activities in Ulm, which were perceived as positivistic—even after their own differentiated description of their epistemological position (Thomä & Kächele, 1975).

It is striking that these polarizations can also be observed internationally. Zaretsky (2004, pp. 475ff.), for example, notes that in the 1970s a (natural) scientific and a philosophical tradition within psychoanalysis separated again. According to his analyses, this was an important factor that contributed to the marginalization of psychoanalysis. International psychoanalysis was divided into two differing trends—a "therapeutic" one, as quasi-medical treatment of the mentally ill with an empirical (positivistic) orientation on the one hand, and a "philosophical" one with a "critical hermeneutic" orientation, on the other hand. At the SFI, these divisions and the associated positions of epistemology were intensively discussed in the 1970s and led, for example, to the definition of psychoanalysis as a "science between the sciences" by Alfred Lorenzer (1974, p. 121) or to the characterization as a therapeutic method committed to an "emancipatory interest in knowledge," which had to constantly re-analyze its "scientist self-understanding" by Jürgen Habermas (1968, 1971).

But as important as these debates about an adequate understanding of the epistemological and methodological positions of psychoanalysis were for the understanding of psychoanalysts themselves, in Germany, they played hardly any role in connection with the evaluations of the Scientific Advisory Board for Psychotherapy from the 1990s until today and therefore also not in the decision as to whether longer psychoanalytical treatments are accepted by health insurance funds.

The decline of Freud's cultural theory

Until the end of the 1960s, the Freudian psychoanalysis reached so many people because it felt like dealing with the great themes of human life—with love and aggression, sexuality, creativity and death, "discomfort in culture," war and peace, etc. Margarete and Alexander Mitscherlich also understood how to express contemporary topics such as the "inability to mourn" and thus initiated a broad discourse in the German post-war period.

It is interesting that these political writings committed to Enlightenment first were met with great interest among the student movement of 1968. In Frankfurt, Mitscherlich's lectures became iconic. But soon the relationship between the students and activists with not only the Mitscherlich's but most of the established psychoanalysts of this older generation cooled down—or even turned into mutual distrust (cf. Hoyer, 2008). In Zurich, for example, the leaders of the student movement were almost predominantly psychoanalysts of the younger generation, such as Berthold Rothschild, Emilio Modena, Peter Passett, and others. The lecture on Wilhelm Reich's "Masspsychology and ego-analysis" by Rothschild during the anti-fascist week in the large auditorium of the university, was one of the highlights of the movement in 1971. But even here the conflicts with the established generation of psychoanalysts became evident. In Zurich, the conflicts between the young generation of psychoanalysts and the established ones in the Swiss Society escalated. This led to a splitting in the Zurich group with far-reaching consequences to this day (cf. Kurz, 1993; Leuzinger-Bohleber & Plänkers, in press).

Not only in Zurich or Frankfurt, but also in Paris, Berkley, and New York, the students and activists increasingly placed their hopes on a political culture and organizations that would change society as a whole and no longer on psychoanalysis. The focus on individuals was considered bourgeois or a "side contradiction." Group therapies (cf. Richter, Foulkes, Horn, etc.) and approaches to institutional theory became more and more attractive. Some of them were also associated with the antipsychiatric movement, which gained broad influence and, among other things, changed psychiatric institutions to a large extent. H.E. Richter and other psychoanalysts succeeded in appointing many psychoanalysts to the newly founded psychosomatic chairs at German universities and encouraging them to become involved in social psychology. Only one generation later most of the successors on these psychosomatic chairs are no longer psychoanalysts, but mainly cognitive-behavioral therapists. In 2019, for example, the last psychoanalytic chair at the University of Frankfurt and thus one of the cities with the most prolific psychoanalytic tradition in Europe will disappear—a sad development for psychoanalysis.

Not only in Germany—but also in many Western societies, psychoanalysis became rather marginalized in the last decades. Zaretsky (2004) describes this development:

> As one great slope of the psychoanalytic edifice disappeared into psychopharmacology, the other slid into identity politics. One effect was to absorb psychoanalysis into new "recognition" or "other-directed" paradigms that were unpsychological and antipsychological.
>
> (Zaretsky, 2004, p. 337)

Thus not much remained of psychoanalysis. Although references to (Lacanian) psychoanalysis popped up in most postmodern cultural theories, in gender and queer theory, deconstruction asf. (cf. Nancy Chodorov, Judith Butler, and others) the connection remained mostly superficial. But even in these discourses psychoanalysis increasingly lost its influence and thereby on society and culture as a whole. It gradually turned into an indispensable but "quiet" voice in the loud chatter.

Loss of importance of psychoanalysis in medicine: the advance of pharmacological treatments and evidence-based medicine

The relationship between psychoanalysis and medicine was complicated from the very beginning. In the U.S., psychoanalysis was closely related to medicine and psychiatry. Until the 1990s, for example, only physicians were allowed to receive full psychoanalytic training (see e.g., Wallerstein, 2001; Kernberg, 2006 and many others). Psychoanalysis in the US gained a unique political influence and an amazing social power: American psychiatry in the 1950s and 60s was almost exclusively in the hands of psychoanalysts. Nonetheless—seen retrospectively—this leaning of the ego psychologists towards a positivistic understanding of science in psychiatry created a paradoxical situation: "Ironically, as we saw, the more the U.S. ego psychologists claimed the mantle of the medical model, the more their critics attacked them as unscientific." (Zaretsky, 2004, p. 334). This can be observed in various discourses, e.g., about the *Diagnostic and Statistical Manual of Mental Disorders* (DSM), in which the influence of psychodynamic thinking disappeared more and more, from version to version, as well as in the emergence of hegemonic "evidence-based medicine." The solely positivistic understanding of research spread in connection with the rapid development of pharmacological treatment of mental disorders, which were perceived by society as "cheaper," "more efficient" and "scientific." This development pushed psychoanalysis more and more out of psychiatry. While in the 1980s a pluralistic approach to methods was still preferred— often a combination of pharmacological, psychodynamic and psychosocial treatment—the fierce controversies triggered by Grünbaum and other "Freud bashers" in the 1990s led to a complete denial of the scientific basis of psychoanalysis and to a predominance of CBT in psychiatric clinics and universities.

Freud bashing and the attack on psychoanalysis in times of evidence-based medicine

In the 1990s in Germany, the danger that psychoanalysis would lose its health insurance accreditation after Klaus Grawe et al.'s attack (1994) in their book *Von der Konfession zur Profession* (From confession to profession, 1997), forced psychoanalysts to critically reconsider their rejection of empirical psychotherapy research. Studies of that kind are as old as psychoanalysis itself (see e.g., Coriat, 1917; Fenichel, 1930; Alexander & Wilson, 1935), but have been little-noticed by the mainstream of psychoanalysis (cf. e.g., Wallerstein, 2001; Fonagy, 2001; Leuzinger-Bohleber, Arnold & Kächele, 2019). Outcome research existed internationally but was a divisive issue in psychoanalytical community—especially in Germany.

To mention just one example: in order to counter the aforementioned political threat, in the early 1990s, the German Psychoanalytic Association (DPV) decided to conduct a large, representative, retrospective study to investigate the long-term effects of psychoanalysis and psychoanalytic long-term treatment—the so-called DPV follow-up study. In total, 402 former patients were investigated with a combination of quantitative and qualitative methods. At that time, it was crucial for the acceptance of this first outcome study of a psychoanalytical society that the methods took into account the epistemological and sociological concerns outlined above and, for example, did not influence the ongoing treatments. Therefore, only a retrospective study was possible. With the quantitative methods, we were able to show that more than 80% of the former patients had improved in symptom-load, quality of life and social relationships at least three years after completion of their long-term treatment. These results were important for the dialogue on the outcome of psychoanalytic long-term treatments. However, for the psycho-analysts involved, the results of the psychoanalytic follow-up interviews were far more interesting. More than 200 former patients had three psychoanalytic follow-up interviews, which led to new insights into the short- and long-term outcomes of psychoanalysis and sparked many controversial discussions within the DPV (cf. Leuzinger-Bohleber et al., 2003). However, it was a bitter pill for many of the researchers and clinicians involved in the DPV follow-up study that this elaborate and methodologically inventive study was hardly noticed by the world of evidence-based medicine mainly because it was a ret-rospective study.

This ignorance was due to apparently not meeting the criteria of outcome research today and the so-called "gold standard": the randomized controlled trial (RCT). These criteria—randomization of patients, precisely described inclusion criteria, blind raters, standardized measuring instruments, manual-ized therapy procedures checked for their adherence, as well as the exact description of samples, drop-outs and applied statistical procedures—must be met in order for a study to be recognized both in the world of psychotherapy research and in health care systems. It is interesting from a historical and soci-ological point of view that in the DPV the LAC Study (see Leuzinger-Bohleber et al. in this volume), which tried to meet all the criteria mentioned above, would not have been possible without the follow-up study in the 1990s. Only this concrete experience had convinced many clinicians of the DPV that an outcome study, which satisfies the criteria of evidence-based medicine does not lead to a nemesis of psychoanalytic treatments. In fact, it can open a space in which the outcome of psychoanalysis can be looked at from different (even epistemological) perspectives. This means the associated demanding theoretical and epistemological questions must not be ignored even in a study meeting the criteria of evidence-based medicine, as foreign and unfavorable to psychoanalysis they might seem. Many of these questions and epistemolog-ical challenges can be critically discussed (at least in short)—even in the main publications of such studies (see e.g., Leuzinger-Bohleber et al., 2019a, 2019b; Kaufhold et al., 2019). In other words: we have continuously tried to link the therapeutic considerations of chronic depression with sociological and cultural–critical reflections, and therefore as far as possible within the framework of an empirical study—to combine the two traditions in psychoanalysis described above, the scientific and the philosophical one.

Can outcome research save the future of psychoanalysis?

Looking into some facets of the traumatic history of psychoanalysis may lead to the assessment that it is by no means guaranteed that good outcome research will save the future of psychoanalysis as a scientific discipline. Social and cultural processes that determine the position of psychoanalysis in the health care systems, the universities, and the academic world as well as the media and in the public are extremely complex and can only be influenced to a limited extent—of course not by a particular type of research alone. We can only mention that some of today's social changes are worrying many of us and there might be more at stake than the future of psychoanalysis: the resurrection of right-wing extremism and nationalism, the growth of populist movements and the associated splits in many countries, global terrorism. It all seems to be endangering the Enlightenment project, with which psychoanalysis is so closely linked. The philosopher and historian of science Michael Hampe (2019) therefore pleads vehemently for a Third Enlightenment:

> It could be that we are currently not primarily in a crisis of democracy, but rather an erosion of enlightened culture has taken place, which affects the way democracies "function". If this is the case, we cannot afford any illusions and must strive for another enlightenment movement. [...] The first Enlightenment, promoted by Socrates in Athens in the 5th century bc, recognized the argument as a better solution than violence. The second Enlightenment, from the 16th to the 18th century, discovered that humans do not have to be completely at the mercy of natural and social powers, that they can set out on the path of emancipation with the help of reason. The Third Enlightenment that lies before us is about the realization that we live in a *complex world* in which there are coincidences as well as necessities and also human beings as factors influencing reality. Human action and its historical consequences take place within this tension....
>
> (Hampe, 2019, p. 10/11, translated by MLB)

Psychoanalysis and its future indeed are embedded in these social changes. Nevertheless, many of us have the dream that the potential for Enlightenment that lies within psychoanalysis will be re-discovered in the near future. But is also on us to find our place and hold our ground.

On the other hand—and on a very different level—in the US and Europe, psychoanalysis as an therapeutic offer in the health care system only has a future if we conduct comparative outcome studies and show, according to the criteria of evidence-based medicine, that its treatments lead to success measured by these very criteria. In the meantime, many research groups and psychoanalytical institutions have devoted themselves to conducting and supporting empirical psychotherapy studies. For example, the Open Door Review of the IPA (Leuzinger-Bohleber, Arnold, & Kaechele, 2019) or Liliengren and Bräcke (2019) show that a large number of empirical psychotherapy studies are now available and can be used as arguments.

In this volume, many studies and meta-analyses are summarized, which shows that psychoanalysis have faced these challenges for several decades, so that even the *Guardian* (2016) talked about the "revenge of Freud" based on the new abundance of evidence, especially on the outcome of short-term psychoanalytic therapies. However, whether this is sufficient to save the (institutional) future of psychoanalysis remains an open question as to how the current professional political struggles in Germany in connection with a new psychotherapist law teach us.

To make a long story very short: of course in psychoanalysis it is always a central matter of protecting our unique way and Freud's famous "*Junktim von Heilen und Forschen*" (Freud, 1927a, German: p. 293, English: p. 256)—the conjunction between cure and research, which can only take place in the safe, trusting space of the professional, therapeutic relationship and can not be accelerated, economized nor medialized. At the same time, however, psychoanalysis—like every scientific discipline—must be accessible to criticism from outside and must be committed to extra-clinical proof of its outcome if it is to remain a therapeutic treatment method in the (statutory) health care system and to face up to academic discourses. A further tension arises from the fact that the specific research object of psychoanalysis is the pathogenic, tabooed causes of individual and collective behavior, which first of all cause resistance of those affected. On the one hand, psychoanalysis is in danger of adapting too much to a prevailing zeitgeist, and thus of losing its credibility, its authenticity as a "science of the unconscious." At the same time, however, it must beware of withdrawing from communication with the non-psychoanalytical world and the public on burning social issues and denying existing dependencies on the scientific community, politics, and media. This would sooner or later lead to scientific and social marginalization.

Overview of the contributions of this volume

This volume consists of three parts: The contributions to Part I discuss the grand scheme of things and the state of the art in psychoanalytic outcome research. Part II contains exemplary research projects that are discussed from a clinical perspective, illustrating the dialogue between researchers and clinicians. In Part III, several psychoanalysts review the importance of critical thinking and research in psychoanalytic education.

As a second introductory chapter Mark Solms, the third editor of this volume, elaborates three central questions of psychoanalytic outcome research: (A) How does the emotional mind work, in health and disease? (B) On this basis, what does psychoanalytic treatment aim to achieve? (C) How effective is it? He summarizes the core scientific claims of psychoanalysis and rebuts the prejudice that it is not "evidence-based." Solm's chapter is an extensive version of a paper that was published in the *British Journal of Psychiatry* (2018).

"Researchers and clinicians alike are seeking new knowledge about improving outcomes in psychotherapy. But, as the contributions of this volume indicate, challenges often arise in appreciating the meaning of changing advances in our field," is the starting point of Robert Emde in Chapter 2

"Five advances in psychoanalytic thinking and their implications for outcome research." Emde is one of the best-known empirical, conceptual, and clinical researchers in psychoanalysis with groundbreaking contributions, especially to psychoanalytical development and prevention research. Over the decades, he has built bridges between researchers and clinicians, was one of the co-founders of the Sandler Conferences and, together with John Clarkin, the long-standing chair of the Research Training Program of the International Psychoanalytical Association. He discusses five areas in advances in psychoanalytic thinking: (1) A two-person psychology, (2) A developmental orientation, (3) A larger view of unconscious functioning, (4) Embodied experience, and (5) An integrative stance. He thus outlines the major trends in psychoanalysis and its research in recent decades and draws conclusions for today's outcome research. He concludes that the time of horse racing is over and contemporary psychotherapy research should focus on answering the questions: *How does it work, in what ways, for whom and under what circumstances and relationship conditions?* Emde formulates a plea for person-centered medicine and psychotherapy and discusses some possibilities for development in this direction. He closes with a reflections on the use of "outcome" as a term, which is not only about relief of suffering, discomfort, and symptoms in the consulting room or upon completion of treatment; even more, it is about the relief of misery and self-imposed problems in times afterwards—in a life of love and work with others.

Jonathan Shedler's chapter "Where is the evidence for 'evidence-based' therapy?" was published widely received and discussed in 2018, because he brilliantly deconstructs the myth of evidence-based therapy. He argues that behind the "evidence-based" therapy movement lies a master narrative, which hardly ever met their own criteria, but has become a justification for all-out attacks on traditional talk therapy. Therefore, Shedler concludes his contribution with concrete hints for readers (including politicians from the health care sector), which should facilitate a critical, non-mystifying reception of empirical studies.

Juan Pablo Jiménez and Carolina Altimir reflect in their chapter on "Developing an innovative, scientific, clinically sensitive approach to investigate the psychoanalytic process," in favor of an interdisciplinary dialogue between psychoanalysis and related disciplines, especially psychotherapy process research. Psychoanalysis needs to broaden interdisciplinary dialogue as in a "two-way street," within the framework of epistemological pluralism. In 100 years of clinical research and 40 years of empirical research, the concept of psychoanalytic process continues to elude a consensual definition, probably because the problem and methodology is not well defined. This chapter advances a research program for the study of psychoanalytic processes that centers on the dyadic and interactional nature of the analytical work, and on the relationship between the implicit (unconscious) and the explicit (conscious) levels of the analytic endeavor. The authors propose that this research program be articulated around three methodological approaches: (1) The use of systematic case studies; (2) The adoption of the events paradigm in order to access the salient phenomena of the psychoanalytic process, and (3) A micro-analytic approach to the specific phenomena occurring within relevant sequences of interaction.

Horst Kächele starts his contribution "From case study to single case research: the specimen case Amalia X" summarizing the long tradition of case studies in psychoanalysis. To this day, clinicians around the world hold fast to the fact that the communication of complex clinical observations can most likely be done by narratives, which means by detailed case presentations. Kächele lists the fundamental, in many respects devastating criticism of this tradition by Arnold Grünbaum (1984), particularly his so-called "tally argument"—that psychoanalysis has nothing to offer in the sense of "scientific evidence of causalities." In the following section some of Edelson's (1984) counterarguments and their further development in positions of many contemporary psychoanalysts are reconstructed. He then proposes an approach to empirical, systematic single case research and presents the work of The Ulm Psychoanalytic Process Research Study Group and their study on a specimen case named "Amalia X."

In Chapter 6 Simone Hauck emphasizes "The importance of psychoanalytic research to contemporary medicine." After years of a narrow focus on diseases and on the development of precise techniques for specific health problems, contemporary medicine is moving toward a person-centered approach and a comprehensive understanding of health and well-being. In her view, psychoanalysis should regain a leading role when findings from health care research are beginning to strengthen the fundamental role of relationships between caregivers and patients—e.g., in the effectiveness of and compliance with treatment. On the other hand, there is growing attention to the higher rates of mental health problems among doctors and medical students demanding a broader understanding of what happens in the minds of professionals and how they deal with factors such as disease, death, and human suffering. In this sense, the advance of science clearly shows the importance of phenomena that psychoanalysis has been studying in clinical settings for over 100 years.

The meta-analyses by Falk Leichsenring and his team were milestones in the fight for recognition of outcomes of psychoanalytic treatments and led to fierce controversies, particularly with representatives of cognitive-behavioral therapy. Unfortunately, the costs of re-printing their new meta-analysis (Steinert, Munder, Rabung, Hoyer, & Leichsenring, 2017) in this volume were too high, so we are using an earlier paper of the same group. In their chapter "Evidence for psychodynamic psychotherapy in specific mental disorders: a systematic review" Leichsenring and Klein review the empirical evidence for psychodynamic therapy for specific mental disorders in adults. According to the results presented here, there is evidence from randomized controlled trials (RCTs) that psychodynamic therapy is efficacious in common mental disorders, including depressive disorders, anxiety disorders, somatoform disorders, personality disorders, eating disorders, complicated grief, posttraumatic stress disorder (PTSD), and substance-related disorders.

Chapter 8 "Clinical Discussion of *Psychodynamic Therapy: A Meta-Analysis Testing Equivalence of Outcome*" by Harriet Wolfe, the incoming president of the International Psychoanalytical Association (IPA), touches on general problems in connection with meta-analyses on treatment outcomes. She then discusses an important topic, which is neglected in all psychotherapeutic schools, namely, how to deal with non-responsive patients. In a courageous, open manner, she speaks of therapeutic experience with a patient with whom after a serious accident the therapy stagnated. In a very sensitive way she reflects on whether and how she could refer the patient to another therapist, possibly a cognitive-behavioral therapist, without evoking the feeling of rejection. From a clinical perspective, it would be helpful to have research on non-responders, she argues, and to be able to predict whether a patient's response to treatment might change with a different psychotherapy.

As discussed it remains a difficult and controversial question how the outcome of psychoanalyses may best be evaluated. At present, we can draw upon the findings of numerous studies investigating the outcome of short-term psychoanalytic therapies. By contrast, due to the challenging epistemo-logical, methodological as well as practical problems, there is still a lack of studies on long-term psychoanalytic therapies. Therefore the LAC Study, summarized by Leuzinger-Bohleber and her team in this volume, has com-pared the outcomes of *long-term* psychoanalytic and cognitive-behavioral therapies for chronically depressed patients. It is the first to compare the long-term effectiveness of cognitive-behavioral (CBT) and psychoanalytic treatment (PAT) of chronically depressed patients with a study design that investigates the influence of treatment preference in contrast to randomized assignment. The aim of the study was to compare those two treatments according to their long-term and short-term effects on different outcome variables regarding depressive symptoms, relapse rate, level of psychosocial outcome variables. However, psychoanalytic treatment does not focus exclusively on reducing psychopathological symptoms; it also seeks to bring "structural" change, i.e., changes in the patients' inner world. These changes have been investigated in the LAC Study via Operationalized Psychodynamic Diagnostics (OPD) and set in relation to symptom changes. The findings show that indeed the two therapies, CBT and PAT, differ statistically in respect to "structural change" achieved as well as its influence on the reduc-tion of depressive symptoms three years after start of treatment. To our knowl-edge, this is the first empirical study that shows differences in the dimension of "structural change" and its impact on the patients.

In her "Discussion of the LAC Study," Esther Dreifus-Kattan first examines from a clinician's point of view why empirical studies are important. She emphasizes the question of why structural changes require long-term treatments that were stimulating and inspiring for her as a practicing psychoanalyst. The main part of her chapter is devoted to a detailed case vignette: she reports from her art therapy group at UCLA with patients suffering from depression due to severe cancer. She describes the three-year art therapy with Henri, a 69-year-old man diagnosed with myeloma, the blood cancer with the poorest prognosis. Dreifus-Kattan illustrates the therapeutic process with impressive paintings of the patient and gives a remarkable insight into how psychoanalyst and group members help the patient to deal with his illness and impending death.

John F. Clarkin, Reed Maxwell, and Julia F. Sowislo in their chapter "Comparative psychotherapy research focused on the treatment of borderline personality disorder," claim that if psychoanalytic treatment wants to maintain a position of respect and influence in the field of psychotherapy, outcome studies that are persuasive to the scientific community and the general public must be accomplished. In their contribution, they report on research on treatment of personality disorders with the aim of obtaining a specific psychoanalytic therapy as the method of choice. The key features of their Transference Focused Therapy (TFP) treatment model for personality pathology include: (1) Structuring the treatment with an oral contract, (2) A focus on disturbed interpersonal behaviors both in relationship to the therapist (transference) and in the patients' current daily interactions, (3) Utilization of the process of interpretation to examine and modify internal representations of self and others, and (4) Real-world changes in interpersonal behavior particularly in the areas of work, friendships and intimate/love relations. After a precise description of the borderline personality disorder, the authors briefly compare their treatment approach with the Dialectical Behavioral Therapy (Linnehan) and Mentalized Based Treatment by Fonagy and his team.

Richard D. Lane, in his chapter "Memory reconsolidation, emotional arousal and the process of change in psychoanalysis" builds a bridge between the recent neuroscientific, cognitive and psychiatric memory research and psychoanalytical outcome research. The discovery that long-term memories are malleable—a phenomenon known as memory reconsolidation—has created new opportunities to understand the process of change in psychoanalysis, he argues. Advances in memory science have implications for the process of change because a key function of memory is to guide future behavior in situations that resemble those from the past. The author reviews a new theory of enduring change that applies to a variety of modalities, including cognitive-behavioral therapy, emotion-focused psychotherapy, and psychoanalysis. The core idea is that enduring change results from the updating of prior emotional memories through a process of reconsolidation that incorporates new emotional experiences.

Manfred E. Beutel, Les Greenberg, and Richard D. Lane in their chapter "Emotions in psychodynamic process and outcome research" explore the role of emotion in psychodynamic psychotherapy and outcome even further.

First, a brief overview of recent emotion research is given. In the following section concepts and studies of the Emotion-Focused Therapy (EFT) are presented. The authors argue that there has been little attention in psychoanalytic and psychodynamic psychotherapy on a specific technique for changing emotional processes and their relationships with outcome. The authors discuss the hypothesis that integrating techniques from Emotion-Focused Therapy could help psychodynamic psychotherapists in identifying, addressing and changing emotional processes and thus contribute to successful treatment outcomes—particularly in patients who have difficulties accessing their emotions.

Clara Raznoszczyk Schejtman, in her chapter "Discussion from a clinical perspective," elaborates three different topics: (1) Clinical psychoanalysis, outcome research, and pluralism, (2) The role of affect in development, psychopathology and clinical work, and (3) Present and future dialogue amongst researchers and clinicians and the training of new generations. She refers to theoretical discourses, research traditions and clinical practice in South America as well as some of her teaching experiences at the University of Buenos Aires. Particularly interesting is her transfer on her own developmental research on early mother–child interactions. She points out that it was precisely empirical infant research and baby observation that led to contemporary treatment techniques—not only being used in short-term therapies, but also in long-term psychoanalysis—in which the central role of affects in the transference relationship between the analysand and the analyst has been established for decades.

Linda S. Goodman in her chapter "A clinician's view of research, critical thinking, and culture in psychoanalytic education" deals with one of the central concerns of this book—bridging the gap between clinicians and researchers. She begins with an impressive "Psychoanalytic classroom vignette," which offers an insight into the practice of a teaching psychoanalyst who tries to combine "clinical wisdom" with openness and curiosity towards empirical research. Goodman pronounces that the intertwining of clinical education, critical thinking, and research may be the greatest challenge as well as a chance for psychoanalysis as an innovative scientific discipline. She merges these thoughts with a very personal description of her experiences as an analyst and her commitment to changes in psychoanalytical training at the NCP and in the ApsA.

In his chapter "Teaching empirical research in psychodynamic psychotherapy: how to make research *really* matter," Joshua Pretsky formulates a passionate plea for the integration of empirical research in the training of analysts, psychotherapists, and psychiatrists. He begins with very personal comments on his own educational biography and attributes it above all to various influential personalities who stimulated his interest in research and motivated him to develop an attitude of openness, curiosity, and critical thinking—especially towards authorities, but also a self-understanding of being a "lifelong learner." In a very touching and open way he describes his positive but in some respects irritating experiences during his own training analysis, in which he often wished for a more active, focused, and emotionally engaging stance. In the second part of his contribution, Pretsky reflects on his teaching experiences in various institutional contexts (teaching psychiatric residents, psychotherapy, and psychoanalysis students, etc.), describing eight different areas that he considers useful for teaching and thus offers a wide range of ideas, concepts, and didactic considerations.

Morris Eagle, at the beginning of his chapter "The role of critical thinking and research in psychoanalytic education: clinician-research," soberingly and at the same time concerned, states that the debate regarding the enhancement of critical thinking and the integration of research findings is not new in psychoanalysis. He discusses some examples from these debates, e.g., on the importance of countertransference and therefore agrees with Kernberg, who sees research as an indispensable part of the psychoanalytical training. However, he emphasizes what research actually means. In the following sections, Morris Eagle deals in an elaborate and clear way with various forms of research in psychoanalysis. The reader gains an impression of the author's own years of teaching and research experiences as well as observations and debates as President of the Division of Psychoanalysis (Division 39) of the American Psychological Association. His reflections lead to basic epistemological and methodological problems of research, e.g., the question of ecological validity and the difference between "experimental psychology" and "correlational psychology." Eagle formulates a conclusion that is of great relevance to the subject matter of this book: the greater the number of individual difference variables studied in an ongoing research program, the less gap between researcher and clinician. He closes his chapter with a vehement plea for an opening and corresponding changes in psychoanalytic training, which he sees as crucial for the future of this discipline.

Notes

1 There are numerous papers discussing different aspects of the relationship between clinicians and (empirical) researchers in psychoanalysis. To mention just a few here: Bachrach et al., 1985, 1991; Boesky, 2002, 2005; Chiesa, 2005; Colombo & Michels, 2007; Dahl et al., 1988; Emde & Fonagy, 1997; Fonagy, 2001a, 2015; Galatzer-Levy, 1997; Hauser, 2002; Haynal, 1993; Holt. 2003; Jones, 1993; Wallerstein, 2001; Waldron, 1997. Overview: see e.g., Leuzinger-Bohleber, 2010; Leuzinger-Bohleber; Arnold, & Kächele, 2019.

2 M. Leuzinger-Bohleber has been responsible for the research program in the field of basic research and psychotherapy research from 2001 to 2016 at the Sigmund-Freud-Institut in Frankfurt a.M. This chapter is based on former papers on this subject, e.g., Leuzinger-Bohleber, 2010; 2011; 2015b; Leuzinger-Bohleber & Plänkers, in print.

3 To our knowledge, there is no comprehensive historical paper yet available on this subject, neither for Germany nor for the IPA. Some parts are covered in Bohleber (2010).

4 Whose experimental work and creativity inspired much later the research group around Wolfgang Leuschner in the 1990s at the Sigmund-Freud-Institut in Frankfurt

a.M. to investigate e.g., the influence on subliminal stimulations in the experimental dream laboratory trying to test Freud's dream theory experimentally.

5 Nonetheless, it is interesting to note that some of the first outcome studies were carried out in Berlin (cf. Alexander & Wilson, 1935; Fenichel, 1930).

6 Mitscherlich's year in London in 1958 and his teaching analysis with Paula Heimann and the supervisions with Balint also had a great influence on him. In a letter to Ernst Klett (23.2.59, EKA) Mitscherlich traces the development of psychoanalysis since 1933. Citing Jones (1936), he says that the National socialists had completely liquidated psychoanalysis. With the foundation of the DPV in 1950, the reconstruction of psychoanalysis had begun, which was completed with the opening of the Sigmund-Freud-Institut as the first government-funded institute for psychoanalysis and psychosomatic medicine in Europe.

7 Thomä was influenced by his one year Fulbright stipend at Yale Psychiatric Institute in 1955 where he learned a critical scientific attitude from Theodor Lidz and others. Returning to Mitscherlich's Psychosomatic Clinic in Heidelberg he worked on his systematic case monograph on Anorexia nervosa (German 1961, English 1967). He trained with M. Balint based on a fellowship at the British Institute, from where he brought home his lasting interest on the therapist's role in the psychoanalytic process. This led him—together with Horst Kächele—to work on a detailed study of processes based on tape recordings at the University of Ulm starting in 1970. The psychoanalytic group in Ulm has become one of the best-known representatives of empirical process and outcome research in Germany with an international reputation (see below).

8 Cf. the three biographies published on his 100th birthday by Martin Dehli (2007): *Leben als Konflikt. Zur Biographie von Alexander Mitscherlich*, by Tobias Freimüller (2007): Alexander Mitscherlich. *Gesellschaftsdiagnosen und Psychoanalyse nach Hitler* and the most detailed of them by Timo Hoyer (2008): *"Im Getümmel der Welt" – Alexander Mitscherlich – Ein Portrait*.

9 Horst Kächele led the important "Collaborative Research Program 129: Psychotherapeutic Processes" supported by the German Research Foundation with many empirical projects on outcome and process in psychoanalytic treatments (see e.g., Kächele, Novak, & Traue, 1989). The work of his research group was highly appreciated internationally (Horst Kächele was e.g., president of the Society for Psychotherapy Research 1991–1992).

References

Alexander, F., & Wilson, G.W. (1935). Quantitative dream studies—A methodological attempt at a quantitative evaluation of psychoanalytic material. *Psychoanal Q.*, 4, 371–407.

Allers, R. (1922). Über psychoanalyse. In: Stransky, E. & Dattner, B. (Eds.). *Über Psychoanalyse. Einleitender Vortrag von Rudolf Allers mit anschließender Aussprache im Verein für angewandte Psychopathologie und Psychologie in Wien* (pp. 2–47). Berlin: Karger.

Bachrach, H.M., Galatzer-Levy, R., & Skolnikoff, A. (1991). On the efficacy of psychoanalysis. *Journal of the American Psychoanalytic Association*, 39, 871–916.

Bachrach, H.M., Weber, J.J., & Solomon, M. (1985). Factors associated with the outcome of psychoanalysis (clinical and methodological considerations): Report of the Columbia Psychoanalytic Center Research Project. *International Review of Psycho-Analysis*, 12, 379–389.

Boesky, D. (2002). Why don't our institutes teach the methodology of clinical psychoanalytic evidence? *Psychoanalytic Quarterly*, 71: 445–475.

Boesky, D. (2005). Psychoanalytic controversies contextualized. *Journal of the American Psychoanalytic Association*, 53, 835–863.

Bohleber, W. (2010). Die Entwicklung der Psychoanalyse in Deutschland nach 1945. Vortrag auf der Tagung der DPG und DPV: 100 Jahre Internationale Psychoanalytische Vereinigung (IPV) – 100 Jahre institutionalisierte Psychoanalyse in Deutschland, Berlin, 7.3.2010.

Bohleber, W. (2019). Über Brüche in der Theoriebildung – Ein Beitrag zur Generationengeschichte der Psychoanalyse in Deutschland 1945–1995. Abraham lecture, May 25, 2019 (will be published in the *Jahrbuch für Psychoanalyse*).

Chiesa, M. (2005). Can psychoanalytic research integrate and improve knowledge for clinical practice? Some reflections and an example. *Scandinavian Psychoanalytic Review*, 28, 31–39.

Colombo, D., & Michels, R. (2007). Can (should) case reports be written for research use? *Psychoanalytic Inquiry*, 27, 640–649.

Coriat, I. (1917). Some statistical results of the psychoanalytic treatment of the psychoneuroses. *Psychoanalytic Review*, 4, 209–216.

Dahl, H., Kächele, H., & Thomä, H. (Eds.) (1988). *Psychoanalytic Process Research Strategies*. Berlin: Springer.

Dehli, M. (2007). *Leben als Konflikt. Zur Biographie von Alexander Mitscherlich*. Göttingen: Wallstein.

Emde, R.N., & Fonagy, P. (1997). An emerging culture for psychoanalytic research? *International Journal of Psycho-Analysis*, 78, 643–651.

Falzeder, E. (2010). *Die Gründungsgeschichte der IPV und der Berliner Ortsgruppe*. Vortrag auf der Tagung der DPG und DPV: 100 Jahre Internationale Psychoanalytische Vereinigung (IPV) – 100 Jahre institutionalisierte Psychoanalyse in Deutschland, Berlin, 6.3.2010.

Fenichel, O. (1930). Statistischer Bericht über die therapeutische Tätigkeit 1920–1930. In: *Zehn Jahre Berliner Psychoanalytisches Institut* (pp. 13–19). Wien: Verlag Internationale Psychoanalyse.

Fonagy, P. (2001a). The talking cure in the cross fire of empiricism—The struggle for the hearts and minds of psychoanalytic clinicians: Commentary on papers by Lester Luborsky and Hans H. Strupp. *Psychoanalytic Dialogues*, 11, 647–658.

Fonagy, P. (2001b). *The open door review* (1st ed.). London: The International Psychoanalytical Association.

Fonagy, P. (2015). The effectiveness of psychodynamic psychotherapies: An update. *World Psychiatry*, 14(2), 137–150. doi:10.1002/wps.20235.

Freimüller, T. (2007). *Alexander Mitscherlich. Gesellschaftsdiagnosen und Psychoanalyse nach Hitler*. Göttingen: Wallstein.

Freud, S. (1900). *Interpretation of dreams*. Standard Edition Vol. V. London: Hogarth.

Freud, S. (1926e). *The question of lay analysis*. Standard Edition Vol. XX: 183–250. London: Hogarth.

Freud, S. (1927a). *Postscript to the question of lay analysis*. Standard Edition Vol. XX: 251–258. London: Hogarth.

Freud, S. (1927a). *Nachwort zur "Frage der Laienanalys."* GW XIV, 287–296.

Galatzer-Levy, R. (1997). Psychoanalytic research: An investment in the future. *Journal of the American Psychoanalytic Association*, 45, 9–12.

Gay, P. (1988). *Freud: A life for our time*. New York: Norton.

Grawe, K., Donati, R., & Bernauer, F. (1994). *Psychotherapie im Wandel. Von der Konfession zur Profession*. Göttingen: Hogrefe.

Grawe, K., Donati, R., & Bernauer, F. (1997). *Psychotherapy in transition – from speculation to science*. Seattle: Hogrefe – Huber Publications.

Habermas, J. (1968). *Erkenntnis und Interesse*. Frankfurt: Suhrkamp.

Habermas, J. (1971). *Knowledge and human interests*. Translated by J.J. Shapiro. Boston: Beacon Press.

Hampe, M. (2019). *Die Dritte Aufklärung*. Berlin: Nicolai Publishing & Intelligence.

Hartmann, H., Pappenheim, M., & Stransky, E. (1931). *I. Internationale Tagung für angewandte Psychopathologie und Psychologie. Wien 5.–7. Juni, 1930*. Berlin: Karger.

Hauser, S.T. (2002). The future of psychoanalytic research: Turning points and new opportunities. *Journal of the American Psychoanalytic Association*, 50, 395–405.

Haynal, A. (1993). *Psychoanalysis and the sciences: Epistemology – history*. Berkeley: The University of California Press.

Holt, R.R. (2003). New directions for basic psychoanalytic research: Implications from the work of Benjamin Rubinstein. *Psychoanalytic Psychology*, 20, 195–213.

Hoyer, T. (2008). *Im Getümmel der Welt: Alexander Mitscherlich, ein Porträt*. Göttingen: Vandenhoeck & Ruprecht.

Jones, E. (1936). The future of psycho-analysis. *International Journal of Psycho-Analysis*, 17, 269–277.

Jones, E.E. (1993). How will psychoanalysis study itself? *Journal of the American Psychoanalytic Association*, 41, Suppl., 91–108.

Jones, E., Jones, K., & Meili-Dworetzki, G. (1960). *Das Leben und Werk von Sigmund Freud* (Vol. 3). Bern: Huber.

Kaufhold, J., Bahrke, U., Kallenbach, L., Negele, A., Ernst, M., Keller, W., … Beutel, M. (2019). Wie können nachhaltige Veränderungen in Langzeittherapien untersucht werden? *PSYCHE*, 73(2), 106–133.

Kächele, H., Novak, P., & Traue, H.C. (1989). Psychotherapeutische Prozesse: Struktur und Ergebnisse. Der Sonderforschungsbereich 129: 1980–1988. *Zeitschrift für Psychosomatische Medizin und Psychoanalyse*, 35, 364–382.

Kernberg, O.F. (2006). The pressing need to increase research in and on psychoanalysis. *International Journal of Psycho-Analysis*, 87, 919–926.

Kurz, T. (1993). Aufstieg und Abfall des Psychoanalytischen Seminars Zürich von der Schweizerischen Gesellschaft für Psychoanalyse. *Luzifer-Amor*, 6(12), 7–54.

Leuzinger-Bohleber, M. (2010). Psychoanalysis as "science of the unconscious" in the IPA centenary. *News of the International Psychoanalytical Association*, 18, Special Edition, 24–26.

Leuzinger-Bohleber, M. (2011). Von der "one man army" zur interdisziplinären Forschung. Zur Forschung in der Klinischen- und Grundlagenabteilung am Sigmund-Freud-Institut heute. In: Leuzinger-Bohleber, M.; Haubl, R. (Eds.). *Psychoanalyse: interdisziplinär – international – intergenerationell.* Zum 50-jährigen Bestehen des Sigmund-Freud-Instituts (pp. 21–61). Göttingen: Vandenhoeck & Ruprecht.

Leuzinger-Bohleber, M. (2015a). *Finding the body in the mind. Psychoanalysis, neurosciences and embodied cognitive science in dialogue.* London: Karnac.

Leuzinger-Bohleber, M. (2015). Development of a plurality during the one hundred-year-old history of research of psychoanalysis. Introduction. In: Leuzinger-Bohleber, M.; Kächele, H. (Eds.). *An open door review of outcome and process studies in psychoanalysis,* 3rd edition (pp. 18–32). Berlin: IPA.

Leuzinger-Bohleber, M., Stuhr, U., Rüger, B., & Beutel, M. (2003). How to study the 'quality of psychoanalytic treatments' and their long-term effects on patient's well-being. A representative, multi-perspective follow-up study. *International Journal of Psycho-Analysis,* 84, 263–290.

Leuzinger-Bohleber, M., Hautzinger, M., Fiedler, G., Keller, W., Bahrke, U., Kallenbach, L., … Beutel, M. (2019a). Outcome of psychoanalytic and cognitive-behavioural long-term therapy with chronically depressed patients: A controlled trial with preferential and randomized allocation. *Can J Psychiatry,* 64(1), 47–58. doi:10.1177/0706743718780340.

Leuzinger-Bohleber, M., Kaufhold, J., Kallenbach, L., Negele, A., Ernst, M., Keller, W., … Beutel, M. (2019b). How to measure sustained psychic transformations in long-term treatments of chronically depressed patients: Symptomatic and structural changes in the LAC Depression Study of the outcome of cognitive-behavioural and psychoanalytic long-term treatments. The *International Journal of Psychoanalysis,* 100(1), 99–127. doi:10.1080/00207578.2018.1533377.

Leuzinger-Bohleber, M., Arnold, S.E.A., & Kächele, H. (2019). *Open door review of clinical, conceptual, process and outcome studies.* Retrieved from: www.opendoorreview.com/.

Leuzinger-Bohleber, M., & Plänkers, T. (in press). The struggle for a psychoanalytic research institute: the evolution of Frankfurt's Sigmund-Freud-Institute. Accepted for publication in the *International Journal of Psychoanalysis.*

Lorenzer, A. (1974). *Die Wahrheit der psychoanalytischen Erkenntnis* (p. 121). Frankfurt am Main: Suhrkamp.

Luyten, P., Mayes, L.C., Fonagy, P., Target, M., & Blatt, S.J. (Eds.). (2015). *Handbook of psychodynamic approaches to psychopathology.* New York: The Guilford Press.

Liliengren, P., & Bräcke, F.S (2019). Comprehensive compilation of randomized controlled trials (RCTs) involving psychodynamic treatments and interventions. *University College, Stockholm, Sweden.*

Lorenzer, A. (1974). *Die Wahrheit der psychoanalytischen Erkenntnis.* Frankfurt am Main: Suhrkamp.

Makari, G. (2008). *Revolution in mind: The creation of psychoanalysis.* Melbourne: Melbourne Univ. Publishing.

Mitscherlich, A. (1948). *Freiheit und Unfreiheit in der Krankheit. Das Bild des Menschen in der Psychotherapie.* Hamburg: Claassen & Goverts.

Mitscherlich, A., & Mielke, F. (1949). *Doctors of infamy. The story of the Nazi medical crimes.* New York: Henry Schuman.

Mitscherlich, A., & Mielke, F. (1960). *Medizin ohne Menschlichkeit: Dokumente des Nürnberger Ärzteprozesses*. Frankfurt: Fischer Bücherei.

Plänkers, T. (2010). Fluctuat nec mergitur. Ein Blick auf die Geschichte des Sigmund-Freud-Instituts. In Leuzinger-Bohleber, M.; Haubl, R. (Eds.). *Psychoanalyse: interdisziplinär – international – intergenerationell*. Zum 50-jährigen Bestehen des Sigmund-Freud-Instituts. (pp. 81–99). Göttingen: Vandenhoeck & Ruprecht.

Schröter, M. (2019). Im Zwischenreich. Akademische Psychiatrie und Psychoanalyse in Wien 1918–1932. *PSYCHE* 73(4), 264–290. doi:10.21o6/ps-73-4-264.

Stransky, E., & Dattner, B. (Hg.) (1922). *Über Psychoanalyse. Einleitender Vortrag von Rudolf Allers mit anschließender Aussprache im Verein für angewandte Psychopathologie und Psychologie in Wien*. Berlin: Karger.

Thomä, H. (1961). *Anorexia nervosa. Geschichte, Klinik und Theorie der Pubertätsmagersucht*. Bern/Stuttgart: Huber/Klett.

Thomä, H. (1967). *Anorexia nervosa*. New York: International University Press.

Thomä, H., & Kächele, H. (1975). Problems of metascience and methodology in clinical psychoanalytic research. *The Annual of Psychoanalysis*, 3, 49–119.

Waldron, S., JR. (1997). How can we study the efficacy of psychoanalysis? *Psychoanal Q.*, 66, 283–322.

Wallerstein, R.S. (2001). The generations of psychotherapy research: An overview. *Psychoanalytic Psychology*, 18, 243–267.

Whitebook, J. (2010). Sigmund Freud – A philosophical physician. Lecture at the 11th Joseph Sandler Research Conference: Persisting shadows of early and later trauma. Frankfurt am Main.

Young-Bruehl, E., & Schwartz, M. (2011). Warum die Psychoanalyse keine Geschichte hat. *PSYCHE*, 65(2), 97–118.

Zaretsky, E. (2004). *Secrets of the soul: Psychoanalysis, modernity, and personal life*. New York: Vintage Books.

Chapter I

The scientific basis of psychoanalysis

Introductory remarks

Mark Solms

My aim is to set out what we psychoanalysts may consider to be the core scientific claims of our discipline.[1] Such stock-taking is necessary due to widespread misconceptions among the public, and disagreements among ourselves regarding specialist details, which obscure a bigger picture upon which we can all agree. Agreement on our core claims, which enjoy strong empirical support, will enable us better to defend them against the prejudice that psychoanalysis is not "evidence-based."

I shall address three questions: (A) How does the emotional mind work, in health and disease? (B) On this basis, what does psychoanalytic treatment aim to achieve? (C) How effective is it? My arguments in relation to these questions will be:

A Psychoanalysis rests upon three core claims about the emotional mind that were once considered controversial but which are now widely accepted in neighbouring disciplines.
B The clinical methods that psychoanalysts use to relieve mental suffering flow directly from these core claims, and are consistent with current scientific understanding of how the brain changes.
C It is therefore not surprising that psychoanalytic therapy achieves good outcomes—at least as good as, and in some important respects better than, other evidence-based treatments in psychiatry today.

A

Our three core claims about the emotional mind, I submit, are the following: (1) The human infant is not a blank slate; *like all other species, we are born with a set of innate needs.* (2) *The main task of mental development is to learn how to meet these needs in the world*, which implies that mental disorder arises from *failures* to achieve this task. (3) *Most of our methods of meeting our emotional needs are executed unconsciously*, which requires us to return them to consciousness in order to change them.

These core claims could also be described as *premises*, but it is important to recognize that they are *scientific* premises, because they are testable and falsifiable. As I proceed, I will elaborate these premises, adding details, but I want to differentiate between the core claims themselves and the specifying details. The details are *empirical*. Whether they are ultimately upheld or not does not affect the core claims. Detailed knowledge changes over time, but core claims are foundational. Everything we do in psychoanalysis is predicated upon these three claims. If *they* are disproven, the core scientific presuppositions upon which psychoanalysis (as we know it) rests will have been rejected. But as things stand currently, in 2018, they are eminently defensible, strongly—indeed increasingly—supported by accumulating and converging lines of evidence in neighbouring fields. This continues to justify Kandel's (1999) assertion that "Psychoanalysis still represents the most coherent and intellectually satisfying view of the mind."

I turn now to each of the proposed three claims.

CLAIM 1. *The human infant is not a blank slate; like all other species, we are born with a set of innate needs.* These needs are regulated autonomically up to a point, beyond which they make "demands upon the mind to perform work," as Freud (1915) put it. Such *mental* demands constitute his "id." They are ultimately *felt* as affects. That is why affect is so important in psychoanalysis. The affect broadcasting a need releases reflexive or instinctual behaviours, which are hard-wired *predictions* (action plans) that we execute in order to meet our needs—e.g., we cry, search, freeze, flee, attack. Universal agreement about the number of innate needs in the human brain has not been achieved,[2] but most mainstream taxonomies (e.g., Panksepp, 1998) include at least a subset of the following *emotional* ones:[3]

- We need to engage with the world—since all our biological appetites (including bodily needs like hunger and thirst) can only be met there.[4] This is a *foraging* or seeking instinct. It is felt as interest, curiosity and the like. (It coincides roughly but not completely with Freud's concept of "libido"; see Solms, 2012.)
- We need to find sexual partners. This is felt as *lust*. This instinct is sexually dimorphic (on average) but male and female inclinations exist in both genders. (Like all other biological appetites, lust is channelled through seeking.)
- We need to escape dangerous situations. This is *fear*.
- We need to destroy frustrating objects (things that get between us and satisfaction of our needs). This is *rage*.
- We need to attach to caregivers (those who look after us). Separation from attachment figures is felt not as fear but as *panic*, and loss of them is felt as *despair*. (The whole of "attachment theory" relates to this need, and the next one.)
- We need to *care* for and nurture others, especially our offspring. This is the so-called maternal instinct, but it exists (to varying degrees) in both genders.

- We need to *play*. This is not as frivolous as it appears; play is the medium through which social hierarchies are formed ("pecking order"), in-group and out-group boundaries are maintained, and territory is won and defended.

CLAIM 2. *The main task of mental development is to learn how to meet our needs in the world.* We do not learn for its own sake; we do so in order to establish optimal *predictions* as to how we may meet our needs in a given environment. This is what Freud (1923) called "ego" development. Learning is necessary because even innate predictions have to be reconciled with lived experience. Evolution predicts how we should behave in, say, dangerous situations in general, but it cannot predict all possible dangers (e.g., electrical sockets); each individual has to learn *what* to fear and *how best* to respond to the variety of actual dangers. The most crucial lessons are learned during critical periods, mainly in early childhood, when we are—unfortunately— not best equipped to deal with the fact that our innate predictions often *conflict* with one another (e.g., attachment vs rage, curiosity vs fear).[5] We therefore need to learn *compromises*, and we must find *indirect* ways of meeting our needs. This often involves *substitute-formation*. Humans also have a large capacity for *delaying* gratification and for satisfying their needs in *imaginary* and *symbolic* ways.

It is crucial to recognize that *successful predictions entail successful emotion regulation, and vice-versa.* This is because our needs are *felt.* Thus successful avoidance of attack reduces fear, successful reunion after separation reduces panic, etc., whereas unsuccessful attempts at avoidance or reunion result in *persistence* of the fear or panic, etc.

CLAIM 3. *Most of our predictions are executed unconsciously.* Consciousness (short-term "working memory") is an extremely limited resource, so there is enormous pressure to consolidate learnt solutions to life's problems into long-term memory, and ultimately to *automatize* them (for review see Bargh & Chartrand, 1999, who conclude that only 5% of goal-directed actions are conscious). Innate predictions are effected automatically from the outset, as are those acquired in the first two years of life, before the preconscious ("declarative") memory systems mature (cf. infantile amnesia). Multiple unconscious ("non-declarative") memory systems exist, such as "procedural" and "emotional" memory, which operate according to different rules. These stereotyped systems (cf. the repetition compulsion) bypass thinking (i.e., the secondary process) and define the system unconscious.

The following fact is of utmost importance. *Not only successful predictions are automatized.* With this simple observation, we overcome the unfortunate distinction between the "cognitive" and "Freudian" unconscious (Solms, 2017). Sometimes a child has to make the best of a bad job in order to focus on the problems which it *can* solve. Such illegitimately or prematurely automatized predictions (i.e., *wishes* as opposed to realistic *solutions*) are called "the repressed." In order for predictions to be updated in light of experience, they need to be "reconsolidated"; that is, *they need to enter consciousness again*, in order for the long-term traces to become *labile* once more (Nader et al., 2000; Sara, 2000; Tronson & Taylor, 2007). This is sometimes difficult to achieve, however; not least because procedural memories are "hard to learn and hard to forget" and some emotional memories—which can be acquired through just a single exposure—appear to be indelible; but also because *the essential mechanism of repression entails resistance to reconsolidation despite prediction errors.* The theory of reconsolidation is very important for understanding the mechanism of psychoanalysis. This leads to my second argument, concerning our treatment.

B

My second argument is that the *clinical methods that psychoanalysts use to relieve mental suffering flow from the above core claims*, which are consistent with current understanding of how the brain changes. The argument unfolds over three steps:

a   *Psychological patients suffer mainly from feelings.* The essential difference between psychoanalytic and psychopharmacological methods of treatment is that we believe feelings *mean something.* Specifically, feelings represent unsatisfied needs. (Thus, a patient suffering from panic is afraid of losing something, a patient suffering from rage is frustrated by something, etc.) This truism applies regardless of etiological factors; even if one person is constitutionally more fearful, say, than the next, or cognitively less capable of updating predictions, their fear still means something. To be clear: *emotional disorders entail unsuccessful attempts to satisfy needs.* That is, psychological symptoms (unlike physiological ones) involve *intentionality.*

b   The main purpose of psychological treatment, then, is to *help patients learn better ways of meeting their needs.* This, in turn, leads to *better emotion regulation.* The psychopharmacological approach, by contrast, suppresses unwanted feelings. We do not believe that drugs that treat feelings directly can *cure* emotional disorder; drugs are symptomatic (not causal) treatments. To cure an emotional disorder, the patient's failure to meet underlying need/s must be addressed, since this is what is *causing* the symptoms. However, symptomatic relief is sometimes necessary before patients become accessible to psychological treatment, since most forms of psychotherapy require collaborative work between patient and therapist (see below). It is also true that some types of psychopathology *never* become accessible to psychotherapy. We must also concede that patients just want to feel better; they do not want to work for it.

c   *Psychoanalytical* therapy differs from other forms of psychotherapy in that it *aims to change deeply automatized predictions*, which—to the extent that they are consolidated into non-declarative memory—*cannot be reconsolidated in working memory*. Non-declarative (i.e., unconscious) predictions are *permanently* unconscious. Psychoanalytic technique[6] therefore focuses on:

- Identifying the *dominant emotions* (which are consciously felt but not always recognized as arising from specific needs and predictions).
- These emotions reveal the *meaning* of the symptom. That is, they lead the way to the particular *automatized predictions* that gave rise to the symptom.
- The pathogenic predictions *cannot be remembered directly* for the very reason that they are automatized (i.e., non-declarative). Therefore, the analyst identifies them *indirectly*, by bringing to awareness the *repetitive patterns of behaviour* derived from them.
- Reconsolidation is thus achieved through reactivation of non-declarative traces via their *derivatives* in the present (this is called "transference" interpretation). Automatized predictions cannot be retrieved into working memory, but patients *can* be made aware of the here-and-now *enactments* of those predictions. This is the essence of psychoanalytical cure.
- Such reconsolidation is nevertheless *difficult to achieve*, mainly due to the ways in which non-declarative memory systems work (they are "hard to learn, hard to forget" and in some respects "indelible") but also because repression entails intense resistance to the reactivation of insoluble problems. For all these reasons, psychoanalytic treatment takes time—and frequent sessions—to facilitate "working through." Working through entails numerous repetitions of transference interpretations in relation to ongoing derivates of repressed predictions, while new (and crucially, better) predictions are slowly consolidated. (Funders of psychological treatments need to learn how learning works.)

C

My third argument is that *psychoanalytic therapy achieves good outcomes*—at least as good as, and in some respects better than, other evidence-based treatments in psychiatry today. This argument unfolds over four stages:

a   *Psychotherapy in general is a highly effective form of treatment.* Meta-analyses of psychotherapy outcome studies typically reveal effect sizes of between 0.73 and 0.85. (An effect size of 1.0 means that the average treated patient is one standard deviation healthier than the average untreated patient.) An effect size of 0.8 is considered a large effect in psychiatric research, 0.5 is considered moderate, and 0.2 is considered small. To put the efficacy of psychotherapy into perspective, recent antidepressant medications achieve effect sizes of between 0.24 (tricyclics) and 0.31 (SSRIs).[7] The changes brought about by psychotherapy, no less than drug therapy, are of course visualizable with brain imaging (see Beauregard, 2014).

b   *Psychoanalytic psychotherapy is equally effective as other forms of psychotherapy* (e.g., CBT). This has recently been demonstrated conclusively by comparative meta-analysis (Steinert et al., 2017). However, there is evidence to suggest that *the effects last longer—and even increase—after the end of the treatment*. Shedler's (2010) authoritative review of all randomized control trials to date reported effect sizes of between 0.78 and 1.46, even for diluted and truncated forms of psychoanalytic therapy.[8] An especially methodologically rigorous meta-analysis (Abbass et al., 2006) yielded an overall effect size of 0.97 for general symptom improvement with psychoanalytic therapy. The effect size increased to 1.51 when the patients were assessed at follow-up. A more recent meta-analysis by Abbass et al. (2014) yielded an overall effect size of 0.71 and the finding of maintained and increased effects at follow-up was reconfirmed.

This was for *short-term* psychoanalytic treatment. According to the meta-analysis of De Maat et al. (2009), which was less methodologically rigorous than the Abbass studies, *longer-term* psychoanalytic psychotherapy yields an effect size of 0.78 at termination and 0.94 at follow-up, and *psychoanalysis* proper achieves a mean effect size of 0.87 at termination and 1.18 at follow-up. This is the overall effect; the effect size that she found for symptom improvement (as opposed to personality change) at termination was 1.03 for long-term therapy, and for psychoanalysis it was 1.38. Leuzinger-Bohleber et al.'s subsequent study (2019a, b; and in this volume) shows even bigger effect sizes: between 1.62 and 1.89 after three years of treatment. These are enormous effects. Follow-up data are, of course, not yet available from this ongoing study. The consistent trend toward *larger effect sizes at follow-up* (where the effects of other forms of psychotherapy, like CBT, tend to *decay*) suggests that psychoanalytic therapy sets in motion processes of change that continue even after therapy has ended (cf. "working through," discussed above). This is called the "sleeper effect."

It is important to recognize that these findings concern symptom improvement only. Psychoanalytic treatments are not directed primarily at symptomatic relief but rather at what might be called personality change. Not surprisingly, therefore, psychoanalytic treatments achieve much better results than other treatments on *this* outcome measure. In Leuzinger et al.'s ongoing study, for example, almost twice as many patients receiving psychoanalytic treatment vs CBT reached their criteria for "structural change" after three years (60% vs 36%; Leuzinger-Bohleber et al., 2019ab; and in this volume).

c   The therapeutic techniques that predict best treatment outcomes *make good sense in relation to the psychodynamic mechanisms outlined above*. These techniques are (Blagys & Hilsenroth, 2000):

• *unstructured*, open-ended dialogue between patient and therapist
• identifying *recurring themes* in the patient's experience

- linking the patient's *feelings* and perceptions to *past experiences*
- drawing attention to *feelings* regarded by the patient as *unacceptable*
- pointing out ways in which the patient *avoids* feelings
- focusing on the *here-and-now therapy relationship*
- drawing connections between the *therapy relationship and other relationships*.

It is highly instructive to note that these techniques lead to the best treatment outcomes, regardless of the "brand" of therapy that the clinician espouses. In other words, these same techniques (or at least a subset of them; see Hayes et al., 1996) predict optimal treatment outcomes in CBT too, even if the therapist believes they are doing something else.

d   It is therefore perhaps not surprising that psychotherapists, irrespective of their stated theoretical orientation, tend to choose psychoanalytic psychotherapy for themselves! (Norcross, 2005)

Conclusion

I am well aware that the claims I have summarized here do not do justice to the full complexity and variety of views in psychoanalysis, both as a theory and a therapy. I am saying only that these are our *core* claims, which underpin all the details, including those upon which we are yet to reach agreement. If we can agree on just these few claims, underpinning the arguments presented in this chapter, we are much better placed to explain our point of view to neighbouring disciplines and to the public. I believe that these claims and arguments are eminently defensible, in light of available scientific evidence, and that they make simple good sense.

However, it is far too soon to rest on our laurels. There is a pressing need, in particular, for more outcome studies focused on the symptomatic and structural effects of long-term psychoanalysis (versus low-frequency and short-term psychoanalytic psychotherapies).

A major disadvantage that we suffer in comparison with psychopharmacological and CBT researchers is an almost total lack of financial support for psychoanalytic outcome studies from statutory sources. If we are going to overcome the prejudice that feeds this lack of support—namely the self-fulfilling (and false, see Shedler, 2015; and in this volume) claim that psychoanalysis is not evidence-based—then psychoanalytic institutions will have to fund such studies themselves.

Notes

1 My introductory comments to this book are based on an article I recently published in the *British Journal of Psychiatry* (Solms, 2018). This is an expanded version of that article.

2 The taxonomy of innate needs is an empirical question of the kind I mentioned earlier; it does not affect the basic claim that we *are* born with a set of innate needs,

which are felt as affects and which trigger stereotyped predictions. I am well aware that the taxonomy I cite below differs from Freud's. Unlike many of his followers, Freud (1920) accepted that biology might well "blow away the artificial fabric of our hypotheses [about drives]."

3 Panksepp (1998) distinguishes between bodily, emotional and sensory needs, which correspond roughly with the terms "drive," "instinct" and "reflex." Here I am focusing on the *emotional* needs—which are felt as separation distress, rage, etc.— not the *bodily* ones—which are felt as hunger, thirst, etc.—or *sensory* ones—which are felt as pain, disgust, etc. My focus is somewhat arbitrary, but I am highlighting the category of needs that most commonly gives rise to psychopathology.

4 The fact that we can only meet our needs by engaging with others is why life is difficult. You cannot successfully copulate with yourself, attach to yourself, etc., although this does not stop us from trying! (The psychoanalytic theory of "narcissism" arises from these simple facts.)

5 This is why childhood, and the quality of parental guidance, are so important in psychoanalysis.

6 See Blagys & Hilsenroth, 2000; Smith & Solms, 2018.

7 See Turner et al., 2008; Kirsch et al., 2008.

8 I would like to thank Jonathan Shedler for his generous help with this chapter.

References

Abbass, A.A., Hancock, J.T., Henderson, J., & Kisely, S. (2006). Short-term psycho-dynamic psychotherapies for common mental disorders. *Cochrane Database of Systematic Reviews*, 4, Article No. CD004687. doi:10.1002/14651858.CD004687.pub3.

Abbass, A.A., Kisely, S.R., Town, J.M., Leichsenring, F., Driessen, E., De Maat, S., Gerber, A., Dekker, J., Rabung, S., Rusalovska, S., & Crowe, E. (2014). Short-term psychodynamic psychotherapies for common mental disorders (Review). *Cochrane Database of Systematic Reviews*, 7.

Bargh, J., & Chartrand, T. (1999). The unbearable automaticity of being. *American Psychologist*, 54, 462–479

Beauregard, M. (2014). Functional neuroimaging studies of the effects of psychotherapy. *Dialogues Clin Neurosci.*, 16, 75–81.

Blagys, M.D., & Hilsenroth, M.J. (2000). Distinctive activities of short-term psycho-dynamic-interpersonal psychotherapy: A review of the comparative psychotherapy process literature. *Clinical Psychology: Science and Practice*, 7, 167–188.

de Maat, S., de Jonghe, F., Schoevers, R., & Dekker, J. (2009). The effectiveness of long-term psychoanalytic therapy: A systematic review of empirical studies. *Harvard Review of Psychiatry*, 17, 11–23.

Freud, S. (1915). Instincts and their vicissitudes. *Standard Edition*, 14.

Freud, S. (1920). Beyond the pleasure principle. *Standard Edition*, 19.

Freud, S. (1923). The ego and the id. *Standard Edition*, 19.

Hayes, A.M., Castonguay, L.G., & Goldfried, M.R. (1996). Effectiveness of targeting the vulnerability factors of depression in cognitive therapy. *Journal of Consulting and Clinical Psychology*, 64, 623–627.

Kandel, E. (1999). Biology and the future of psychoanalysis: A new intellectual framework for psychiatry revisited. *Am J Psychiatry*, 156, 505–24.

Kirsch, I., Deacon, B.J., Huedo-Medina, T.B., Scoboria, A., Moore, T.J., & Johnson, B.T. (2008). Initial severity and antidepressant benefits: A meta-analysis of data submitted to the Food and Drug Administration. *PLoS Med*, 5, e45. doi:10.1371/journal.pmed.0050045.

Leuzinger-Bohleber, M., Hautzinger, M., Fiedler, G., Keller, W., Bahrke, U., Kallenbach, L., … Beutel, M. (2019a). Outcome of psychoanalytic and cognitive-behavioural long-term therapy with chronically depressed patients: A controlled trial with preferential and randomized allocation. *Can J Psychiatry*, 64(1), 47–58. doi:10.1177/0706743718780340.

Leuzinger-Bohleber, M., Kaufhold, J., Kallenbach, L., Negele, A., Ernst, M., Keller, W., … Beutel, M. (2019b). How to measure sustained psychic transformations in long-term treatments of chronically depressed patients: Symptomatic and structural changes in the LAC Depression Study of the outcome of cognitive-behavioural and psychoanalytic long-term treatments. *The International Journal of Psychoanalysis*, 100(1), 99–127. doi:10.1080/00207578.2018.1533377.

Nader, K., Schafe, G.E., & Le Doux, J. (2000). Fear memories require protein synthesis in the amygdala for reconsolidation after retrieval. *Nature*, 406, 722–726.

Norcross, J.C. (2005). The psychotherapist's own psychotherapy: Educating and developing psychologists. *American Psychologist*, 60, 840–850.

Panksepp, J. (1998). *Affective neuroscience*. Oxford University Press.

Sara, S.J. (2000). Retrieval and reconsolidation: Toward a neurobiology of remembering. *Learn. Mem.* 7, 73–84.

Shedler, J. (2010). The efficacy of psychodynamic psychotherapy. *American Psychologist*, 65, 98–109.

Shedler, J. (2015). Where is the evidence for 'evidence-based' therapy? *Journal of Psychological Therapies in Primary Care*, 4, 47–59.

Smith, R., & Solms, M. (2018). Examination of the hypothesis that 'repression is premature automatization': A psychoanalytic case report and discussion. *Neuropsychoanalysis*, 19. https://doi.org/10.1080/15294145.2018.1473045.

Solms, M. (2012). Are Freud's 'erogenous zones' sources or objects of libidinal drive? *Neuropsychoanalysis*, 14, 53–56.

Solms, M. (2017). What is 'the unconscious,' and where is it located in the brain? A neuropsychoanalytic perspective. *Annals of the New York Academy of Sciences*, 1406, 90–97.

Solms, M. (2018). The scientific standing of psychoanalysis. *British Journal of Psychiatry – International*, 15, 5 8.

Steinert, C., Munder, T., Rabung, S., Hoyer, J., & Leichsenring, F. (2017). Psychodynamic therapy: As efficacious as other empirically supported treatments? A meta-analysis testing equivalence of outcomes. *American Journal of Psychiatry*, doi: 10.1176/appi.ajp.2017.17010057.

Tronson, N.C., & Taylor, J.R. (2007). Molecular mechanisms of memory reconsolidation. *Nat Rev Neurosci*, 8, 262–275.

Turner, E., Matthews, A., Linardatos, E., Tell, R., & Rosenthal, R. (2008). Selective publication of antidepressant trials and its influence on apparent efficacy. *N Engl J Med*, 358, 252–260.

Part I

Outcome research

State of the art

Five advances in psychoanalytic thinking and their implications for outcome research

Robert N. Emde

Today we have compelling needs about making connections—connections involving ongoing research, on the one hand, and connections involving ongoing clinical application, on the other. Researchers and clinicians alike are seeking new knowledge about improving outcomes in psychotherapy. But, as the contributions of this volume indicate, challenges often arise in appreciating the meaning of changing advances in our field. Further, at times it seems we may even lose awareness about changing background perspectives in the scope of recent psychoanalytic thinking. I believe this lack of awareness of context may sometimes be a problem—interfering both with our making connections and with appreciating clinical meaning. In other words, to put it more positively, considering a broader context may help us to evaluate the extent of adaptive outcomes in psychotherapy—perhaps seeing new needs, accomplishments and opportunities.

Because of this, it seems appropriate to review five areas of advances in psychoanalytic thinking that I believe arise both from clinical experience and commonly accepted research. When brought forward, they build upon each other and may seem self-evident to many, but surprising to others. Featured in previous Sandler conference discussions, they represent major changes in perspective that, although they frame much of current useful practice, they also involve areas of meaning that need more exploration for the future of psychoanalysis. Thus, as I will emphasize, they highlight ongoing needs for inclusion in psychotherapy outcome research as well as clinical work. The five areas of advances in psychoanalytic thinking I will review comprise (1) a two-person psychology, (2) a developmental orientation, (3) a larger view of unconscious functioning, (4) embodied experience and (5) an integrative stance.

A two-person psychology

The first of these advances is that *psychoanalysis is now regarded as a two-person psychology*. The view is now widely accepted, reflected in training and in clinical discussions, that a core of what happens in psychoanalytic therapy depends upon the activation of transference and counter-transference experiences, with the dynamics of what happens in their interactions, over time. Psychotherapy research has shown, for example, that a most important variable influencing outcomes of treatment is whether, at the beginning of consultation, a patient likes the therapist, feels understood and, further, research has shown the importance of the responsiveness and "match" in the minds of both patient and analyst during treatment, as influencing outcomes (Silberschatz 2017; Watson, Steckley, & McMullen 2014; Kantrowitz 1995; Lyons-Ruth 1999). Overall, it seems that relationship factors, although not typically measured, are now being given more attention as influencing favorable outcomes across psychoanalytic therapy. More widely, it has been pointed out that all mental health therapies in general involve the effect of human relationships on other relationships. One could go on citing data from recorded analyses from the Ulm process research (Kächele & Thomä 1993; Leuzinger-Bohleber, Arnold & Kächele 2019) but implications seem clear: as we consider future collaborative studies of psychoanalytic work, assessments need to include those of the therapist/analyst as well as those of the patient as we think about outcomes. Study assessments of each partner need to occur before, during and after treatment, and, if possible during therapeutic interactions. Discussions in this volume indicate that, with advances in technology assessments could occur soon for psychoanalytic work, during and after sessions, as well as for brain functioning in a relatively non-intrusive way. And there is more. Neuroscientists have increasingly realized that the human brain, to be understood, must be studied in its social context, not in isolation. Brain structure exists as a result of adaptive functioning that has occurred over evolutionary time and during ontogeny and is wired to be social (Iacoboni 2008).

A developmental orientation

This brings us to a second advance. *Psychoanalysis is now more fully appreciated as developmental.* It is future oriented. While psychoanalytic theory at its origins and core has been developmental (Freud 1905/1953), this has been largely understood as the past influencing the present. Now there is more. Much has been and is being learned about psychodynamic and psychobiological processes in development (Emde 1988, 2005). Psychoanalytic therapy itself takes place over time and is oriented not only for understanding the past and helping with processes of adaptation in the present but, vitally, also for healthy adaptation in the future—again, outside of the consultation room and beyond the periods of treatment. Psychoanalytic psychotherapy is about prevention as well as recovery (Emde & Leuzinger-Bohleber 2014; Emde 2011). And, appropriately, within the purview of thinking more about the two-person psychology of psychoanalysis, this orients us to goals for psychotherapy of improving healthy adaptive functioning outside of the relationship experience within therapy—to meaningful ongoing social relationships in family, work and beyond.

A larger view of unconscious functioning

A third major advance is that *psychoanalytic psychology now includes a larger view of unconscious and conscious mental functioning*. Its theory now includes but goes beyond its original theory of unconscious conflict involving the dynamics of defense and repression (Leuzinger-Bohleber, Arnold, & Solms 2016). As is discussed throughout the contributions of this volume, unconscious mental functioning is now appreciated to involve adaptive domains of skill-based procedural and implicit knowledge and these domains are importantly included in neuropsychological assessments, including those of executive functioning and their emotional connections. Emotions function as adaptive organizers of consciousness and plans, not primarily as disorganizers, as was previously thought (Solms 2019). I would also point out that a major therapeutic factor in infant–parent psychotherapy and in ages beyond has been identified as relational, involving unconscious functioning and has been conceptualized by the Boston Psychotherapy Change Group as "implicit relational knowing" (Stern et al. 1998; Lyons-Ruth 1999). Importantly, this implies that adaptive emotional configurations of the therapeutic relationship experience are learned and go forward in time. This is intended to occur in mental representations and actions, outside of consulting rooms, to be applied usefully in other life relationships. Such learned, unconscious relationship skills resulting from psychotherapy, comprise an area that is rarely assessed or considered in our discussions.

Embodied experience

A fourth advance in thinking consists of a wider appreciation that *psychoanalytic psychology is embodied* (Lakoff & Johnson 2008; Leuzinger-Bohleber, Emde & Pfeifer 2013). Consciousness and mental processes are influenced by our sensori-motor experiences, emotions and bodily states, healthy and otherwise, (including "metaphors we live by," as explicated by Lakoff & Johnson 2008). Such embodied states, importantly, are embedded in social relationships, going forward in time. They are also vital for understanding clinical engagement and consciousness in psychotherapy sessions and in for understanding the experiences of relationships beyond. Increasingly, we are appreciating how such experiential states as fatigue, emotional dysfunction and suffering and variations in somatic feedback influence relationships, development and consciousness over time. Accordingly, the experience of changes in psychotherapy are necessarily embodied and to be understood as such—for patient, and therapist, during consultations and outcomes.

An integrative stance

A fifth major advance is that psychoanalytic thinking aspires to be *integrative*. Psychoanalysis, in its explorations and therapeutics, is not simply "analysis."

As noted above, it involves making new connections and being mindful of adaptive meanings with the bodily self and others as they emerge. That is, it involves synthesis as well as analysis, emergence of new connections and possibilities as well as old problematic repetitions. Whereas, in the past, psychoanalysis was limited by its isolation from other academic disciplines, there is now a major shift in the context of thinking. Psychoanalysis as a psychology now aspires to connect—integrating its knowledge and findings about therapeutics within the larger context of thinking about relational adaptations, ongoing development, unconscious conflict, and embodiment with that of other scientific and health disciplines—in this way contributing to clinical as well general knowledge. As this volume illustrates, psychoanalytic research and clinical discourse is now interdisciplinary. Due to this advance in perspective and attitude, we can now draw together and make use of what experienced psychotherapists and their patients have learned, across disciplines and beyond their original theories of training. Further, clinicians can now join researchers in seeking general knowledge across numbers and domains in order to understand what works for whom under what circumstances and how—an aim that is guided, but not constrained, by disciplinary theory.

Implications for outcomes research

As has been proclaimed, the days of horse racing are over—that means doing research studies that merely look at comparing overall efficacies of two or more forms of treatment. Evidence shows that psychoanalytic psychotherapy works beneficially, as does cognitive-behavioral and some other forms of systematic psychotherapy. But more fully: *How do they work, and in what ways and for whom and under what circumstances and relationship conditions?* These questions are ones, in today's parlance, for understanding the clinical applications of big data research for "personalized medicine." In other words, if we compare two or more conditions or types of psychotherapy, over time, to what extent can we better understand the times and the embodied mechanisms of adaptive change (Leuzinger-Bohleber, Kallenbach, & Schoett 2016)? To the extent we can pursue this aspirational stance, the hope is that clinicians will then be able to apply findings from the research of the many (using big data) to individual patients (in their practices).

The above hope is furthered by the integrative stance of psychoanalysis that includes the other advances in thinking. Paradoxically, just as psychoanalysis is more than "analysis," involving the development of synthesis and new meanings, it is also true that psychoanalysis is more than the usual sense of "psycho," involving many levels of biological experience. And, powerfully, assessments are now becoming available for understanding changes in healthy regulatory processes at micro-momentary levels of functioning as well as for levels involving stress and other connected and enduring adaptive relationship experiences with therapist and with meaningful others in family, workplace and elsewhere.

At this point, let us draw together some of the clinical implications of our changes in psychoanalytic thinking for future outcomes research. First, as implied, "outcomes" cannot be cross-sectional; they need to be understood and studied over time. Outcomes are dynamic, changing according to development. They are relational and they vary according to epigenetic challenge and life circumstances. These occur in addition to transference–countertransference interactions and interpretations. And presumably, with treatment, a dynamic developmental future-oriented process will change in a more adaptive direction as a positive outcome. Thus outcomes need to be assessed and understood at multiple times during therapy and afterwards. Second, if we compare two different types or conditions of psychotherapy, we need to assess the therapist over time in the two-person process as well as the patient. Third, outcomes of treatment, over time, need to include assessments of adaptive meaningful relationships of the patient in family, work and other life settings. Fourth, as this volume indicates, along the lines of an integrative psychology, research involving psychoanalytic outcomes, needs to make increasing use of opportunities provided by contemporary discoveries in the developmental neurosciences, and systems biology, taking advantage of changes in biomarkers, that underpin consciousness, unconscious conflict and adaptive behavior. As indicated, meaningful research now can go beyond merely looking at comparing overall efficacies of treatment. Opportunities now present themselves, with advances in assessments of biomarkers for stress, psychoneuroimmunology, brain imaging, as well as for assessments of lived experiences including feelings, conscious and unconscious meaning in addition to assessments of cognitive processes, plans and behavior. And, powerfully, assessments are now becoming available for understanding changes in healthy regulatory processes at micro-momentary levels of functioning as well as for levels involving connected and enduring adaptive relationship experiences with therapist and with meaningful others in family, workplace and elsewhere.

A final reflection. The use of "outcome" as a term needs to be thought about more deeply. Outcome is not only about relief of suffering, discomfort and symptoms in the consulting room or upon completion of treatment; even more, it is about relief of misery and self-imposed problems in times afterwards—in a life of love and work with others. Assessments of outcome for psychotherapy require longitudinal study, to see if there are changes among the patient's adaptive experiences involving connections and meaning. And to remind us of a key point: outcomes of research trials are valuable mainly if they are connected with sharing increased knowledge about what works for whom within treatment and how, across disciplines. This is not only in line with our five advances in psychoanalytic thinking, but joins in our collaborative passions of benefitting individual patients working with their therapists. We want to learn and improve what we do. In thinking deeply about outcomes, we have a lot to learn from each other.

References

Emde, R.N. (1988). Development terminable and interminable: II. Recent psycho-analytic theory and therapeutic considerations. *International Journal of Psycho-Analysis*, 69, 283–296.

Emde, R.N. (2005). A developmental orientation for contemporary psychoanalysis. In G. Gabbard, E. Person, A. Cooper (Eds.) *Textbook of psychoanalysis* (pp. 117–130). Washington: American Psychiatric Publishing Inc.

Emde, R.N. (2011). Regeneration und Neuanfang: Perspektiven einer entwicklungs-bezogenen Ausrichtung der Psychoanalyse. *Psyche* 65 (9): 778–807. (English manuscript title: Recovery and new beginnings: Prospects for the developmental orientation of psychoanalysis).

Emde, R.N., & Leuzinger-Bohleber, M. (Eds.). (2014). *Early parenting and prevention of disorder: Psychoanalytic research at interdisciplinary frontiers*. London: Karnac Books.

Freud, S. (1905/1953). Three essays on the theory of sexuality. In J. Strachey (Ed. and Trans.). *The standard edition of the complete psychological works of Sigmund Freud* (Vol. 7, pp. 125–245). London: Hogarth Press.

Iacoboni, M. (2008). *Mirroring people: The new science of how we connect with others*. New York: Farrar, Straus and Giroux.

Kantrowitz, J.L. (1995). The beneficial aspects of the patient–analyst match. *International Journal of Psycho-analysis*, 76, 299–313.

Kächele, H., & Thomä, H. (1993). Psychoanalytic process research: Methods and achievements. *J. Amer. Psychoanal. Assn.*, 41S (Supplement), 109–129.

Lakoff, G., & Johnson, M. (2008). *Metaphors we live by*. Chicago: University of Chicago Press.

Leuzinger-Bohleber, M., Arnold, S., & Solms, M. (Eds.). (2016). *The unconscious: A bridge between psychoanalysis and cognitive neuroscience*. London/New York: Routledge.

Leuzinger-Bohleber, M., Arnold, S.E.A., & Kächele, H. (2019). Open door review of clinical, conceptual, process and outcome studies. Retrieved from: www.opendoorreview.com/.

Leuzinger-Bohleber, M., Kallenbach, L., & Schoett, M.J. (2016). Pluralistic approaches to the study of process and outcome in psychoanalysis. The LAC depression study: A case in point. *Psychoanalytic Psychotherapy*, 30(1), 4–22.

Leuzinger-Bohleber, M., Emde, R.N., & Pfeifer, R. (Eds.). (2013). *Embodiment: Ein innovatives Konzept für Entwicklungsforschung und Psychoanalyse*. Göttingen: Vandenhoeck & Ruprecht.

Lyons-Ruth, K. (1999). The two-person unconscious: Intersubjective dialogue, enactive relational representation, and the emergence of new forms of relational organization. *Psychoanalytic Inquiry*, 19(4), 576–617.

Silberschatz, G. (2017). Improving the yield of psychotherapy research. *Psychotherapy Research*, 27, 1–13.

Solms, M. (2019). APsaA's major new research initiative will further the scientific basis of psychoanalysis. *The American Psychoanalyst*, 33 (1).

Stern, D.N., Sander, L.W., Nahum, J.P., Harrison, A.M., Lyons-Ruth, K., Morgan, A.C., … & Tronick, E.Z. (1998). Non-interpretive mechanisms in psychoanalytic therapy: The 'something more' than interpretation. *International Journal of Psycho-Analysis*, *79*, 903–921.

Watson, J.C., Steckley, P.L., & McMullen, E.J. (2014). The role of empathy in promoting change. *Psychotherapy Research*, *24*, 286–298.

Chapter 3

Where is the evidence for "evidence-based" therapy?[1]

Jonathan Shedler

"Evidence-based therapy" has become a marketing buzzword. The term "evidence based" comes from medicine. It gained attention in the 1990s and was initially a call for critical thinking. Proponents of evidence-based medicine recognized that "We've always done it this way" is poor justification for medical decisions. Medical decisions should integrate individual clinical expertise, patients' values and preferences, and relevant scientific research (Sackett, Rosenberg, Gray, Haynes, & Richardson, 1996).

But the term evidence based has come to mean something very different for psychotherapy. It has been appropriated to promote a specific ideology and agenda. It is now used as a code word for manualized therapy—most often brief, one-size fits-all forms of cognitive behavior therapy (CBT). "Manualized" means the therapy is conducted by following an instruction manual. The treatments are often standardized or scripted in ways that leave little room for addressing the needs of individual patients.

Behind the "evidence-based" therapy movement lies a master narrative that increasingly dominates the mental health landscape. The master narrative goes something like this: "In the dark ages, therapists practiced unproven, unscientific therapy. Evidence-based therapies are scientifically proven and superior." The narrative has become a justification for all-out attacks on traditional talk therapy— that is, therapy aimed at fostering self-examination and self-understanding in the context of an ongoing, meaningful therapy relationship.

Here is a small sample of what proponents of "evidence-based" therapy say in public. "The empirically supported psychotherapies are still not widely practiced. As a result, many patients do not have access to adequate treatment" (Hollon, Thase, & Markowitz, 2002) (emphasis added). Note the linguistic sleight-of-hand: if the therapy is not "evidence based" (read, manualized), it is inadequate. Other proponents of "evidence-based" therapies go further in denigrating relationship-based, insight-oriented therapy: "The disconnect between what clinicians do and what science has discovered is an unconscionable embarrassment" (Mischel, 2008).

The news media promulgate the master narrative. The *Washington Post* ran an article titled "Is your therapist a little behind the times?" which likened traditional talk therapy to pre-scientific medicine when "healers commonly used ineffective and often injurious practices such as blistering, purging and bleeding." *Newsweek* sounded a similar note with an article titled, "Ignoring the evidence: Why do psychologists reject science?"

Note how the language leads to a form of McCarthyism. Because proponents of brief, manualized therapies have appropriated the term "evidence-based," it has become nearly impossible to have an intelligent discussion about what constitutes good therapy. Anyone who questions "evidence-based" therapy risks being branded anti-evidence and anti-science.

One might assume, in light of the strong claims for "evidence-based" therapies and the public denigration of other therapies, that there must be extremely strong scientific evidence for their benefits. There is not. There is a yawning chasm between what we are told research shows and what research actually shows.

Empirical research actually shows that "evidence-based" therapies are ineffective for most patients most of the time. First, I discuss what empirical research really shows. I then take a closer look at troubling practices in "evidence-based" therapy research.

Part I: What research really shows

Research shows that "evidence-based" therapies are weak treatments. Their benefits are trivial. Most patients do not get well. Even the trivial benefits do not last. This may be different from what you have been taught. It is incompatible with the master narrative. I will not ask you to accept my word for any of this. That is why I will discuss and quote primary sources.

In the beginning

The gold standard of evidence in "evidence-based" therapy research is the randomized controlled trial. Patients with a specific psychiatric diagnosis are randomly assigned to treatment or control groups and the study compares the groups.

The mother of all randomized controlled trials for psychotherapy is the National Institute of Mental Health (NIMH) Treatment of Depression Collaborative Research Program. It was the first large-scale, multisite study of what are now called "evidence based" therapies. The study included three active treatments: manualized CBT, manualized interpersonal therapy, and antidepressant medication. The control group got a placebo pill and clinical management but not psychotherapy. The study began in the mid-1970s and the first major findings were published in 1989.

For the last quarter of a century, we have been told that the NIMH study showed that CBT, interpersonal therapy, and antidepressant medication are "empirically validated" treatments for depression. We have been told that these treatments were proven effective. I focus here on CBT because the term evidence-based therapy most often refers to CBT and its variants.

The primary outcome measure in the NIMH study was the 54-point Hamilton Depression Rating Scale. The difference between the CBT treatment group and the placebo control group was 1.2 points.(Elkin et al., 1989) The 1.2-point difference between the CBT and control group is trivial and clinically meaningless. It does not pass the "So what?" test. It does not pass the "Does it matter?" test. It does not pass the "Why should anyone care?" test.

How could there be such a mismatch between what we have been told versus what the study actually found? You may be wondering whether the original researchers did not present the data clearly. That is not the case. The first major research report from the NIMH study was published in 1989 in Archives of General Psychiatry (Elkin et al., 1989). The authors wrote: "There was limited evidence of the specific effectiveness of interpersonal psychotherapy and none for cognitive behavior therapy" (emphasis added). That is what the original research article reports.

In 1994, the principal investigator wrote a comprehensive review of what we learned from the study, titled "The NIMH Treatment of Depression Collaborative Research Program: Where we began and where we are." (Elkin, 1994). Writing in careful academic language, the principal investigator stated, "What is most striking in the follow-up findings is the relatively small percentage of patients who remain in treatment, fully recover, and remain completely well throughout the 18-month follow-up period." The percentage is so small that it "raises questions about whether the potency of the short-term treatments for depression has been oversold" (Elkin, 1994).

What was that percentage, actually? It turns out that only 24% of the patients got well and stayed well. In other words, about 75%—the overwhelming majority—did not get well. How can this be? We have been told the opposite for one-quarter of a century. We have been told that manualized CBT is powerful and effective.

Statistically significant does not mean effective

The word significant gives rise to considerable misunderstanding. In the English language, significant is a synonym for important or meaningful. In statistics, significant is a term of art with a technical definition, pertaining to the probability of an observed finding.[2] "Statistically significant" does not indicate that findings are of scientific import (a point emphasized in a recent statement by the American Statistical Association: Wasserstein and Lazar (2016)). They absolutely do not mean that patients get well or even that they improve in any clinically meaningfully way.

There is a mismatch between the questions studies of "evidence-based" therapy tend to ask versus what patients, clinicians, and health care policymakers need to know. Studies are conducted by academic researchers who often have little or no clinical practice experience, who may not appreciate the challenges and complexities therapists and patients face in real-world practice. Writing in *American Psychologist*, eminent CBT researcher Alan Kazdin (2006) noted, "Researchers often do not know if clients receiving an evidence-based treatment have improved in everyday life or changed in a way that makes a difference" (emphasis added).

Major misunderstandings arise when researchers "disseminate" research findings to patients, policymakers, and practitioners. Researchers speak of "significant" treatment benefits, referring to statistical significance. Most people understandably, but mistakenly, take this to mean that patients get well or at least meaningfully better.

Few other disciplines emphasize "significance" instead of actual change. When there is a meaningful treatment benefit, investigators emphasize that, not "significance." If a drug is effective in lowering blood pressure, we report how much it lowers blood pressure. If we have an effective weight loss program, we report that the average person in the program lost 20 pounds, or 30 pounds, or whatever. If we have a drug that lowers cholesterol, we report how much it lowers cholesterol. We would not focus on statistical significance. When researchers focus on statistical significance, something is being hidden.

I am embarrassed that when I first wrote about the NIMH depression study, I assumed that the 1.2-point difference between the CBT group and the placebo control group was statistically significant, even if clinically irrelevant (Shedler, 2015). I assumed this was why the study was widely cited as scientific evidence for CBT. When I subsequently examined the primary sources more closely, I discovered that the 1.2-point difference on the depression rating scale was not even statistically significant. It was difficult to wrap my head around the notion that widespread claims that the study provided scientific support for CBT had no basis in the actual data. This seems to be a case where the master narrative trumped the facts.

Research continues, treatment benefits do not

The NIMH findings were published more than 25 years ago. Surely, research findings for CBT must have improved over time. Let's jump ahead to the most recent state-of-the-art randomized controlled trial for depression (Driessen et al., 2013). The study included 341 depressed patients randomly assigned to 16 sessions of manualized CBT or 16 sessions of manualized psychodynamic therapy. The two treatments did not differ in effectiveness. The study was published in 2013 in the *American Journal of Psychiatry*. The authors wrote, "One notable finding was that only 22.7% of the patients achieved remission" (Driessen et al., 2013).] They continued, "Our findings indicate that a substantial proportion of patients … require more than time-limited therapy to achieve remission." In other words, about 75% of patients did not get well. It is essentially the same finding reported in the NIMH study one-quarter of a century earlier.

The appropriate conclusion to be drawn from both of these major studies is that brief manualized therapies are ineffective for most depressed patients most of the time.

I have described the earliest major study and the most recent. What about the research in between? The findings are largely the same. The research is summarized in a review paper in *Psychological Bulletin* by Drew Westen and colleagues (Westen, Novotny, & Thompson-Brenner, 2004). The paper is a detailed, comprehensive literature review of manualized CBT for depression and anxiety disorders.

The researchers found that the average patient who received manualized CBT for depression remained clinically depressed after treatment, with an average Beck Depression Inventory score greater than 10. What about conditions besides depression? How about panic disorder? Panic seems to be the condition for which brief, manualized CBT works best. However, the average patient who received "evidence-based" treatment for panic disorder still had panic attacks almost weekly and still endorsed four of seven symptoms listed in the *Diagnostic and Statistical Manual of Mental Disorders*, 4th edition. These patients did not get well either.

Another finding was that the benefits of manualized "evidence-based" therapies are temporary. Treatment outcome is typically measured the day treatment ends. But when patients are followed over time, treatment benefits evaporate. The majority of patients who receive an "evidence-based" therapy—more than 50%—seek treatment again within six to 12 months for the same condition. This finding should give investigators pause. It would also be a mistake to conclude that those who do not seek additional treatment are well. Some may have gotten well. Many may have simply given up on psychotherapy.

Even ardent CBT advocates have acknowledged that manualized CBT offers lasting help to few. Writing in Psychological Science in the Public Interest, eminent CBT researcher Steven Hollon noted "Only about half of all patients respond to any given intervention, and only about a third eventually meet the criteria for remission.... Moreover, most patients will not stay well once they get better unless they receive ongoing treatment."[3] Ironically, this was written by the same researcher who declared other forms of psychotherapy "inadequate." Sadly, such information reaches few clinicians and fewer patients. I wonder what the public and policy makes would think if they knew these are the same treatments described publicly as "evidence-based," "scientifically proven," and "the gold standard."

Part 2: A closer look at research practices

In this section, I address some research practices behind the claims for manualized, "evidence-based" therapies. I address the following issues: First, most patients are never counted. Second, the control groups are shams. Third, manualized, "evidence-based" therapy has not shown superiority to any other form of psychotherapy. Fourth, data are being hidden.

Most patients are never counted

In the typical randomized controlled trial for "evidence-based" therapies, about two-thirds of the patients are excluded from the studies a priori (Westen et al., 2004). Sometimes exclusion rates exceed 80%. That is, the patients have the diagnosis and seek treatment, but because of the study's inclusion and exclusion criteria, they are excluded from participation. The higher the exclusion rates, the better the outcomes (Westen & Morrison, 2001). Typically, the patients who are excluded are those who meet criteria for more than one psychiatric diagnosis, or have personality pathology, or are considered unstable, or who may be suicidal. In other words, they are the patients we treat in real-world practice. The patients included in the research studies are not representative of any real-world clinical population.

Here is some simple arithmetic. Approximately two-thirds of patients who seek treatment are excluded from the research studies. Of the one-third who are treated, about one-half show improvement. This is about 16% of the patients who initially presented for treatment. But this is just patients who show "improvement." If we consider patients who actually get well, we are down to about 11% of those who originally sought treatment. If we consider patients who get well and stay well, we are down to 5% or fewer. In other words, scientific research demonstrates that "evidence-based" treatments are effective and have lasting benefits for approximately 5% of the patients who seek treatment. Here is another way to look at it. The iceberg represents the patients who seek treatment for a psychiatric condition—depression, generalized anxiety, and so on. The tip of the iceberg represents the patients described in the "evidence-based" therapy research literature. All the rest— the huge part of the iceberg below the water—do not get counted. The research methods render them invisible.

Control groups are shams

Second point: the control group is usually a sham. What do I mean? I mean that "evidence-based" therapies are almost never compared to legitimate alternative therapies. The control group is usually a foil invented by researchers committed to demonstrating the benefits of CBT. In other words, the control group is a fake treatment that is intended to fail.

A state-of-the-art, NIMH-funded study of posttraumatic stress disorder (PTSD) provides a good illustration of a sham control group (Gilboa-Schechtman, Shafran, & Foa, 2011). The study focused on "single incident" PTSD. The patients were previously healthy. They developed PTSD after experiencing a specific identifiable trauma. The study claims to compare psychodynamic

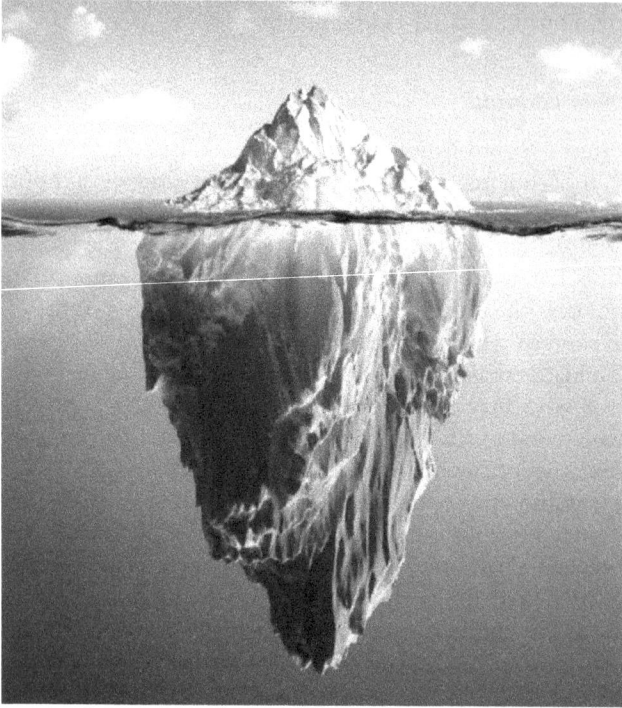

Figure 3.1 Most patients are never counted. (Courtesy of iStock by Getty Images, St. Louis, Missouri).

therapy with a form of CBT called prolonged exposure therapy. It claims to show that CBT is superior to psychodynamic therapy. This is what it says in the discussion section: "[CBT] was superior to [psychodynamic therapy] in decreasing symptoms of PTSD and depression, enhancing functioning ... and increasing overall improvement."

That is what was communicated to the media, the public, and policymakers. If you read the fine print and do a little homework, things look very different. Who were the therapists who provided the "psychodynamic" treatment? Were they experienced, qualified, psychodynamic therapists? No. It turns out that they were graduate students. They received two days of training in psychodynamic therapy from another graduate student—a graduate student in a research laboratory committed to CBT. In contrast, the therapists who provided CBT received five days of training by the developer of the treatment, world-famous author and researcher Edna Foa. That is not exactly a level playing field.

But that was the least of the problems. The so-called psychodynamic therapists were prohibited from discussing the trauma that brought the patient to treatment. Imagine that—you seek treatment for PTSD because you have experienced a traumatic event, and your therapist refuses to discuss it. The therapists were trained to change the topic when patients brought up their traumatic experiences.

If a clinician practiced this way in the real world, it could be considered malpractice. In "evidence-based" therapy research, that is considered a control group, and a basis for claims that CBT is superior to psychodynamic therapy.[4] Even with the sham therapy control condition, the advantage of CBT still disappeared at long-term follow up—but you would have to sift through the results section with a fine-toothed comb to know this.

The "superiority" of evidence-based therapy is a myth

In case you are thinking the PTSD study is unusual—perhaps cherry-picked to make a point—that is not the case. There is a comprehensive review of the psychotherapy research literature that addresses this very question (Wampold et al., 2011). It focused on randomized controlled trials for both anxiety and depression. The researchers examined studies that claimed to compare an "evidence-based" therapy with an alternative form of psychotherapy. The researchers examined more than 2500 abstracts. After closer examination, they winnowed that down to 149 studies that looked like they might actually compare an "evidence-based" therapy with another legitimate form of therapy. But when they finished, there were only 14 studies that compared "evidence-based" therapy with a control group that received anything resembling bona fide psychotherapy. These studies showed no advantages whatever for "evidence-based" therapies.

Many studies claimed to use control groups that received "treatment as usual." But "treatment as usual" turned out to be "predominantly 'treatments' that did not include any psychotherapy" (Wampold et al., 2011). I am not interpreting or paraphrasing. This is a quotation from the original article. In other words, "evidence-based" therapies were not compared with other forms of legitimate psychotherapy. They were compared and found "superior" to doing nothing. Alternatively, they were compared with control groups that received sham psychotherapy where therapists had their hands tied—as in the PTSD study described above.

This literature review was published in a conservative scholarly journal and the authors stated their conclusions in careful academic language. They concluded, "Currently, there is insufficient evidence to suggest that transporting an evidence-based therapy to routine care that already involves psychotherapy will improve the quality of services." In somewhat plainer English, "evidence-based" therapies are not more effective than any other form of psychotherapy. That is what the scientific literature actually shows. That is not just my opinion. It is the official scientific policy conclusion of the American Psychological Association (Campbell, Norcross, Vasquez, & Kaslow, 2013).

Data are suppressed

"Publication bias" is a well-known phenomenon in research. Publication bias refers to the fact that studies with positive results—those that show the outcomes desired by the investigators—tend to get published. Studies that fail to show the desired outcome tend not to get published. For this reason, published research can provide a biased or skewed picture of actual research findings. There is a name for this phenomenon, it is called the "file-drawer effect." For every published study with positive results, how many studies with negative results are hidden in researchers' file drawers? How can you prove there are file drawers stuffed with negative results? It turns out there is a way to do this. There are statistical methods to estimate how many unpublished studies have negative results that are hidden from view.

A team of researchers tackled this question for research on CBT for depression (Cuijpers, Smit, Bohlmeijer, Hollon, & Andersson, 2010).

They found that the published benefits of CBT are exaggerated by 75% owing to publication bias. How do you find out something like this? How can you know what is hidden in file drawers? You know by examining what is called a funnel plot. The idea is actually quite simple. Suppose you are conducting a poll—"Are US citizens for or against building a border wall with Mexico?"—and you examine very small samples of only three people. The results can be all over the place. Depending on the three people you happen to select, it may look like 100% of citizens favor a wall or 100% oppose it. With small sample sizes, you see a wide scatter or range of results. As sample sizes get larger, the findings stabilize and converge.

If you graph the findings—in this case, the relationship between sample size and treatment benefit—you get a plot that looks like a funnel (Figure 3.2, left).

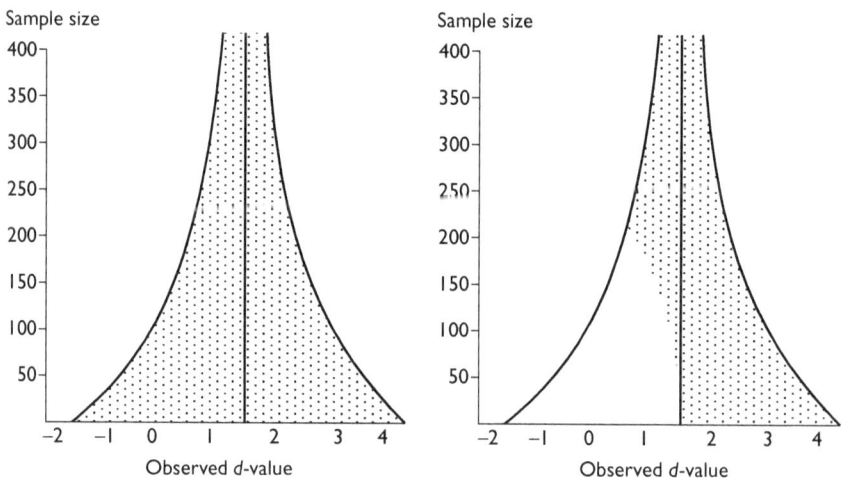

Figure 3.2 Sample funnel plot.

Studies with smaller sample sizes show more variability in results, and studies with larger sample sizes tend to converge on more similar values. That is what it should look like if data are not being hidden. In fact, what it looks like is something like the graph on the right (see Figure 3.1). The data points that are supposed to be in the lower left area of the graph are missing.[5]

What "evidence-based" is supposed to mean

What is "evidence-based" supposed to mean? I noted earlier that the term originated in medicine. Evidence-based medicine was meant to be the integration of:

a   Relevant scientific evidence,
b   Patients' values and preferences, and
c   The individual experience and clinical judgment of practitioners (Figure 3.2) (APA Presidential Task Force on Evidence-Based Practice, 2006; Sackett et al., 1996).

What has happened to these ideas in psychotherapy? "Relevant scientific evidence" no longer counts, because proponents of "evidence-based" therapies ignore evidence for therapies that are not manualized and scripted. In 2010, I published an article in *American Psychologist* titled, "The efficacy of psychodynamic psychotherapy" (Shedler, 2010). The article demonstrates that the benefits of psychodynamic therapy are at least as large as those of therapies promoted as "evidence based"—and, moreover, the benefits of psychodynamic therapy last. Subsequent research replicates and extends these findings. Yet proponents of

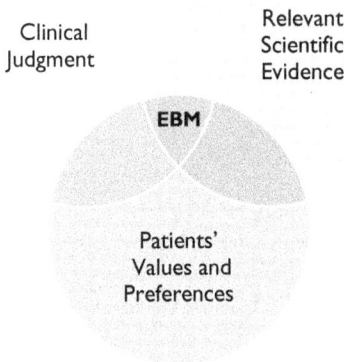

Figure 3.3 Illustration of evidence-based medicine (EBM).

Source: Adapted from Sackett, D.L., Rosenberg, W.M., Gray, J.A., et al. Evidence based medicine: what it is and what it isn't. *BMJ* 1996; 312(7023): 71–2; with permission.

"evidence-based" therapy often disregard such evidence. "Evidence based" does not actually mean supported by evidence, it means manualized, scripted, and not psychodynamic. What does not fit the master narrative does not count.

"Patients' values and preferences" also do not count, because patients are not adequately informed or offered meaningful choices. They may be offered only brief manualized treatment and told it is the "gold standard." This serves the financial interests of health insurers, who have an economic incentive to shunt patients to the briefest, cheapest treatments (Bendat, 2014). Patients who know nothing of therapy aimed at self-reflection and self-understanding, or who have heard it only denigrated as inadequate or unscientific, are hardly in a position to exercise informed choice.

"Clinical judgment" also no longer matters, because clinicians are often expected to follow treatment manuals rather than exercise independent judgment. They are increasingly being asked to function as technicians, not clinicians.[5] One could argue that "evidence based," as the term is now applied to psychotherapy, is a perversion of every founding principle of evidence-based medicine.

Facts and alternative facts

The information in this chapter may seem at odds with virtually all other respectable scholarly sources. Why should you believe me? You should not believe me. You should not take my word for any of this—or anyone else's word. I will leave you with three simple things to do to help sift truth from hyperbole. When somebody makes a claim for a treatment, any treatment, follow these three steps:

- Step 1: Say, "Show me the study." Ask for a reference, a citation, a PDF. Have the study put in your hands. Sometimes it does not exist.
- Step 2: If the study does exist, read it—especially the fine print.
- Step 3: Draw your own conclusions. Ask yourself: Do the actual methods and findings of the study justify the claim I heard?

If you make a practice of following these simple steps, you may make some shocking discoveries.

Notes

1 This is a reprint of the article printed in *Psychiatric Clinics of North America* (Volume 41, Issue 2, June 2018; pp. 319–329). Reprinted with permission.
2 More precisely, "the probability under a specified statistical model that a statistical summary of the data (e.g., the sample mean difference between two compared groups) would be equal to or more extreme than its observed value" (Wasserstein & Lazar, 2016).
3 Shockingly, when a letter to the editor called the researchers on the fact that the sham therapy control condition was not psychodynamic therapy, they doubled down and insisted it was (Gilboa-Schechtman et al., 2010; Wittmann, Halpern, Adams, Ørner, & Kudler, 2011).

4 There was public outcry when research revealed the extent of publication bias in clinical trials for antidepressant medication (Turner, Matthews, Linardatos, Tell, & Rosenthal, 2008). The bias was widely attributed to the influence of the pharmaceutical industry and conflicts of interest of investigators with financial ties to pharmaceutical companies. However, the publication bias for antidepressants medication pales in comparison with the publication bias for "evidence-based" therapy.

5 Lest the reader think this a misrepresentation or caricature, consider that prominent proponents of manualized therapy advocate treatment by minimally trained paraprofessionals. The journal *Psychological Science in the Public Interest*, the house organ of the Association for Psychological Science, published the following:

> Many of these [evidence-based] interventions can be disseminated without highly trained and expensive personnel.… CBT is effective even when delivered by nondoctoral therapists or by health educators with little or no prior experience with CBT who received only a modest level of training … manuals and workbooks are available on user-friendly websites.
>
> (Baker, McFall, & Shoham, 2008)

The devaluation of clinical expertise inherent in these statements requires no interpretation.

References

APA Presidential Task Force on Evidence-Based Practice. (2006). Evidence-based practice in psychology. *The American Psychologist*, *61*(4), 271.

Baker, T.B., McFall, R.M., & Shoham, V. (2008). Current status and future prospects of clinical psychology: Toward a scientifically principled approach to mental and behavioral health care. *Psychological Science in the Public Interest*, *9*(2), 67–103. doi:10.1111/j.1539-6053.2009.01036.x.

Bendat, M. (2014). In name only? Mental health parity or illusory reform. *Psychodynamic Psychiatry*, *42*(3), 353–375. doi:10.1521/pdps.2014.42.3.353.

Campbell, L.F., Norcross, J.C., Vasquez, M.J., & Kaslow, N.J. (2013). Recognition of psychotherapy effectiveness: The APA resolution. *Psychotherapy*, *50*(1), 98.

Cuijpers, P., Smit, F., Bohlmeijer, E., Hollon, S.D., & Andersson, G. (2010). Efficacy of cognitive–behavioural therapy and other psychological treatments for adult depression: Meta-analytic study of publication bias. *British Journal of Psychiatry*, *196*(3), 173–178. doi:10.1192/bjp.bp.109.066001.

Driessen, E., Van, H.L., Don, F.J., Peen, J., Kool, S., Westra, D., … Dekker, J.J.M. (2013). The efficacy of cognitive-behavioral therapy and psychodynamic therapy in the outpatient treatment of major depression: A randomized clinical trial. *American Journal of Psychiatry*, *170*(9), 1041–1050. doi:10.1176/appi.ajp.2013.12070899.

Elkin, I. (1994). Treatment of depression collaborative research program: Where we began and where we are. In A.E. Bergin & S. Garfield (Eds.), *Handbook of psychotherapy and behavior change: An empirical analysis* (4th ed., pp. 114–139). New York: Wiley.

Elkin, I., Shea, M.T., Watkins, J.T., Imber, S.D., Sotsky, S.M., Collins, J.F., … Parloff, M.B. (1989). National Institute of Mental Health Treatment of Depression collaborative research program: General effectiveness of treatments. *JAMA Psychiatry*, *46*(11), 971–982. doi:10.1001/archpsyc.1989.01810110013002.

Gilboa-Schechtman, E., Foa, E.B., Shafran, N., Aderka, I.M., Powers, M.B., Rachamim, L., ... Apter, A. (2010). Prolonged exposure versus dynamic therapy for adolescent PTSD: A pilot randomized controlled trial. *Journal of the American Academy of Child & Adolescent Psychiatry*, *49*(10), 1034–1042. doi:https://doi.org/10.1016/j.jaac.2010.07.014.

Gilboa-Schechtman, E., Shafran, N., & Foa, E.B. (2011). Drs. Gilboa-Schechtman et al. reply. *Journal of the American Academy of Child & Adolescent Psychiatry*, *50*(5), 522–524. doi:https://doi.org/10.1016/j.jaac.2011.03.003.

Hollon, S.D., Thase, M.E., & Markowitz, J.C. (2002). Treatment and prevention of depression. *Psychological Science in the Public Interest*, *3*(2), 39–77. doi:10.1111/1529-1006.00008.

Kazdin, A.E. (2006). Arbitrary metrics: Implications for identifying evidence-based treatments. *American Psychologist*, *61*(1), 42–49. doi:10.1037/0003-066X.61.1.42.

Mischel, W. (2008). Connecting clinical practice to scientific progress. *Psychological Science in the Public Interest*, *9*(2), i–ii. doi:10.1111/j.1539-6053.2009.01035.x.

Sackett, D.L., Rosenberg, W.M.C., Gray, J.A.M., Haynes, R.B., & Richardson, W.S. (1996). Evidence based medicine: What it is and what it isn't. *BMJ*, *312*(7023), 71–72. doi:10.1136/bmj.312.7023.71.

Shedler, J. (2010). The efficacy of psychodynamic psychotherapy. *American Psychologist*, *65*(2), 98–109. doi:10.1037/a0018378.

Shedler, J. (2015). Where is the evidence for "evidence-based" therapy? *The Journal of Psychological Therapies in Primary Care*, *4*(1), 47–59.

Turner, E.H., Matthews, A.M., Linardatos, E., Tell, R.A., & Rosenthal, R. (2008). Selective publication of antidepressant trials and its influence on apparent efficacy. *New England Journal of Medicine*, *358*(3), 252–260. doi:10.1056/NEJMsa065779.

Wampold, B.E., Budge, S.L., Laska, K.M., Del Re, A.C., Baardseth, T.P., Flückiger, C., ... Gunn, W. (2011). Evidence-based treatments for depression and anxiety versus treatment-as-usual: A meta-analysis of direct comparisons. *Clinical Psychology Review*, *31*(8), 1304–1312. doi:https://doi.org/10.1016/j.cpr.2011.07.012.

Wasserstein, R.L., & Lazar, N.A. (2016). The ASA's statement on p-values: Context, process, and purpose. *The American Statistician*, *70*(2), 129–133. doi:10.1080/00031305.2016.1154108.

Westen, D., & Morrison, K. (2001). A multidimensional meta-analysis of treatments for depression, panic, and generalized anxiety disorder: An empirical examination of the status of empirically supported therapies. *J Consult Clin Psychol*, *69*(6), 875–899. doi:10.1037/0022-006X.69.6.875.

Westen, D., Novotny, C.M., & Thompson-Brenner, H. (2004). The empirical status of empirically supported psychotherapies: Assumptions, findings, and reporting in controlled clinical trials. *Psychological Bulletin*, *130*(4), 631–663. doi:10.1037/0033-2909.130.4.631.

Wittmann, L., Halpern, J., Adams, C.B.L., Ørner, R.J., & Kudler, H. (2011). Prolonged exposure and psychodynamic treatment for posttraumatic stress disorder. *Journal of the American Academy of Child & Adolescent Psychiatry*, *50*(5), 521–522. doi:https://doi.org/10.1016/j.jaac.2011.03.005.

Chapter 4

Developing an innovative, scientific, clinically sensitive approach to investigate psychoanalytic process

Juan Pablo Jiménez and Carolina Altimir

Psychoanalysis must espouse diverse sources and strategies of gaining psychoanalytic knowledge

Since Freud abandoned the idea of constructing a psychoanalytic theory based on the biology of his time, psychoanalysis focused on the construction of a hermeneutical metapsychology based on accumulated clinical experience. The metapsychology thus constructed has many epistemological problems that are still under discussion (Jiménez 2006). However, the revolution of the last decades in neurosciences offers psychoanalysis a second opportunity to step into the scientific mainstream in the attempt to understand the mind–brain relationship (Jiménez 2017). A constructive interdisciplinary dialogue may allow movement towards a global, albeit partial and complex under-standing that covers from the molecular levels of the brain to the symbolic levels of the mind. This implies for psychoanalysis to open theory building beyond hermeneutics to include scientific strategies of collecting information. We cannot go into details of the contemporary epistemological controversy in psychoanalysis (see Jiménez & Altimir 2019). Our contention is that psychoanalytic theory construction must adopt diverse sources and strategies of collecting information. The discussion must move from a monistic epistemological position to the conception of a psychoanalysis that takes advantage of hermeneutics and science, i.e., to an epistemological and meth-odological pluralism, under the guiding question, *which method of research—clinical, empirical, quantitative or qualitative, conceptual, etc.—can be used to brighten which particular psychoanalytic problem or question*. Certainly, all methods have pros and cons; the complexity of the mind/brain requires that we accept uncertainties and partial knowledge. Scientific research is, by its very nature, an ongoing process of knowledge acquisition. The empirical implications derived from a stance that advocates for a pluralistic and interdisciplinary dia-logue between psychoanalysis, related disciplines, and psychotherapy process research involve an attempt to bridging the gap between a hermeneutic and a scientific position. Thus, the research-minded clinician, or the clinical oriented researcher, tries to keep him/herself in a middle ground. On the one hand, he/she cannot dismiss clinical material as a primary and valuable source of information for understanding psychotherapy and psychoanalysis. On the other hand, he/she cannot deny the contribution of systematic and valid observations of the clinical situation.

Outcome research and process-outcome research in psychotherapy and psychoanalysis

In recent decades, and the topic of this book is an example of this, there has been growing interest in demonstrating the efficacy and effectiveness of psychoanalytic treatment. Taken together, these studies offer considerable evidence for the efficacy and effectiveness of brief psychodynamic treatments and long-term psychodynamic treatments in a variety of disorders, although it is also clear that more such studies are needed. The interest in process-outcome studies, however, is more modest in comparison. Outcomes studies, while important in justifying the value of psychoanalytic treatment to society, say little or nothing about the mechanisms of therapeutic change and do not illuminate psychoanalytic practice. What is the gain for clinicians in knowing that psychoanalytic therapy is just as effective—or more effective—than other therapies or medications for treating certain disorders? In fact, the field of psychotherapy research is increasingly interested in learning more about mechanisms of change (Kazdin 2009), knowledge that can enrich an "evidence-based therapeutic practice" beyond "brands," and contribute to answer the question of "what works for whom" under what circumstances (Roth & Fonagy 2004). On the other hand, we believe that process-outcome research is the path that links theory-driven "top-down" research, guided by psychoanalytical concepts, and "bottom-up" research that does justice to *real* psychoanalytical practice.

The theoretical and practical centrality of the concept of psychoanalytic process

During presentations of clinical material in psychoanalytic meetings we often listen to the affirmation "That is not analysis!" The irony of this is that we psychoanalysts—in more than a century of existence of the psychoanalytic movement have not yet reached a consensual definition of what is essentially psychoanalytic in a particular treatment. In spite of this, we are not afraid to err in saying that we all share the idea that "psychoanalytic process" is a salient aspect of the psychoanalytic treatment. However, there is no agreement about the concept of "psychoanalytic process" itself at hand. Several authors in a similar tenor repeat the following statement by Abrams in 1987:

> The psychoanalytic process conceptualizes what is fundamental to the investigative and clinical potential of psychoanalysis. Yet, it is hard to

imagine any term more burdened by ambiguity, controversy and diversity of usage, … it has become a Babel, a shibboleth, and a weapon.

(Abrams 1987, p. 441)

Searching for agreement, the Committee on Psychoanalytic Education (COPE) of the American Psychoanalytic Association established in 1984 a study group to develop a consensual definition for the concept of psychoanalytic process. To facilitate the success of this venture, a group of 11 analysts was chosen for having a similar "mainstream" orientation. They met biannually for five years. Despite the assertion by its leader (Boesky 1990) that the group had a unified set of assumptions about the process, the only complete consensus within the group was that no consensus was reached on the psychoanalytic process. Individual members published their findings separately. So, based on the research procedures employed by traditional psychoanalytic inquiry, the only conclusion authors have reached is that each analytic process is unique, ideographic, and therefore different and incomparable to any other, or to any other analytic dyad (Foehl 2010).

Despite these difficulties, in most psychoanalytic institutes of the IPA candidates must demonstrate "psychoanalytic process" in their treatment reports to achieve graduation. If this is so, if the concept of psychoanalytic process is central, both in theory and practice, and yet there is no consensual definition of it, we are facing a serious problem for psychoanalysis as an academic and professional discipline.

Traditional research strategies on psychoanalytic process have reached a dead end

The search for a consensual definition of the psychoanalytic process through traditional clinical research has reached an impasse. Similarly, the strategies for the operationalization of the concept and its empirical validation have not achieved the consensus sought. In the face of this, eminent psychoanalytical researchers such as Luborsky, Spence, Vaughan, Dahl, Ablon and Jones, etc., have provided ideas, concepts and methods of measurement. Thomä and Kächele and the Ulm's group—with whom one of us (JPJ) reached a PhD degree during the late eighties—investigated the psychoanalytic process systematically with empirical methodology for 40 years. However, Tuckett, in 2004, asserted that psychoanalytic process still eludes definition and now, despite a good deal of psychoanalytic research, we too cannot identify substantial progress in empirically validating the concept of psychoanalytic process. This stalemate prevents the generation of new statements about the workings and mechanisms of analytic process and change.

In view of this, Schachter and Kächele (2017) conclude that it is not possible either to define or to measure the traditional concept "psychoanalytic process" and propose therefore to change strategy and focus on a detailed observation and description of the analyst–patient interaction using modern technologies such as videotaping. These authors advance the idea that the reason for the stalemate is that psychoanalytic theory, in its eagerness to discard the effect of suggestion on therapeutic change, has been for 100 years trapped by the monadic conception that the psychoanalytic process is an entelechy, which emerges dissociated from the influence of the analyst's person.

We support the conception that although it is true that the specific subjective reality and intimate experience of each analytic dyad is unique and particular to the reality co-constructed by both participants and their shared history, mirrored in the so called implicit relational knowledge, it is no less true that systematic observation and description of particular intersubjective, intimate and idiosyncratic experiences, can also allow the possibility of making generic statements regarding the main characteristics of a particular phenomenon. This is what teaches us the productive discipline of mother–infant research and its predecessor, attachment research.

The relational turn in contemporary psychoanalysis and a new approach to investigate analytic interaction

Perhaps the most important change in psychoanalytic theorizing of the last decade is the shift from a one-person psychology to a two-person psychology. This means a move from the intrapsychic, monadic realm to the interaction between patient and therapist, to the interpersonal and intersubjective, dyadic field. The leading research question is now: *What's going on here between patient and therapist?* It is a Copernican turn in the direction of questioning, away from the top-down theory-driven perspective to the bottom-up observational perspective. Thirty years ago, Daniel Stern asserted that "interactions between patient and analyst instantiate the defensive exclusions or contradictions of the patient's implicit procedural knowing, including the resort to defensive distortion or exclusion of affective information" (Stern 1985, p. 853). In this vein, Daniel Stern coined the concept of *moment of meeting*, meaning the shared moments, mutually understood by patient and therapist that create a shared implicit knowledge about their relationship; these experientially shared moments are crucial for therapeutic change insofar they create a new intersubjective state that modifies the relation and rearranges the patient's implicit knowledge about relationships.

The discovery of what is called "implicit relational knowledge" adds another layer to the relational turn in psychoanalysis, in this case a turn to what might be called the experiential realm of the therapeutic relationship. Even though interpretive work can bring about changes, these can only be achieved if the implicit doing-something-together and the implicit relational knowledge, which has been modified, frame and seal the flow of explicit understanding. This experiential turn to which we are referring comes from studies into the micro-processes of regulation and self-regulation in the mother–infant dyad and their application to the interaction in the therapeutic relationship, where these micro-processes are also at play (Beebe & Lachmann 2002). Following Blatt and Behrends (1987), the psychoanalytic process can be better understood as a series of unfolding interaction, both at conscious and unconscious levels, between patient and therapist, with moments of *experienced* compatibilities and incompatibilities, moments of meeting, understanding, and mutuality versus moments of separation and misunderstanding (Luyten, Blatt, & Mayes 2012).

Considering the above, we believe that the difficulty of the dialogue between psychoanalysis and related disciplines also lies in some problems in which empirical science has not lived up to psychoanalytic conception. We see two major problems that should be addressed in an innovative psychoanalytic research paradigm:

1 Empirical research has not done justice to the "dyadic nature of the construction of experience" in psychoanalytic therapy. Although the idea of defining empirical variables based on relational concepts may seem obvious, in practice a great amount of research efforts interested in the therapeutic relationship nevertheless draw findings that do not account for the relational essence of this phenomenon. This is probably a consequence of the traditional praxis in scientific research of "dividing in order to study" and then establishing *post hoc* associations. In any case, as a result, the "in-between" processes of the intersubjective encounter between therapist and patient remain concealed behind the more "static" or *post hoc* associations.

2 The second matter that an innovative research program should address is the empirical study of the processes that take place between patient and therapist paying special attention to the manifestations of the *implicit domain* of the relational experience. One of the most relevant findings of contemporary neuroscience are the implicit phenomena, i.e., those that are out of consciousness, and account for more than 90% of mental life. Implicit phenomena play a relevant role in the patient-therapist affective communication. Most relational exchanges are strongly based on affective cues that contain specific information about emotional states and cognitive appraisal processes, which are captured and utilized by both participants at the instant. Within this communication, affective signals take place in fragments of seconds, so that the speed and density of the information that is being exchanged does not allow the central control of cognition, that is, a verbal translation and conscious reflection. An innovative research program must be able to capture the implicit level, the moment-by-moment exchange, and the interactive emotional patterns of facial behavior, gaze, vocalization and orientation of the participant simultaneously.

Modern mother–infant research

Based on the thorough observation and micro-analytic description of the interactions between mother and infant, at the split-second level, mother–infant research have derived in important conclusions regarding the interactive processes involved in the development of the self that have relevant consequences in normal as well as psychopathological development and adult life.

In contrast to traditional psychoanalytic research, mother–infant research has derived *generic* principles about functional and dysfunctional processes in the development of self (for instance, hyper self-regulation or excessive interactive regulation), based on the observation of unique, intimate and idiosyncratic experiences of specific mother–infant dyads, with their one co-created history of interactions, that cannot be "compared," in its uniqueness, to any other. Furthermore, these principles have been extrapolated to the adult analytic situation, thus informing psychoanalytic theory as well.

Our proposal: building bridges between the unformulated, implicit, unconscious and the verbal, explicit, conscious edges in psychoanalysis/ psychotherapy process research

During the last nine years, at the *Millennium Institute for Research on Depression and Personality* (MIDAP) in Santiago de Chile, we have been investigating the psychotherapeutic process according to this new approach. We propose that in order to continue to progress in building psychoanalytic theory that is connected with research, and specifically with research derived from psychoanalytic process "as it is usually delivered by psychoanalysts," there has to be a *change of level* in the approach. Psychoanalytic process research should be inspired in or borrow from the procedures of mother-infant research, and applied to analytic process, *together* with providing a clinically sound context for its analysis and interpretation.

What does this method consist of?

a   **With methods derived from mother–infant research** we study the patient–analyst interaction at the micro-level, specifically those micro-sequences related to the domain of the implicit or sub-symbolic (Bucci 1997), as they relate to psychological states and processes mostly lined to the unformulated or unconscious and therefore can be further linked to several higher-order psychoanalytic concepts. Within this domain of interactions are included: facial affective behavior, vocal quality, vocal rhythm, and body synchrony, among others. Research on facial affective nonverbal behavior of patient and therapist, allows the study of the *dyad in action*. Facial affective behavior is spontaneous and unconscious

(Merten 2005), and represents an observable component of emotional processes (Bänninger-Huber, & Widmer 1999). Therefore, it constitutes an important empirical access to the emotional communication of the interactive partners, but also to elements that belong to the implicit domain of experience. Its emphasis on the affective regulation process highlights the analyst's contribution (Merten 2005; Rasting & Beutel 2005), thus stressing the *interaction as a study unit*. This research field proposes that the communicative meaning of facial affects may have different functions, one of which is to regulate the relationship with the interactive partner by transmitting certain attitudes towards him/her or towards the state of the relationship, with the concomitant expectations about the interaction (Anstadt, Merten, Ullrich, & Krause 1997; Bänninger-Huber 1992; Bänninger-Huber, & Widmer 1999; Merten 1997; Rasting & Beutel 2005). In this context, each emotion involves a specific desire of regulation and when it is expressed, it entails a specific relational offer to the interactive partner (Bänninger-Huber, & Widmer 1999; Benecke, & Krause 2005).

b   **Derived from a long-standing tradition in psychotherapy process research we apply the events paradigm approach.** The study of clinically significant events of therapy constitutes what can be considered the observable manifestations of concepts that are close to psychoanalysis. In other words, these events can be defined as *clinically significant units of meaning*, which are conceptually sound to psychoanalytic theory. Examples of such events are ruptures (which imply a temporal deterioration of the therapeutic alliance, but also contain, according to the underlying theoretical background, a strain in a negotiation between the need of self-definition and relatedness, thus activating several unconscious relational schemes and affective representations in both patient and therapist). Another example can be events of enactment: actually, some ruptures in the therapeutic alliance can be considered enactments in themselves (Safran & Muran 2001).

The research method proceeds identifying in a selected sample of therapeutic sessions significant episodes that have been operationalized, for example, as ruptures and resolutions of the therapeutic alliance (Safran & Kraus 2014) in videotaped sessions of psychoanalytic therapies. The concepts of rupture and resolution of the alliance developed by Safran and Muran (2000, 2001, 2006) highlight the relational basis of the therapeutic alliance and operationalize the mutual regulatory processes through the idea of intersubjective negotiation between the needs of agency or self-definition, and those of relatedness of both patient and therapist (Luyten, Blatt, & Mayes 2012). It can be hypothesized, for example, that introjective patients will show different strategies for resolving ruptures of the therapeutic alliance than anaclitic patients. As a matter of fact, our next research step intend to establish the association between anaclitic and introjective personality configurations, and patients' and therapists' affect regulation strategies displayed during rupture and resolution episodes throughout the analytic process (Altimir & Jiménez 2017). In this way, psychoanalytic concepts of higher order can be significantly linked to observable empirical findings. Safran and Muran have defined the concepts of rupture and resolution strategies so that they are susceptible of objective assessment by third parties through observation (Eubanks, Muran, & Safran 2015), and the action of both patient and therapist can be accounted for simultaneously.

The aim is to identify the underlying emotional states of patient and therapist during different kind of ruptures and resolution of ruptures. The underlying emotional states can be accessed through facial affective behavior, an observable component of emotional processes that is organized at a non-symbolic, non-verbal, unconscious level (Bucci 2007), and to which both members of the dyad react beneath awareness (Schore 2012). Video-taped episodes of different kind of ruptures from face to face therapies are examined using the *Facial Action Coding System* (FACS; Ekman & Friesen 1978) a coding system for the objective description of facial behavior (Ekman, Friesen, & Hager 2002), and of seven basic emotions (joy, anger, contempt, disgust, fear, sadness and surprise). FACS also allows the coding—in face-to-face therapies—of the facial-affective behaviors

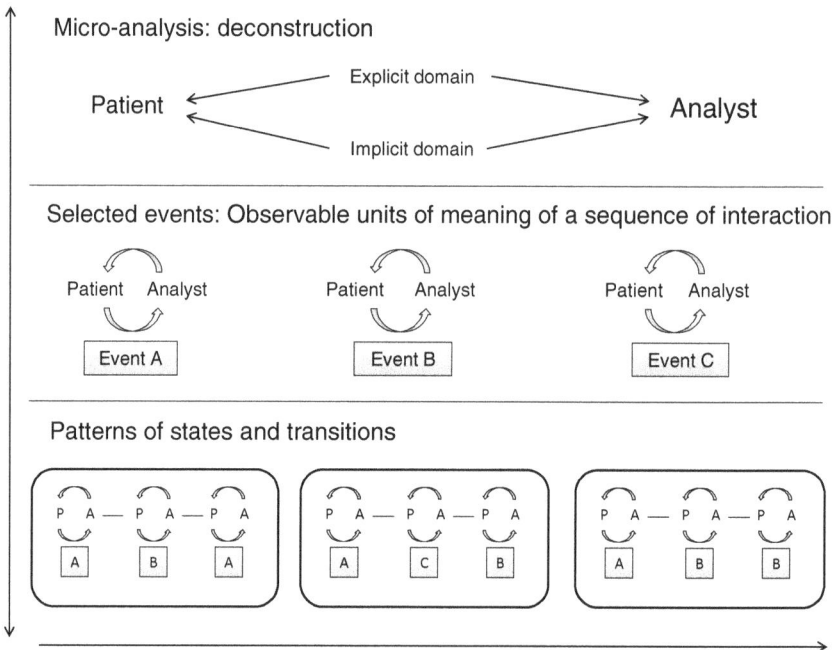

Figure 4.1 Dimensions and approaches of the innovative, scientific, and clinically sensitive research program.

of patients and therapists, of indicators of emotion dysregulation, and emotional involvement (associated to gaze behavior) (Merten, 1997).

The relevance of combining the "bottom-up" approach of mother–infant research, with the events paradigm, is that the latter can provide a context of meaning that can make sense of the "smaller" descriptions (unit of analysis) derived from micro-analysis. A significant sequence of affect regulation between patient and therapist does not have the same meaning and psychological function if it takes place within an enactment, or if it takes place within an event of insight, or a moment of meeting. Furthermore, these micro-sequences of events will not have the same clinical significance and influence whether they take place at the beginning of a process, or when the treatment is well advanced in time. Thus, this implies that context can be considered at different levels of analyses as well, simultaneously.

Final: What does this approach contribute to psychoanalytic theory of change and to clinical practice?

The bottom-up approach to psychoanalytic process research is a contribution to:

*   Theory development as it allows the possibility of making new statements about analytic process sustained on systematic observation on how psychoanalytic treatment is being carried out in practice.
*   Clinical training and supervision, inasmuch as the systematic description of interactions belonging to the micro-level of the therapeutic endeavor constitute an observable proxy of the elements and processes that are linked to psychoanalytic concepts of a higher order, for instance, transference-countertransference matrix, but that can be connected to the moment-to-moment experience of the analytic interaction.
*   In other words, the clinician may have in mind these observable sequences of interaction as indicators of higher-ordered concepts and identify them in his/her practice as they take place, allowing an immediate and adequate intervention.

References

Abrams, S. (1987). The psychoanalytic process: A schematic model. *Int J Psychoanal* 68, 441–452.

Altimir, C., & Jiménez, J.P. (2017). Personality configuration and its association with affect regulation during rupture and resolution episodes of the analytic process. Research application to *Research Advisory Board* (RAB), IPA. Manuscript.

Anstadt, T., Merten, J., Ullrich, B., & Krause, R. (1997). Affective dyadic behavior, core conflictual relationship themes, and success of treatment. *Psychotherapy Research* 7, 397–417.

Bänninger-Huber, E. (1992). Prototypical affective microsequences in psychotherapeutic interaction. *Psychotherapy Research* 2, 291–306.

Bänninger-Huber, E., & Widmer, C. (1999). Affective relationship patterns and psy-chotherapeutic change. *Psychotherapy Research* 9, 74–87.

Beebe, B., & Lachmann, F. (2002). *Infant research and adult treatment. Co-constructing interactions.* New Jersey: The Analytic Press.

Benecke, C., & Krause, R. (2005). Facial affective relationship offers of patients with panic disorder. *Psychotherapy Research* 15, 178–187.

Blatt, S.J., & Behrends, R.S. (1987). Internalization, separation-individuation, and the nature of therapeutic action. *Int J Psychoanal* 68, 279–297.

Boesky, D. (1990). The psychoanalytic process and its components. *Psychoanalytic Quarterly* 59, 550–584.

Bucci, W. (1997). *Psychoanalysis and cognitive science: A multiple code theory.* New York: Guilford.

Ekman, P., & Friesen, W.V. (1978). *Facial action coding system: A technique for the meas-urement of facial movement.* Palo Alto, CA: Consulting Psychologists Press.

Ekman, P., Friesen, W.V., & Hager, J.C. (2002). *The facial action coding system.* Salt Lake City, UT: Research Nexus eBook.

Eubanks, C.F., Muran, J.C., & Safran, J.D. (2015). *Rupture Resolution Rating System (3RS): Manual.* Technical Report.

Foehl, J.C. (2010). The play's the thing. The primacy of process and the persistence of pluralism in contemporary psychoanalysis. *Contemporary Psychoanalysis* 46(1), 48–86.

Kächele, H., Schachter, J., Thomä, H., & The Ulm Psychoanalytic Process Study Group (2009). *From psychoanalytic narrative to empirical single case research. Implications to psychoanalytic practice.* New York: Routledge.

Kazdin, A.E. (2009). Understanding how and why psychotherapy leads to change, *Psychotherapy Research*, 19, 4–5, 418–428.

Luyten, P., Blatt, S.J., & Mayes, L.C. (2012). Process and outcome in psychoanalytic psychotherapy research: The need for a (relatively) new paradigm. In: R.A. Levy, J.S. Ablon, & H Kächele Eds. *Psychodynamic psychotherapy research. Evidence-based practice and practice-based evidence* (pp. 345–359). New York: Humana Press, Springer.

Merten, J. (1997). Facial-affective behavior, mutual gaze, and emotional experience. *Journal of Nonverbal Behavior* 21(3), 179–201.

Merten, J. (2005). Facial microbehavior and the emotional quality of the therapeutic relationship. *Psychotherapy Research* 15, 325–333.

Rasting, M., & Beutel, M. (2005). Dyadic affective interactive patterns in the intake interview as a predictor of outcome. *Psychotherapy Research* 15(3), 188–198.

Roth, A., & Fonagy, P. (2004). *What works for whom. A critical review of psychotherapy research.* 2nd ed. New York: Guilford Press.

Safran, J.D., & Kraus, J. (2014). Alliance ruptures, impasses, and enactments: A rela-tional perspective. *Psychotherapy, American Psychological Association* 51(3), 381–387.

Safran, J.D., & Muran, J.C. (2000). *Negotiating the therapeutic alliance. A relational treat-ment guide.* New York: The Guilford Press.

Safran, J.D., & Muran, J.C. (2001). The therapeutic alliance as a process of intersub-jective negotiation. In Muran JCh (Ed.), *Self-relations in the psychotherapeutic process* (pp. 165–192). Washington, DC: American Psychological Association.

Safran, J.D., & Muran, J.C. (2006). Has the concept of the therapeutic alliance out-lived its usefulness? *Psychotherapy: Theory, Research, Practice, Training* 43, 286–291, doi:10.1037/0033-3204.43.3.286.

Schachter, J., & Kächele, H. (2017). *Nodal points: Critical reflections on contemporary psychoanalytic therapy*. New York: International Psychoanalytic Books.

Schore, A.N. (2012). *The science of the art of psychotherapy*. New York, NY: W.W. Norton & Company.

Stern, D.N. (1985). *The interpersonal world of the infant. A view from psychoanalysis and developmental psychology*. New York: Basic Books.

Tuckett, D. (2004). Presidential address: Building a psychoanalysis based on confidence in what we do. *EPF Bulletin* 58, 5–19.

Chapter 5

From case study to single case research

The specimen case Amalia X

Horst Kächele

Introduction

Throughout the history of psychoanalysis, theories have always hinged on clinical case reports and teaching has focused on the value of such case histories. Freud and many of his followers believed clinical case histories were critical for scientific testing of psychoanalytic theories. In a pivotal review of the problem of psychoanalytic treatment research Wallerstein and Sampson (1971) gave a double message: "The whole corpus of psychoanalysis [...] comprehending the phenomena of both normal and abnormal personality development and functioning, attests brilliantly to the explanatory power of the theory derived from data of the consulting room" (p. 11). However, they continue, it would be clear that "we need at least equally cognizant of the limitations of the case study method as a source of prospective continuing knowledge" (p. 12).

They referred to experimental work in the lab and to systematic observational studies likewise. This statement, in fact, covers two fields of psychoanalytic research: personality theory and treatment theory that both are deeply anchored in the clinical case study method. It is worthwhile to note that early in the 1970s a comprehensive critical-friendly review on the experimental findings of psychoanalytic personality theory was published by the British experimental psychologist Kline (1972) and the psychoanalyst Dahl (1972) published his first systematic-observational study. Three decades later Wallerstein (2002) concluded:

> that we are without warrant [...] to claim the greater heuristic usefulness or validity of anyone of our general theories over the others, other than by the indoctrination and allegiances built into us by the happenstance of our individual trainings, our differing personal dispositions and the explanatory predilections then carried over into our consulting rooms.
>
> (p. 1251)

Likewise, Gabbard and Westen (2003) urge that "we attempt to move from arguing about the *therapeutic action of psychoanalysis* to demonstrating and refining it" (p. 338). Their recommendation to embark on systematic case studies to enhance the field of treatment research already expressed the awareness that to better understand what is going on within the sessions and within the mind of the analyst and his patient, more than retrospective reports were in demand. The best possibility for resolving these differences and for developing some consensus about the fundamental tenets of psychoanalysis rests with empirical-systematic research generating relevant data that can provide a basis for consensual agreement about fundamental psychoanalytic principles.

Looking back, we have to register that Freud was so convinced of the validity of this connection that when he was offered the results of experimental studies confirmatory of his theories he wrote dismissively to Rosenzweig: "I cannot put much value on these confirmations because the wealth of reliable observations on which these assertions rest make them independent of experimental verification. Still, it can do no harm" (quoted in Shakow & Rappaport 1964, p. 129).

However, the idea that clinical case histories provided scientific tests of psychoanalytic theories was criticized from the outset even by those sympathetic to psychoanalysis and certainly by its detractors because of the possible influence of suggestion (Breuer, about his own work with Anna O., in Breuer & Freud 1893–1895, p. 43; and Fliess, in Grünbaum 1984, pp. 32, 130). Von Krafft-Ebing (1896) tried the Breuer–Freud method on a few hysterical patients and found that bringing the causal trauma to light did not suffice to cure the symptom. The shadow of increasing doubt on the scientific value of clinical case histories has continued and later, in response to this, systematic-observational (not experimental) studies of single cases began to be formulated. Critiques notwithstanding, traditional analysts continued to maintain that case-history-based clinical findings are "the real basis of psychoanalysis" (Jones1959, p. 3, quoted by Grünbaum 1984, p. 99).

Freud's seemingly famous, yet somehow resignative statement in the *Studies on Hysteria* (1895) that his "case histories should read like short stories and that, they lack the serious stamp of science" (p. 160) may be made responsible for an unnecessary sharp divide between science and psychoanalysis. But even using Freud's work one may find useful demonstrations what a treasure the archived clinical notes can be.

Take as example the case report on the Ratman (Freud 1909d) and go to E. Zetzel's "Additional notes" from 1966:

> It was my intention when I first undertook this study to base my discussion primarily on the 1909 report published in Freud's collected papers. Fortunately, however, I decided to reread the case history in the Standard Edition. I was surprised and excited by the discovery I made—namely the unique salvage of Freud's daily notes covering the first four months of this analysis…. In striking contrast with the 1909 publication,

there are more than forty references to a highly ambivalent mother-son
relationship in the original clinical notes.

(p. 129)

The message is clear: case reports are artistic condensations created out of raw
data. The question is: what is raw and what is cooked?

For discourse analysts story telling is highly estimated as an important way
of transporting individual experience into shared knowledge (Ehlich 1980).
Thus psychoanalysis became a narrative science using narration aspiring to
narrative truth (Forrester 1980). Freud's writing, Shakow and Rapaport
(1964) already observed:

> is characterized by subtlety and power of language rather than precision
> and organization of propositions. While his case histories and clinical dis-
> cussions are unrivalled to this day, his theoretical formulations still leave
> very much for the reader to unravel.
>
> (p. 7)

The same position was later endorsed by Spence (1982). To highlight the
importance of this methodological decision, imagine the development of chemistry if chemists had evolved the habit of reporting what they had seen in their
test-tubes having performed most exciting experiments: a science of chemistry
based on reported colors, of blue and red and green reactions in the little tubes
after having done this and that. Or imagine a science of musicology with musi-
cians sharing their most personal experiences by writing case histories, or by
letting consumers telling their emotional involvements after a piano concerto.
What is wrong about such an approach? It well could be that one could built a
science of musical experience by collecting a large sample of these reported subjective testimonies. It wouldn't work for chemistry, that's why the alchemist in
vain tried to find the recipe how to make gold. To leave these rather fancy
examples let me remind you of the Brüder Grimm, the two professors from
Göttingen who systematically started out to collect orally transmitted fairy tales.
For a long time there has been a well-developed field of fairy tale research with
highly sophisticated methods to analyze the available large collections from all
over the world (Propp 1968 {1928}). I shall later return to this issue. Today we
encounter prominent authors underscoring that the clinical encounter is best
reported via the narrative mode (Michels 2000). There is growing endorsement
from qualitative oriented researchers that the psychoanalytic case study can and
should be used as a source of epistemic knowledge (Frommer & Langenbach
2001). But knowledge about what? That is the crucial issue!

Grünbaum's critique

Analysts, riding the crest of the popularity of psychoanalysis, may have felt,
like Freud, that they were so certain of the validity of their theories about

personality, about the principles of mental functioning etc. that there was little need for experimental validation. These convictions, however, were challenged by an incisive critique of psychoanalysis by Grünbaum (1984), a professor of the philosophy of science. Psychoanalysts mounted a vigorous response and defense. Grünbaum began his rigorous examination by quoting Freud's (1916/17) earlier statement that:

> After all his [the patient's] conflicts will only be successfully solved and his resistances overcome if the anticipatory ideas he is given tally with what is real in him. Whatever in the doctor's conjecture that is inaccurate drops out in the course of the analysis....
>
> (p. 452)

Grünbaum called this Freud's "tally" argument. One should note that Grünbaum focuses on a basic tenet of psychoanalytic treatment theory that was anchored in psychoanalytic personality theory. He refutes Freud's "tally" argument by contending that: (1) If a correct psychoanalytic interpretation removes the cause of the patient's disturbance or symptoms, then psychoanalytic treatment should be more effective than treatments that do not use such interpretations, but there is no evidence that that is the case; (2) Contemporary psychoanalysts recognize that they do not know what factors have produced therapeutic improvement in an individual patient, and therefore the possibility that the improvement is a function of suggestion and/or a placebo effect cannot be ruled out.

Marmor (1986) similarly states, "No serious scientist today would assert that the success of any therapeutic method constitutes proof of the correctness of the theory on which the therapeutic technique was based" (p. 249). Luborsky and Spence (1978) asserted that "far more is known now [in psychoanalysis] through clinical wisdom than is known through quantitative, objective studies" (p. 350) and add the sobering caveat that psychoanalysts "literally do not know how they achieve their results" (p. 360). Freud had also proposed an argument stating that if the data pieces fit together exactly, like those of a picture puzzle, they almost certainly must be correct. Grünbaum stresses that this argument is spurious because it assumes the independence of the pieces of evidence, but they cannot be independent because of a shared contaminant, the analyst's influence. In addition, the consilience itself is, in part, a function of the cleverness of the analyst and depends on it. The recognition that some of Freud's views, such as his conceptions of femininity and of homosexuality, proved to be erroneous is consistent with the conclusion that putative consilience may be mistaken. Grünbaum noted that when relying on the patient's recall, it is not possible to determine if a reported childhood experience is veridical. Further, even if the experience may be shown to have taken place, we still lack basis for claiming that that the specific childhood experience was the cause of the adult disorder. Here is a key to Freud's scientific credo: to understand how interpretation works leads to claims for the etiology of a disturbance!

The claim that the test of a traditional analyst's interpretation is the therapeutic effect it produces, which served Freud as evidence that it tallies with what is real in the patient's mind, should then also apply to interpretations by Kleinian analysts, self-psychological analysts, relational analysts and perhaps to cognitive behavioral therapists as well. Since what each of them finds in the patient's mind differs qualitatively from what the traditional and other schools find in the patient's mind (see e.g., Pulver 1987a), the tally argument must finally be discarded. Grünbaum cements this conclusion by quoting Marmor (1962): "the patients of each [rival psychoanalytic] school seem to bring up precisely the kind of phenomenological data which confirm the theories and interpretations of their analyst! Thus, each theory tends to be self-validating" (p. 289). This finding suggests how pervasive the effects of the analyst's suggestions can be.

From this everlasting debate different pathways could be taken. Mitchell (1998) noted that after exposure to Grünbaum's critique, psychoanalysts become afflicted with the "Grünbaum Syndrome," which included trying to "remember how analysis of variance works, perhaps even pulling a twenty-year-old statistics book of the shelf and quickly putting it back. There may also be a sleep disturbance and distractions from work" (p. 4). Or we move to a new position by clearly distinguishing between research on personality dynamics and research on treatment dynamics. This leads me to now focusing on the issue of single subject research.

Edelson's defense of single case studies

Edelson (1984) proffered the most spirited, articulate and sophisticated response to Grünbaum's critique of causative inferences based upon clinical case studies. Single subject research (Dukes 1965), he argues, has an advantage over group comparison research in that it is possible to enhance the validity and reliability of variables of interest by individualizing instruments for obtaining data, instead of employing a scattershot approach of a variety of behaviors or states that may be relevant to some members of a group and not to others. Therefore single subject research can focus upon those behaviors, which the investigator has reason to believe are especially relevant to the individual subject. Edelson considers whether statistical tests in single subject research are justifiable since they involve the assumption that observations or measurements are independent:

> One may try to justify the use of statistical methods; develop new statistical methods to deal with the kinds of dependencies which violate the independence assumption; or, eschewing statistical reasoning and methods, seek to achieve effects that are clearly clinically or theoretically

significant, such large effects indeed that it can be argued [... that it] excludes as implausible the alternative hypothesis that this effect is due to chance or random fluctuations produced by extraneous variables.

(1984, p. 69)

Edelson draws a parallel between psychoanalysis and Darwin's development of a methodology enabling him to make causal inferences about natural history. He cites Gould (1986) who argues "that iterated pattern, based on types of evidence so numerous and so diverse that no other coordinating interpretation could stand—even though any item, taken separately could not provide conclusive proof—must be the criterion for evolutionary inference" (Edelson 1984, p. 65). However, he fails to recognize both Darwin's and Gould's observations are entirely independent of each other and of the observer, whereas the analyst's pervasive influence upon the patient undermines the independent nature of the patient's data. One of the fundamental ways the analyst influences the patient's "free association" is by ignoring some of the patient's associations and by selecting others for exploration or comment. Independence is crucial for consilience, and it cannot be found in the consulting room. Edelson questions Grünbaum's claim that there is no way of assessing contamination of the patient's material. He argues that unless there is some evidence the analysand intends consciously to deceive, his conscious feelings, thoughts and perceptions can be included as data. These data, he asserts, are theory laden, but the theory with which they are laden is not psychoanalytic theory but the patient's personal theory, and he therefore contends that with respect to psychoanalytic theory such data are non-theoretical facts. He also believes that it might be possible to reduce the adulteration of data by suggestion to such a degree that it ceases to be a plausible alternative explanatory candidate. He adds:

The disciplined use of psychoanalytic technique which focuses on interpreting defense, rather than providing the analysand with suggestions about what he is defending against, also might cast doubt on a claim that suggestion is a plausible alternative explanation for an outcome observed in a particular single subject research.

(1984, p. 130)

In addition, he proposes that the phenomenon of suggestion itself may be studied and the extent of its influence measured.

I believe Edelson underestimates the pervasiveness of suggestion by the analyst while the recent literature is more cognizant of it and approaches it from different directions. Glover (1952) wrote, "we cannot exclude or have not excluded the transference effect of suggestion through interpretation" (p. 405). Thomä and Kächele (1994a) assert similarly that "The analyst who approaches his object, the analytic process, with a specific conception of a model, influences, by means of his expectations, the occurrence of events which agree with his model" (p. 333). Masling and Cohen (1987) reach an identical conclusion: "All psychotherapists generate clinical evidence that supports their theoretical positions—[and] can be understood as instances of therapists systematically rewarding and extinguishing various client behaviors. Therapists' belief in their theories serves as a self-fulfilling prophecy" (p. 65). Marmor (1962) (quoted earlier) extended this observation to different analytic schools by stating that the sources of the analyst's implicit influences and suggestions are manifold, in part derived from the analyst's subjectivity, which encompasses the analyst's realistic reactions to the patient, the analyst's transference responses to the patient, the analyst's theoretical orientation, the analyst's current, personal concerns about his/her own life, and the analyst's personal values; the influences of the latter have been widely discussed. Many years later Strenger (2005) asserts that "it is unrealistic to believe that a therapist's personal predilection, her sense of what constitutes the central dimension of meaning in life, does not crucially influence each and every one of her interventions" (p. 92).

Edelson (1984) also countered another of Grünbaum's arguments that there was no warrant for concluding that an event remote in time, a childhood experience, could be causative of an adult symptom. He argues: "The pathogen reappears in all its virulence, with increasing frankness and explicitness, in the transference—in a new edition, a new version, a reemergence, a repetition of the past pathogenic events or factors" (p. 95). But recourse to that argument begs the question, since there is no proof that the current "transference" is a repetition of a childhood experience. An unsubstantiated psychoanalytic hypothesis cannot be used to validate psychoanalytic theory. Thus, whether a present "transference" expression is a reappearance of a childhood experience remains a hypothesis requiring independent verification (Schachter 2002). Today many analysts have factually given up the notion of direct causal relevance of early experiences that fueled Grünbaum's criticism. Narrative truth is what is sought for; creating meaning within the present state of mind.

Here, as a postscript to Edelson's views, is a contemporary call to colleagues by Wolitzky, Director of the Ph.D. Program in Clinical Psychology at New York University, that, in contradistinction to Grünbaum, utilizes the criterion of plausibility for assessing the value of a single case report:

> I am interested in collecting a series of case studies, particularly those published in the last two decades, that offer persuasive evidence for the psychoanalytic formulation of phobias, or any other psychoanalytic propositions. The cases should be ones in which enough detail, including some verbatim material (if possible) is provided to make a compelling case.... I want to be clear that to nominate a paper you do not have to feel that the clinical illustration "proves" something, only that the clinical

evidence is persuasive … that the formulation made a good deal of clinical sense to you (i.e., that it was highly plausible, coherent, internally consistent, and not overly speculative). In other words, the formulation should lead to serious consideration for an open-minded skeptic.

(Wolitzky 2007)

Notes on the methodology of single case studies

The methodological basis for systematic-observational studies of single cases in our field had been spelled out in a research primer by the statistician Chassan (1967) who had developed an intensive design in the evaluation of drug efficacy during psychotherapy (Chassan & Bellak 1966). So it is useful to list the pro and cons.

Davison and Lazarus (1994) have listed some positive features of case studies:

- a case study may cast doubt on a general theory
- a case study may provide a valuable heuristic to subsequent and better controlled research
- a case study may permit the investigation, although poorly controlled, of rare but important phenomena
- a case study can provide the opportunity to apply new principles and notions in entirely new ways
- a case study, under circumstances, can provide enough experimenter control over an phenomenon to furnish "scientifically acceptable" information
- a case study can assist in placing "meat" on the "theoretical skeleton."

There are also critical voices on case studies that pertain to all clinical reports we should not leave out:

- a case study is an anecdote and works on narrative persuasion
- a case study is not a documented archival report
- a case study provides mostly an argument by authority
- a case study leads to an inflation of the prevailing theory
- a case study most have exhibits a total non-representativeness of sample
- a case study most likely at best is a mixture of aesthetic and clinical interest
- a case study has most likely only literary and reportorial value.

As a pointer Edelson (1985) proposed six requirements for a systematic-observational—as contrasted to a clinical—case study:

1   There is a clear statement of the hypothesis
2   The phenomena are made intersubjectively accessible
3   Negative instances of the generalization are clearly specified

4   Evidence that the hypothesis has not contaminated the data
5   Formulations alternative to the hypothesis are offered
6   The range of individuals and situations to which the hypothesis applies is
    made explicit.

With such a directory we may move to look at some of the more recent
examples of systematic–observational case studies that have been published
since Wallerstein and Sampson's call for such studies. As a caveat I would like
to note that sometimes it seems to me that more pleas for single case studies
have been made than such studies itself (Donnellan 1978). Even Edelson as
the most prolific combatant has never published such a single case study. As a
healing contrast Leuzinger-Bohleber (1995) has long promoted single case
studies as psychoanalytic research instruments.

   These formalized systematic case studies usually provide a clinical account
and some external measurement operations. The introduction of tape-recording
into the psychoanalytic treatment situation opened a new window onto the
process that for a long time was ardently debated and for most analysts is still
controversial. Audio-recordings of the psychoanalytic dialogue indeed do
pose a number of substantial clinical and ethical problems, although for scientific reasons they provide true progress (Kächele et al. 1988). They allow an
independent, third-person perspective on the psychoanalytic, interpersonal
transaction; with regard to the analyst's and the patient's internal modes of
experiencing they are silent and ideally have to be completed by the participant's testimony. The recording of these cases has opened up access to many
theoretical and technical issues. Single case studies are not confined to tape-
recording; any systematic gathering of treatment relevant material can be used
to document a treatment. Overviews on the methodology have been presented by Fonagy and Moran (1993), Hilliard (1993) and Kazdin (2011).
Fonagy and Moran summarized the goals succinctly:

> Individual case studies attempt to establish the relationship between
> intervention and other variables through repeated systematic observation
> and measurement. [...] The observation of variability across time within
> a single case combines a clinical interest to respond appropriately to
> changes within the patient, and a research interest to find support for a
> causal relationship between intervention and changes in variables of the-
> oretical interest. The attention to repeated observations, more than any
> other single factor, permits knowledge to be drawn from the individual
> case and has the power to eliminate plausible alternative explanations.
>
> (Fonagy & Moran 1993, p. 65)

Hartvig Dahl's (1972) quantitative study on the negative course of a treatment of a former female patient of M. Gill by a young female candidate
deserves to be mentioned here as a prime example. However, little attention

was paid to such a systematic–observational study in the professional environment of the New York Institute where he, for many years, was the director of the research division. His main focus, having been trained at the Menninger Clinic, became the case of Mrs. C, which was the first completely recorded psychoanalytic case.

The case earned public interest when Jones and Windholz (1990) designed their method for systematic inquiry of a complete case. In collaboration with W. Bucci and others this case became a model, for which Luborsky and Spence (1971) had suggested the term "specimen case." Converging evidence for emotional structures was demonstrated (Bucci 1988), but her method, the referential cycle, also demonstrated pattern of discourse in good and troubled hours (Bucci 1997). Alas, the discrepancies between the findings of Jones and Windholz and her studies on the final outcome of the treatment of Mrs. C were never debated or even resolved.

A controlled study of the psychoanalytic treatment of brittle diabetes by Moran et al. (1991) illustrated nicely that blood sugar data and systematic session reports show systematic correlations. Ideal candidates for such psychosomatic correlations that cannot be identified in group statistics are chronic disorders like M. Crohn. Brosig et al. (1997) illustrate this potential by reporting a single case analysis of the course of a psychoanalytic treatment. Schubert (2011), as editor of a first volume of psychoneuroimmunology and psychotherapy, endorses the view that only single case studies will promote the new field.

In the 1950s Lester Luborsky started his systematic work on the context-dependency of somatic and psychological symptoms that he first summarized in 1970. In the final book (1996) he presented a convincing study on the context for stomach ulcer pain from his first experimental subject. The ups and downs of depressive mood shifts using the symptom-context method have shown the fertility of the technique (Peterson et al. 1983).

Quite often we encounter single subject research when new methods are tested. The Shedler-Westen SWAP-tool was implemented by Lingiardi et al. (2006, 2010) and Porcerelli et al. (2007) for personality measurement; the Analytic Process Scales, designed by Waldron et al. (2004), were used to compare a good and poor outcome case (Gazzillo et al. 2014) and Mergenthaler's cycle computer text-analysis software has been tested in a fair number of cases (e.g., Mergenthaler 1998; Mergenthaler & Kächele 1996).

The strength of single case studies is particularly obvious in the context of a collaborative program. Sharing the data base provides an opportunity to refine and sharpen concepts and research perspectives. Such a collaboration has been initiated by Grawe (Bern) and Kächele (Ulm) in the 1990s. Two short-term treatments, a cognitive-behavioral therapy and a psychoanalytic focal therapy, were studied by multiple methods and an impressive group of researchers stemming from various theoretical background (Kächele 1992). The shared interest in methods led to the establishment of method-centered study groups (like CCRT-study group), which in turn stimulated the application of this specific method also in other countries (Ávila-Espada & Mitjavila 2003; López Moreno et al. 2005).

The San Francisco research group of Weiss and Sampson has systematically used the single case approach to explore, describe, test and finally validate the unconscious plan methodology. Testing alternative psychoanalytic explanations of the therapeutic process, they used the case of Mrs. C (Weiss & Sampson 1986) that Jones and Windholz also had studied, and later expanded the range of cases (Pole et al. 2002; Persons et al. 1991; for a summary see Silberschatz 2005).

With the growing acceptance of attachment theory within the psychoanalytic world, the AAI became one of the prime instruments for evaluating structural change (Levy et al. 2006). A representative study by Szecsödy (2008) demonstrates the usefulness of combining process description with annual AAI interviewing. Another single case study explored the change in reflective functioning during psychotherapy as a promising measure (Gullestad & Wilberg, 2011).

So far so good, one might say. We are in a situation where we might say single case research methodology has found its followers. It is a useful device to study in more detail the specific of a treatment. What is missing, in my view, is the step to introduce that degree of open access that Luborsky and Spence (1971) had asked for. We need model cases—specimen cases—that the psychoanalytic community can share.

The Ulm Psychoanalytic Process Research Study Group

For many years the Ulm Psychoanalytic Process Research Study Group has implemented a program to examine the material bases of psychoanalytic therapy. We were and are convinced that only the careful exploration of the patient's interaction with the analyst can illustrate the central aspects of psychoanalytic treatment and enable an experimentally driven theory of the process. Therefore we have undertaken a sustained, multi-level, collaborative examination of what may be described as a "specimen case." Over the course of many years—even decades—studies of various kinds in qualitative and quantitative methodology have been made on the psychoanalytic treatment of our first specimen case named "Amalia X."[1] Clinical vignettes and a psychodynamic summary of the case have been provided in the second volume of Thomä and Kächele's textbook *Psychoanalytic Practice* (1994b) from which I now quote the clinical description of the patient:

> Amalia X (born 1939) was in psychoanalytic treatment (517 sessions) during the early seventies with good results. Some years later she returned to her former therapist for a short period of analytic therapy because of problems with her lover, many years her junior. Twenty-five

years later she consulted a colleague of mine as her final separation from this partner had caused unbearable difficulties and she again asked for circumscribed help.

Amalia X came to psychoanalysis because the severe restrictions she felt on her self-esteem had made her vulnerable to depression in the last few years. Her entire life history since puberty and her social role as a woman had suffered from the severe strain resulting from her hirsutism. Although it had been possible for her to hide her stigma—the virile growth of hair all over her body—from others, the cosmetic aids she used had not raised her self-esteem or eliminated her extreme social insecurity. Her feeling of being stigmatized and her neurotic symptoms, which had already been manifest before puberty, strengthened each other in a vicious circle; scruples from a compulsion neurosis and various symptoms of anxiety neurosis impeded her personal relationships and, most importantly, kept the patient from forming closer heterosexual friendships.

> (Thomä & Kächele 1994b, p. 79)

Given the prevailing paucity of systematic descriptive data on psychoanalytic cases, we have to accept that the various studies performed on the specimen case of Amalia X refer to parts and aspects of the treatment only, and must eventually be integrated so that the relationships among them, and thus the case as a whole may be appreciated. Whether general conclusions can be drawn from our efforts remains an open question. Our principal conviction ultimately leading to the start of this enterprise was the credo that psychoanalysis—like any other scientific field—requires careful descriptive work. This necessary step in research was dubbed the "botanical phase in psychotherapy research" (Grawe 1988, p. 4). Luborsky and Spence's (1971) statement concerning the requirements for specimen cases spells out quite succinctly what is at stake here.

> Ideally, two conditions should be met: The case should be clearly defined as analytic, and the data should be recorded, transcribed and indexed so as to maximize accessibility and visibility.
>
> (p. 426)

The first condition has been met as well as possible, given the existing epistemological problem that there is no consensually agreed definition of psychoanalytic process, by virtue of the fact that a reasonable number of colleagues considered this case as being truly "analytic." The treating analyst had a high reputation in the professional community, although all analysts have to demonstrate the nature of their work in each and every case. Based on the results of studies, it can also be said in retrospect that the treating analyst conformed to the fundamental psychoanalytic rules extant during the seventies. Conforming to a specific method should not be confused with abiding a law.

Rather, I share the view of Gabbard and Westen (2003) that the process should be conducted according to the principle of trial and error. But this stand on this issue is still not consistent with the attitude in the psychoanalytic professional community.

The second condition formulated by Luborsky and Spence (1971) is fulfilled by the utilization in our studies of the *Ulm Textbank* (Mergenthaler & Kächele 1988), in which audio recordings of 517 sessions of this psychoanalytic case are stored and kept available for investigation by members of the scientific community. Through many years of work, more than half the sessions of this case have been transcribed according to the rules of the *Ulm Textbank* (Mergenthaler & Stinson 1992). Most of our investigations would not have been possible without these audio recordings and verbatim transcripts of dialogue. I would like to emphasize the value that audio recordings create for the realization of interdisciplinary research. The accessibility of psychoanalytic dialogue, and the investigation of it by psychoanalytic researchers in collaboration with psychologists, linguists, or other independent scholars, strengthens the interdisciplinary foundation of psychoanalysis. In the past, too often scholars wrote about psychoanalysis without having access to its primary data—a situation that may be compared to discussing of the philosophical ideas of Socrates without actually having read the Platonic dialogues.

The systematic–observational approach: a multi-level observational strategy

Our long-term aim has been to establish ways of systematically describing the various aspects and dimensions of the psychoanalytic processes, and to use the descriptive data obtained in this way to examine process hypotheses. This entailed the generation of general process hypotheses as well as the specification of single case process assumptions.

Specifying how a psychoanalytic process should unfold must go beyond general clinical ideas by considering the kind of material brought forth by each patient and the strategic interventions most appropriate to achieving change in the dimensions of theoretical relevance specified for each particular case. Although our approach excluded the use of non-clinical measures to limit the intrusions on the clinical process,[2] independent psychometric pre-post outcome and follow-up data were used to assess the effectiveness of the psychoanalytic treatment, and have been published in the second volume of Thomä and Kächele (1994b, chap. 9.11.2).

Our methodological approach distinguishes four levels of case research, each working on different material studied at different levels of conceptualization (Kächele & Thomä 1993). These are clinical case study (level I); systematic clinical description (level II); guided clinical judgment procedures (level III) and linguistic and computer-assisted text analysis (level IV). Following Sargent's (1961) recommendations, we chose this multi-level strategy based on our understanding that the gap between clinical understanding and objectification cannot be meaningfully bridged by using only one approach.

The account of this unique single case study has been summarized elsewhere (Kächele et al. 2006); the details on the manifold aspects of the work can be found in Kächele et al. (2009). In view of the paucity of thorough systematic-observational studies of psychoanalytic cases, Werbart (2009) in his careful review expressed the opinion that this work represents a major step in devising a methodology of sound systematic-observational research into the process of analytic treatments. First by demonstrating that it can be done, and then by showing how it can be done, given sufficient dedication and institutional support. Psychoanalytic treatment can be made the focus of objective and methodologically sophisticated research, leading to findings and discoveries that cannot be made by the treating analyst alone. The clinical perspective of the treating analyst is essential but necessarily limited by his or her role as a participant observer of the analytic process. Supplementing this, formal systematic research opens the way to independent understandings of the mechanisms of change in psychoanalysis.

The studies of our specimen case not only support the notion that this analytic treatment led to considerable change in many aspects of the patient's cognitive and emotional functioning, but also demonstrate the usefulness of micro-analytic research techniques that help to identify and conceptualize change processes. The number of descriptive dimensions that are possible and necessary to describe these changes is not small. However, one conclusion can safely be drawn from the studies of our specimen case, which is that change processes exist and can be demonstrated by research methods that are reliable and valid. Both the process of change in psychoanalysis and in the patient's basic psychological capacities take place all along the way, and it is often but not always the case that they can be described in terms of linear trends along the continuum of the treatment.

The case of Amalia X is one of the most intensely studied, perhaps the most intensively studied, of all specimen cases. Almost all of the process hypotheses tested were significant, thereby providing support for the underlying conceptions of psychoanalytic treatment that guided the studies. Although this substantiation is valuable, it is also of interest to consider the limitations of the studies. Except for the hypotheses relating to Amalia X's improvement in acceptance by others, which were not confirmed, in all other instances we found what we expected to find. Whether this may be read as an expression of investigator allegiance (Luborsky et al. 1999) remains open. The transcripts of the raw data are publicly available and any one is invited to check our findings. In any case, the implication is that we need to develop and to address further innovative questions.

Although we have documented substantial changes in various aspects of Amalia X's personality, it remains difficult to pinpoint which were the most important mutative factors in her substantial improvement. Although momentary affective patient–analyst interactions may have mutative effects as we demonstrated in the specimen session 152 of Amalia X (Buchholz et al. 2015), I would conclude that only a longitudinal view of the course of treatment provides the necessary data to assess structural changes in the patient. This emphasizes the extraordinary complexity of attempting to delineate the causes of mutative effects, and reinforces the need for humility in approaching such endeavors. Often the analyst's uncertainty is defended against by compensatory feelings of knowing all about analytic treatment, or, as Jonathan Lear (1998) terms it, "Knowingness."

Having said that, I would like to assert that in the domain of examining mutative factors specifically in psychoanalytic treatment, that single case research has certain advantages compared to group studies. Conversely, concerning assessment of global therapeutic benefit, that group studies seem to have advantages. Indeed, group studies seem to have solidly established the efficacy of psychoanalytic treatment (Leichsenring & Rabung 2008; de Maat et al. 2009; Zimmermann et al. 2015; Leuzinger-Bohleber et al. 2019).

Open questions

Any attempt to study mutative factors in psychoanalytic treatment in particular must deal with the unresolved epistemological problem that there is no consensually agreed definition of "psychoanalytic process" (Vaughan & Roose 1995). This is so vexing that it has been dealt with largely by denial of the problem's existence (Schachter & Kächele 2017).

As I have demonstrated, single case research allows for a number of research methodologies to be implemented in order to conquer the universe each individual analytic couple represents. "The careful scrutiny of the psychoanalytic process through concurrent use of multiple methodologies has created a comprehensive reference text that clinicians can use to improve their understanding of the mechanisms of change," comments Fonagy (2009) on the full-length account of this research enterprise.

I would like to encourage other research groups to single out a carefully documented, tape-recorded case and zoom into the various dimensions. We want to encourage other psychoanalysts to open the privacy of their clinical work in the endeavor to improve clinical work by allowing others in the scientific community to carefully scrutinize their work. To achieve this the establishment of public databases that provide structured information on published single cases is a timely enterprise (Desmet et al. 2013). The next step from single-case studies leads to practice-based knowledge by aggregating and synthesizing case studies (Iwakabe & Gazzola, 2009).

I recommend the training of researchers who are also trained as clinicians, and the training of clinicians who are also trained as researchers, so that they may learn to identify with both the clinical and research tasks. We need analysts and researchers with the ability to support long-term commitment to making slow but cumulative progress. Systematic investigations are dependent on teams supported by institutions which promote cooperation between analysts in practice and full-time researchers. Implementation of such research will help to move psychoanalysis creatively beyond its contemporary crisis.

Notes

1 Since then we have completed a report on the second specimen case Christian Y (Kächele 2009); two more cases are to follow, Franziska X and Gustav Y.
2 In the 1970s—when this case was recorded—extra-clinical interviewing during the analytic treatment was not yet in our mind; today this strategy has shown not to be detrimental to the analytic process (Taubner et al. 2012).

References

Ávila-Espada, A., & Mitjavila, M. (2003). El método del plan de acción latente de la terapeuta (TKLAP). Un nuevo método para predecir la contribución cualitativa del terapeuta al resultado de tratamiento. *Subjetividad y Procesos Cognitivos, 3* (3), 9–36.

Brosig, B., Kupfer, J., Brähler, E., & Eucker, D. (1997). M. Crohn – Einzelfallanalyse eines Therapieverlaufes (M. Crohn – Single case analysis of the treatment course). In P. Kosarz & H.C. Traue (Eds.), *Psychosomatik chronisch-entzündlicher Darmerkrankungen* (pp. 169–184). Bern: Huber.

Bucci, W. (1988). Converging evidence for emotional structures: Theory and method. In H. Dahl, H. Kächele, & H. Thomä (Eds.), *Psychoanalytic process research strategies* (pp. 29–49). Berlin/Heidelberg/New York/Tokyo: Springer.

Bucci, W. (1997). Pattern of discourse in good and troubled hours. *Journal of the American Psychoanalytic Association, 45*(1), 155–188.

Buchholz, M.B., Spiekermann, J., & Kächele, H. (2015). Rhythm and blues. Amalia's 152nd session. From psychoanalysis to conversation and metaphor analysis – and retour. *International Journal of Psychoanalysis, 96,* 877–910.

Chassan, J.B. (1967). *Research design in clinical psychology and psychiatry* (1st ed.). New York: Appleton-Century-Crofts.

Chassan, J.B., & Bellak, L. (1966). An introduction to intensive design in the evaluation of drug efficacy during psychotherapy. In L.A. Gottschalk & A.H. Auerbach (Eds.), *Methods of Research in Psychotherapy* (pp. 478–499). New York: Appleton-Century-Crofts.

Dahl, H. (1972). A quantitative study of psychoanalysis. In R.R. Holt & E. Peterfreund (Eds.), *Psychoanalysis and contemporary science* (pp. 237–257). New York: Macmillan Company.

Davison, G.C., & Lazarus, A.A. (1994). Clinical innovation and evaluation. *Clinical Psychology: Science and Practice, 1,* 157–167.

De Maat, S., de Jonghe, F., Schoevers, R., & Dekker, J. (2009). The effectiveness of long-term psychoanalytic therapy: A systematic review of empirical studies. *Harvard Review of Psychiatry, 17,* 1–23.

Desmet, M., Meganck, R., Seybert, C., Willemsen, J., Geerardyn, F., Dclercq, F., …
   Kächele, H. (2013). Psychoanalytic single cases published in ISI-ranked journals: The
   construction of an online archive. *Psychotherapy and Psychosomatics, 82*, 120–121.
Donnellan, G.J. (1978). Single-subject research and psychoanalytic theory. *Bulletin of
   the Menninger Clinic, 42*, 352–357.
Dukes, W.F. (1965). N = 1. *Psychological Bulletin, 64*, 74–79.
Edelson, M. (1984). *Hypothesis and evidence in psychoanalysis.* Chicago: University of
   Chicago Press.
Edelson, M. (1985). The hermeneutic turn and the single case study in psychoanaly-
   sis. *Psychoanalysis and Contemporary Thought, 8*, 567–614.
Ehlich, K. (Ed.) (1980). *Erzählen im Alltag.* Frankfurt: Suhrkamp.
Fonagy, P. (2009). Blurb statement to Kächele, Schachter, Thomä 2009.
Fonagy, P., & Moran, G. (1993). Selecting single case research design for clinicians.
   In N.E. Miller, L. Luborsky, & J.P. Barber (Eds.), *Psychodynamic treatment research. A
   handbook for clinical practice* (pp. 62–95). New York: Basic Books.
Forrester, J. (1980). *Language and the origins of psychoanalysis.* London: Macmillan.
Freud, S. (1909d). Notes upon a case of obsessional neurosis. *Standard Edition, 10*,
   153–318.
Freud, S. (1916/17). Introductory lectures on psycho-analysis. *Standard Edition, 16*,
   243–463.
Frommer, J., & Langenbach, M. (2001). The psychoanalytic case study as a source of
   epistemic knowledge. In J. Frommer & D.L. Rennie (Eds.), *Qualitative psychother-
   apy research. Methods and methodology* (pp. 50–68). Lengerich: Pabst.
Gabbard, G.O., & Westen, D. (2003). Rethinking therapeutic action. *International
   Journal of Psychoanalysis, 84*, 823–842.
Gazzillo, F., Waldron, S., Genova, F., Angeloni, F., Ristucci, C., & Lingiardi, V.
   (2014). An empirical investigation of analytic process: Contrasting a good and poor
   outcome case. *Psychotherapy, 51*(2), 270–282. doi:10.1037/a0035243.
Glover, E. (1952). Research methods in psychoanalysis. *International Journal of Psycho-
   analysis, 33*, 403–409.
Gould, S.J. (1986). Evolution and the triumph of homology, or why history matters.
   American Scientist, 74 (1), 60–69.
Grawe, K. (1988). Zurück zur psychotherapeutischen Einzelfallforschung (Back to
   single case research). *Zeitschrift für Klinische Psychologie, 17*, 4–5.
Grünbaum, A. (1984). *The foundations of psychoanalysis. A philosophical critique.* Berkeley
   Los Angeles London. University of California Press.
Gullestad, F., & Wilberg, T. (2011). Change in reflective functioning during psychotherapy:
   A single-case study *Psychotherapy Research, 21*(1), 97–111.
Hilliard, R.B. (1993). Single case methodology in psychotherapy process and
   outcome research. *Journal of Consulting and Clinical Psychology, 61*, 373–380.
Iwakabe, S., & Gazzola, N. (2009). From single-case studies to practice-based knowledge:
   Aggregating and synthesizing case studies. *Psychotherapy Research, 19*(4), 601–611.
J, B. (1893–1895). Case I. Fräulein Anna O. Studies on hysteria. *Standard Edition, 2*, 1–47.
Jones, E.E., & Windholz, M. (1990). The psychoanalytic case study: Toward a
   method for systematic inquiry. *Journal of the American Psychoanalytic Association,
   38*(4), 985–1016.

Kächele, H. (1992). Une nouvelle perspective de recherche en psychothérapie: le projet "PEP." *Psychothérapies*, *2*, 73–77.

Kächele, H., Albani, C., Buchheim, A., Hölzer, M., Hohage, R., Mergenthaler, E., … Thomä, H. (2006). The German specimen case Amalia X: Empirical studies. *International Journal of Psychoanalysis*, *87*(3), 809–826.

Kächele, H., Schachter, J., & Thomä, H. (Eds.). (2009). *From psychoanalytic narrative to empirical single case research. Implications for psychoanalytic practice*. New York: Routledge.

Kächele, H., & Thomä, H. (1993). Psychoanalytic process research: Methods and achievements. *Journal of the American Psychoanalytic Association*, *41*, 109–129 Suppl.

Kächele, H., Thomä, H., Ruberg, W., & Grünzig, H.-J. (1988). Audio-recordings of the psychoanalytic dialogue: scientific, clinical and ethical problems. In H. Dahl, H. Kächele, & H. Thomä (Eds.), *Psychoanalytic process research strategies* (pp. 179–194). Berlin Heidelberg New York Tokyo: Springer.

Kazdin, A.E. (2011). *Single-case research designs. Methods for clinical and applied settings*. New York Oxford: Oxford University Press.

Kline, P. (1972). *Fact and fantasy in Freudian theory* (1st ed.). London: Methuen.

Lear, J. (1998). *Open minded: Working out the logic of the soul*. Cambridge, MA: Harvard University Press.

Leichsenring, F., & Rabung, S. (2008). Effectiveness of long-term psychodynamic psychotherapy. A meta-analysis. *JAMA*, *300*(13), 1551–1565.

Leuzinger-Bohleber, M. (1995). Die Einzelfallstudie als psychoanalytisches Forschungsinstrument (The single case study as psychoanalytic research instrument). *Psyche – Zeitschrift für Psychoanalyse*, *49*, 434–480.

Leuzinger-Bohleber, M., Hautzinger, M., Fiedler, G., Keller, W., Bahrke, U., Kallenbach, L., … Beutel, M. (2019). Outcome of psychoanalytic and cognitive-behavioural long-term therapy with chronically depressed patients: A controlled trial with preferential and randomized allocation. *The Canadian Journal of Psychiatry/ La Revue Canadienne de Psychiatrie*, 1–12. doi:10.1177/0706743718780340.

Levy, K.N., Clarkin, J.F., Yeoman, F.E., Scott, L.N., Wassermann, R.H., & Kernberg, O.F. (2006). The mechanisms of change in the treatment of borderline personality disorder with transference focused psychotherapy. *Journal of Clinical Psychology*, *62*(4), 481–501.

Lingiardi, V., Gazzillo, F., & Waldron, S. (2010). An empirically supported psychoanalysis: The case of Giovanna. *Psychoanalytic Psychology*, *27*, 190–218. doi:10.1037/a0019418.

Lingiardi, V., Shedler, J., & Gazillo, F. (2006). Assessing personality change in psychotherapy with the SWAP-200: A case study. *Journal of Personality Assessment*, *86*, 23–32.

López Moreno, C.M., Schalayeff, C., Acosta, S.R., Vernengo, P., Roussos, A.J., & Dorfman Lerner, B. (2005). Evaluation of psychic change through the application of empirical and clinical techniques for a 2-year treatment: a single case study. *Psychotherapy Research*, *15*(3), 199–209.

Luborsky, L., Diguer, L., Seligman, D.A., Rosenthal, R., Krause, E.D., Johnson, S., … Schweitzer, E. (1999). The researcher's own therapy allegiances: A "wild card" in comparisons of treatment efficacy. *Clinical Psychology: Science and Practice*, *6*, 95–106.

Luborsky, L., & Spence, D.P. (1971). Quantitative research on psychoanalytic therapy. In A.E. Bergin & S.L. Garfield (Eds.), *Handbook of psychotherapy and behavior change* (1st ed., pp. 408–438). New York: Wiley & Sons.

Luborsky, L., & Spence, D.P. (1978). Quantitative research on psychoanalytic therapy. In S.L. Garfield & A.E. Bergin (Eds.), *Handbook of psychotherapy and behavior change: An empirical analysis* (2nd ed., pp. 331–368). New York Chichester Brisbane: Wiley & Sons.

Marmor, J. (1962). Psychoanalytic therapy as an educational process. In J. Masserman (Ed.), *Psychoanalytic education* (pp. 286–299). New York: Grune and Stratton.

Marmor, J. (1986). The question of causality. Commentary on Grünbaum: Foundations of psychoanalysis. *Behavioral and Brain Sciences, 9,* 249.

Masling, J., & Cohen, J. (1987). Psychotherapy, clinical evidence and the self-fulfilling prophecy. *Psychoanalytic Psychology, 4,* 65–79.

Mergenthaler, E. (1998). I patterns di Emozione-Astrazione nei trascritti delle verbalizzazioni: un nuovo approccio per la descrizione dei processi in psicoterapia. *Psicoterapia, 12,* 26–38.

Mergenthaler, E., & Kächele, H. (1988). The Ulm Textbank management system: A tool for psychotherapy research. In H. Dahl, H. Kächele, & H. Thomä (Eds.), *Psychoanalytic process research strategies* (pp. 195–212). Berlin/Heidelberg/New York/London/Paris/Tokyo: Springer.

Mergenthaler, E., & Kächele, H. (1996). Applying multiple computerized text-analytic measures to single psychotherapy cases. *The Journal of Psychotherapy Practice and Research, 5,* 307–317.

Mergenthaler, E., & Stinson, C.H. (1992). Psychotherapy transcription standards. *Psychotherapy Research, 2*(2), 125–142.

Michels, R. (2000). The case history. *Journal of the American Psychoanalytic Association, 48,* 355–375.

Mitchell, S.A. (1998). The analyst's knowledge and authority. *Psychoanalytic Quarterly, 67,* 1–31.

Moran, G., Fonagy, P., Kurtz, A., Bolton, A., & Brook, C. (1991). A controlled study of the psychoanalytic treatment of brittle diabetes. *Journal of the American Academy of Child and Adolescent Psychiatry, 30,* 926–935.

Persons, J.B., Curtis, J.T., & Silberschatz, G. (1991). Psychodynamic and cognitive-behavioral formulations of a single case. *Psychotherapy, 28*(4), 608–617.

Peterson, C., Luborsky, L., & Seligman, M.E.P. (1983). Attributions and depressive mood shifts: A case study using the symptom-context method. *The Journal of Abnormal Psychology, 92*(1), 96–103.

Pole, N., Ablon, J., O'Connor, L., & Weiss, J. (2002). Ideal control mastery technique correlates with change in a single case. *Psychotherapy: Theory Research Practice Training, 39,* 88–96.

Porcerelli, J., Dauphin, V.B., Ablon, J.S., & Leitman, S. (2007). Psychoanalysis with avoidant personality disorder: A systematic case study. *Psychotherapy: Theory, Research, Practice, Training, 44,* 1–13.

Propp, V. (1968 (1928)). *Morphology of folktale.* Austin: The American Folklore Society and Indiana University.

Pulver, S.E. (1987a). How theory shapes technique: perspectives on a clinical study. *Psychoanalytic Inquiry, 7*, 141–299.

Sargent, H.D. (1961). Intrapsychic change: Methodological problems in psychotherapy research. *Psychiatry, 24*, 93–108.

Schachter, J. (2002). *Transference, shibboleth or albatross?* Hillsdale, NJ: The Analytic Press.

Schachter, J., & Kächele, H. (2017). Psychoanalytic process: A concept ready for retirement. In J. Schachter & H. Kächele (Eds.), *Nodal points. Critical issues in contemporary psychoanalytic therapy.* New York: IPBOOKS ebook.

Schubert, C. (Ed.) (2011). *Psychoneuro-Immunologie und Psychotherapie.* Stuttgart: Schattauer Verlag.

Shakow, D., & Rapaport, D. (1964). The influence of Freud on American psychology. *Psychological Issues, 4*(1, Whole No. 13), 1–243.

Silberschatz, G. (2005). *Transformative relationships. The control-mastery theory of personality.* New York: Routledge.

Spence, D.P. (1982). Narrative truth and theoretical truth. *Psychoanalytic Quarterly, 51*, 43–69.

Strenger, C. (2005). *The designed self. Psychoanalysis and contemporary identities.* Hillsdale, NJ: The Analytic Press.

Szecsödy, I. (2008). A single-case study on the process and outcome of psychoanalysis. *Scandinavian Archive of Psychoanalysis, 31*, 105–113.

Taubner, S., Koch-Hübner, I., Böllinger, L., Kächele, H., Cierpka, M., Buchheim, A., & Bruns, G. (2012). How does formal research influence psychoanalytic treatments? Clinical observations and reflections from a study on the interface of clinical psychoanalysis and neuroscience. *American Journal of Psychoanalysis, 72*(3), 269–286.

Thomä, H., & Kächele, H. (1994a). *Psychoanalytic practice. Vol. 1 Principles.* New York: Jason Aronson.

Thomä, H., & Kächele, H. (1994b). *Psychoanalytic practice. Vol. 2 Clinical studies.* New York: Jason Aronson.

Vaughan, S., & Roose, S. (1995). The analytic process: Clinical and research definitions. *International Journal of Psychoanalysis, 76*, 343–356.

Von Krafft-Ebing, R. (1896). Zur Suggestions-Behandlung der Hysteria gravis. *Zeitschrift für Hypnotismus, 4*(1), 27–31.

Waldron, S., Scharf, R.D., Hurst, D., Crouse, J., Firestein, S.K., & Burton, A. (2004). What happens in a psychoanalysis? A view through the lens of the Analytic Process Scales. *International Journal of Psychoanalysis, 85*, 443–466.

Wallerstein, R.S. (2002). The trajectory of psychoanalysis: A prognostication. *International Journal of Psychoanalysis, 83*, 1247–1268.

Wallerstein, R.S. Sampson, H. (1971). Issues in research in the psychoanalytic process. *Int. J. Psycho-Anal., 52*, 11–50.

Weiss, J., & Sampson, H. (1986). Testing alternative psychoanalytic explanations of the therapeutic process. In J.M. Masling (Ed.), *Empirical studies of psychoanalytic theories* (pp. 1–26). Hillsdale, NJ: The Analytic Press.

Werbart, A. (2009). Review: Minding the gap between clinical practice and empirical research in psychoanalysis: "From psychoanalytic narrative to empirical single case research: Implications for psychoanalytic practice" by Horst Kächele, Joseph Schachter, Helmut Thoma. *International Journal of Psychoanalysis, 90*, 1459–1466.

Wolitzky, D.L. (2007). The role of clinical inference in psychoanalytic case studies. *American Journal of Psychotherapy*, *61*(1), 17–36.

Zetzel, E.R. (1966). Additional notes upon a case of obsessional neurosis: Freud 1909. *International Journal of Psychoanalysis*, *47*(2), 123–129.

Zimmermann, J., Löffler-Stastka, H., Huber, D., Klug, G., Albabbo, S., Bock, A., & Benecke, C. (2015). Is it all about the higher dose? Why psychoanalytic therapy is an effective treatment for major depression. *Clinical Psychology and Psychotherapy*, *22*, 469–487.

Chapter 6

The importance of psychoanalytic research to contemporary medicine

Simone Hauck

> *It is a very remarkable thing that the [unconscious] of one human being can react on that of the other without passing through the [consciousness].*
>
> (Freud 1915, p. 194)

The imperative to bring research in psychoanalysis and clinical practice closer together is clear and urgent, but one can see the role of research in psychoanalysis from an even broader perspective. There is a clear demand that psychoanalytic knowledge extend beyond the walls of analytic clinical offices and institutes, providing informed theories and hypothesis that can reach not only psychiatric circles in general but also medicine and allied fields.

Psychoanalysis can be one of the protagonists at this moment when the findings of research in the health area are showing ever more clearly the fundamental role of the relationship between caregivers and patients in the effectiveness of treatment. This is not only due to the question of the importance of the therapeutic alliance when it comes to compliance with treatment, but also to the direct impact of the relationship upon factors such as response to treatment (of any kind), time of hospitalization, and the efficacy of the immunity system, among many other factors (Kelley, Kraft-Todd, Schapira, Kossowsky, & Riess, 2014). It would be unfortunate if psychoanalytic knowledge failed to occupy its place in this scenario since the advance of science clearly shows the importance of phenomena that psychoanalysis has been studying for over 100 years and concerning which it has accumulated vast experience. Psychoanalysis emerged from roots in neurology and has taken into account phenomena that, at the time Freud gradually developed the psychoanalytic theory, could not be understood with older scientific tools. It is very likely that, if Freud were alive today, he would probably not miss this opportunity for reconciliation.

There have been debates over what active ingredients contribute to changes in patients in the course of psychotherapy/psychoanalysis since the early beginnings of investigation in this area, but the issue remains without conclusive answers (Mulder, Murray, & Rucklidge, 2017). Many researchers have indicated the need to construct new methodologies that can grasp the complexity inherent to the phenomena studied. The therapeutic encounter may be considered a complex system where countless variables interact with one another in different directions and levels. The characteristics and interventions of therapists, together with characteristics and attitudes of patients and the atmosphere resulting from the interactions between them, be they verbal or nonverbal, conscious or unconscious, indicate a universe of possibilities. Many parts of these interconnected relationships can be understood, but the most complex dimension of the phenomena cannot be taken as a simple linear system of cause and effect, nor through partial approaches (only the therapist or only the patient; only what is explicit or only what is implicit).

The quest for new viewpoints and new tools to understand the mechanisms and action involved is a necessity. Moreover, the search for a pluralistic perspective would probably be the best path, based on the understanding that the chasm between clinical phenomena and the requisites of empirical science cannot be spanned through a single approach. This approach to research follows Freud's position of looking for what is behind the phenomena observed, the unknown, which cannot be seen. This is surely a difficult and complex task that calls for initiatives like many described in this book. Current knowledge must be taken beyond what is "visible," looking for joint efforts from different areas, references and methods.

Research has long been focused on comparisons between different modalities of psychotherapy. Nonetheless, even though such research evidences efficacy, and often shows effectiveness, similar results are seen from different techniques and very little clarification is produced as to how they operate, thus contributing very little to clinical practice (Shedler, 2010). In an article published in 2017 in *The Lancet Psychiatry*, Multer and colleagues stated that even though it can be said that psychotherapies are efficacious, we cannot assure that they are validated. In their words, "As with other constructs, validation of psychotherapy would require evidence not only that the approach is beneficial as expected, but also that the benefits arise through the mechanisms postulated by the approach and in the behaviors enacted by therapists" (Mulder et al., 2017, p. 3). In this sense, methodologies that deal with what goes on, in fact, moment by moment, in an analytic process can greatly contribute, through evaluations that are based on the interaction of the therapeutic dyad, considering implicit communication that can be analyzed parallel to explicit communication in analysis (or in any other relationship). Such tools can be of great value to the field (see Jiménez in this volume) and this methodology can be expanded as research tools and scientific techniques evolve in neurobiological, clinical and neuroimaging research.

Omissions committed by psychoanalysts and the absence of its contributions could lead to a loss of precious time for science. Much time has already been lost, for decades, involving dichotomies among "teams" such as specific versus nonspecific factors, and between psychoanalytic therapy versus cognitive behavioral therapy. In terms of research, what should be asked is what works, whom does it work for, and how and under what circumstances does it work. One example of a possible consequence of omission by a psychoanalytic approach in the field of research may have been the fact that, for a long period, cognitive-behavioral therapy stood as the gold standard of therapies based on evidence. Recently some authors have insisted, however, that quantity is not quality. When controlled for "researcher bias," that is, the researcher's chosen therapy, some papers have shown that less than 20% of the studies on behavioral therapy could be described as having quality (Leichsenring & Steinert, 2017). An excessively critical position of psychoanalysis concerning research may have also brought about a counter-reaction, which broadened the distance between fields for many years. In the current scenario, medical and health care research in general have come to recognize the importance of therapeutic relationships, focusing on patient-centered and more comprehensive approaches to address health problems and the attainment of well-being. In this environment, attempts at approximation between psychoanalytic research and theory could contribute considerably to advances that could have been hoped for at the beginning.

One might recall that, according to Bion, one of the main objectives of psychoanalysis is exactly to broaden viewpoints and possibilities. Certainly, the constructs derived from clinical observation and the development of meta-psychology can produce important knowledge about the human mind. Much will be lost, however, if there is no feedback or re-approximation by inverting the paradigm for bottom-up observations and some convergence of these two lines. It is easy to get lost if one is not checking to see whether a given hypothesis really occurs in practice and if it can be generalized.

Research on development through observations on the specific aspects of interaction between mother (or other caregiver) and baby have produced indisputable progress in our understanding of how mental activities develop. Much of what goes on in clinics may well go through very similar processes, thus broadening mental functions or even generating functions that were not previously present and that could not be developed during the early stages of life. Therefore, the use of techniques similar to those applied in mother-infant research can be appropriate. However, there is a specific character of the analytic setting because psychoanalysts and psychodynamic therapists deal with a potentially more difficult task, in the sense that there is already implicit knowledge of the repercussions of relationships that patients have had during their whole lives up to that point. It is difficult and complex to change implicit knowledge, as the task involves experiences that are beyond theoretical understanding and awareness at older ages when the brain is less plastic than it was in early childhood.

Research that leads to further understandings as to how interactions operate and promote change in psychodynamic settings can directly and indirectly contribute to the broader field referred to as the "patient-doctor relationship." As an example, one can consider Helen Riess's work on communication between clinicians and their patients, which was inspired on her own experience as a volunteer in a study by one of her students on nonverbal aspects of interactions with patients (based on examination of the synchronicity of biomarkers). Riess has developed a model for teaching how to detect and express nonverbal factors to medical students. This model, which has proved to be effective, is known as E.M.P.A.T.H.Y: "E" is for eye contact; "M" is for muscle facial expression; "P" for posture; "A" for affect; "T" for tone of voice; "H" for hearing the whole patient; and "Y" for your response (Riess, 2011; Riess & Kraft-Todd, 2014). It is very clear how close this is to variables that have been studied in psychoanalysis since its beginning. It would also seem important to note that the aspect entitled "observe your emotional response"—letter "Y"—used as a tool in medical training, is similar to the current concept and understanding of the use of countertransference in psychoanalysis. In this sense, broadening and validating psychoanalytic theory and techniques benefit not only the field of psychoanalysis itself. At present, there is a strong possibility that medicine will move toward a more comprehensive medicine, in opposition to the strong technicism and over-specialization seen in recent decades. Such a trend could place psychoanalysis in a position to contribute enormously to psychiatry and medicine, based on its long experience with the therapeutic relationship and intersubjectivity as well as, with the analytic field.

Another topic being widely debated in current medical literature is the issue of physicians becoming ill during their training (Brazeau et al., 2014; Dyrbye et al., 2014; Pacheco et al., 2017; Puthran, Zhang, Tam, & Ho, 2016). Among other factors, there is the question of the price of empathy (Gleichgerrcht & Decety, 2013; Smith, Norman, & Decety, 2017). A broader understanding of what is known as "empathy," of course, has much to do with nonverbal communication. Psychoanalysis has long studied these phenomena and their specific aspects, based on clinical work. The development of methodology that can capture nonverbal communication in analytic processes may be one of the opportunities to develop tools to be used in teaching not only psychoanalysts and psychotherapists, but physicians and health professionals in general.

Another important aspect is the movement of psychiatric diagnoses towards a trans-diagnostic character. By considering the therapeutic relationship as the object being studied, one can diverge from classifications based solely on phenomenological observations and not be restricted to current diagnostic classifications. For example, despite being valid attempts that have brought advances to the field of psychiatry, diagnostic systems like the DSM have been questioned and, together with dichotomies of the x-versus-y type, have been held responsible for the inertia evident in research in the area of mental health. To be brief, the fact is that a search for common causes in diagnostic categories led to the final conclusion that there is no specific neurobiological substrate for the majority of the varying diagnoses, there being much more that is common, than different, among mental disorders. Research and ensuing interventions are migrating toward a dimensional rather than a categorical model.

The psychoanalytic encounter is a complex phenomenon where conscious and unconscious (explicit and implicit) factors, common and specific factors of technique, and many others, take place simultaneously and interact in complex and non-exclusive ways. In this sense, evolution in methodologies may well lead, for example, to the development of instruments that will make it possible to detect "minute by minute" interactions in chosen sessions of a single treatment, and in different treatments, generating data that could be used in analyses such as Machine Learning (ML). The advantage of ML is the possibility of simultaneously analyzing great numbers of variables (known as Big Data) without presupposing causality or linearity. This type of evolution in analysis of data possibilities may enable researchers to study very complex and non-linear phenomena of human interaction that have been observed in clinical settings by psychoanalysis for decades.

Another interesting question is the supportive–expressive continuum: How far can the mind of a patient go without losing its capacity to regulate affect in a healthy way? What is the role of the analyst as she or he "moves in the continuum" either through verbal interventions strictly speaking or through nonverbal language to aid in a process of affect regulation, thus broadening this capacity toward, for example, broader reflective capacity? In states of great arousal, one loses the ability to mentalize, using this term here to refer to a specific definition of reflective function. Possibly what puts a patient's "ability to think" back on the track has much more to do with nonverbal factors involving the therapist's attitude. Making a bridge with fundamental questions in psychoanalytic theory, the entire process discussed up to this point constantly brings to my mind Bion's concept of containing function and the process of transforming Beta elements (pre-reflective perception and related brain areas) into Alpha elements (reflective function associated with midline structures). A further question is what constitutes a good enough mother/therapist/analyst for Winnicott. Without going too far into this aspect, several current evolutions and hypotheses in neuroscience indicate brain zones involved in "pre-reflective" empathy or "simulation," where one feels "in fact" feelings of others and one's own feelings, versus others' zones that correspond to reflective empathy such as thinking about one's own and others' states and feelings, more cognitive, mentalization. These are independent functions up to a point but they constantly interact with one another (Adolphs, 2009; Keysers & Gazzola, 2007; Luyten & Fonagy, 2015). On reflecting about these two functions, we might ask ourselves, for example, whether it is possible to completely mentalize things that are not felt? On the other hand, feelings, operating on their own, can be toxic (including for the therapist and health professionals in general). The inclusion of implicit factors in research will make it possible to understand better how these factors interact and complement one another and how they are "learned and apprehended" in the analytic process. Maybe science is about to understand how "Beta" is transformed into "Alpha" in the analytic process. And this understanding may be of great importance for enhancing effectiveness of health treatments and contributing to a better quality of life for health professionals.

References

Adolphs, R. (2009). The social brain: neural basis of social knowledge. *Annu Rev Psychol*, *60*, 693–716. doi:10.1146/annurev.psych.60.110707.163514.

Brazeau, C.M., Shanafelt, T., Durning, S.J., Massie, F.S., Eacker, A., Moutier, C., … Dyrbye, L.N. (2014). Distress among matriculating medical students relative to the general population. *Acad Med*, *89*(11), 1520–1525. doi:10.1097/ACM.0000000000000482.

Dyrbye, L.N., West, C.P., Satele, D., Boone, S., Tan, L., Sloan, J., & Shanafelt, T.D. (2014). Burnout among U.S. medical students, residents, and early career physicians relative to the general U.S. population. *Acad Med*, *89*(3), 443–451. doi:10.1097/ACM.0000000000000134.

Freud, S. (1915). The standard edition of the complete psychological works of Sigmund Freud: On the history of the psycho-analytic movement, papers on metapsychology and other works. London: The Hogarth Press and The Institute of Psycho-Analyses; Translation from the German under the General Editing of James Strachey in collaboration with Anna Freud assisted by Alix Strachey and Alan Tyson – Volume XIV (1914–1916).

Gleichgerrcht, E., & Decety, J. (2013). Empathy in clinical practice: how individual dispositions, gender, and experience moderate empathic concern, burnout, and emotional distress in physicians. *PLoS ONE*, *8*(4), e61526. doi:10.1371/journal.pone.0061526.

Kelley, J.M., Kraft-Todd, G., Schapira, L., Kossowsky, J., & Riess, H. (2014). The influence of the patient–clinician relationship on healthcare outcomes: a systematic review and meta-analysis of randomized controlled trials. *PLoS ONE*, *9*(4), e94207. doi:10.1371/journal.pone.0094207.

Keysers, C., & Gazzola, V. (2007). Integrating simulation and theory of mind: from self to social cognition. *Trends Cogn Sci*, *11*(5), 194–196. doi:10.1016/j.tics.2007.02.002.

Leichsenring, F., & Steinert, C. (2017). Is cognitive behavioral therapy the gold standard for psychotherapy?: the need for plurality in treatment and research. *JAMA*, *318*(14), 1323–1324. doi:10.1001/jama.2017.13737.

Luyten, P., & Fonagy, P. (2015). The neurobiology of mentalizing. *Personal Disord*, *6*(4), 366–379. doi:10.1037/per0000117.

Mulder, R., Murray, G., & Rucklidge, J. (2017). Common versus specific factors in psychotherapy: opening the black box. *Lancet Psychiatry*, *4*(12), 953–962. doi:10.1016/S2215-0366(17)30100-1.

Pacheco, J.P., Giacomin, H.T., Tam, W.W., Ribeiro, T.B., Arab, C., Bezerra, I.M., & Pinasco, G.C. (2017). Mental health problems among medical students in Brazil: a systematic review and meta-analysis. *Rev Bras Psiquiatr, 39*(4), 369–378. doi:10.1590/1516-4446-2017-2223.

Puthran, R., Zhang, M.W., Tam, W.W., & Ho, R.C. (2016). Prevalence of depression amongst medical students: a meta-analysis. *Med Educ, 50*(4), 456–468. doi:10.1111/medu.12962.

Riess, H. (2011). Biomarkers in the psychotherapeutic relationship: the role of physiology, neurobiology, and biological correlates of E.M.P.A.T.H.Y. *Harv Rev Psychiatry, 19*(3), 162–174. doi:10.3109/08941939.2011.581915.

Riess, H., & Kraft-Todd, G. (2014). E.M.P.A.T.H.Y.: a tool to enhance nonverbal communication between clinicians and their patients. *Acad Med, 89*(8), 1108–1112. doi:10.1097/ACM.0000000000000287.

Shedler, J. (2010). The efficacy of psychodynamic psychotherapy. *Am Psychol, 65*(2), 98–109. doi:10.1037/a0018378.

Smith, K.E., Norman, G.J., & Decety, J. (2017). The complexity of empathy during medical school training: evidence for positive changes. *Med Educ, 51*(11), 1146–1159. doi:10.1111/medu.13398.

Research and clinical practice in dialogue

Chapter 7

Evidence for psychodynamic psychotherapy in specific mental disorders

A systematic review

Falk Leichsenring and Susanne Klein

In this chapter,[1] the available evidence for psychodynamic psychotherapy (PDT) in adults is reviewed. The focus will be on randomized controlled trials (RCTs), which are regarded as the "gold standard" for demonstrating treatment efficacy. Previous reviews have been undertaken, for example, by Fonagy, Roth, and Higgitt (2005), Leichsenring, Klein, and Salzer (2014), Shedler (2010), and Gerber et al. (2011). Shedler (2010) came to the conclusion that effect sizes of PDT are as large as those reported for other forms of psychotherapy that are regarded as "empirically supported." In addition, he found that effects of PDT were stable or tended to improve after the end of treatment. In a quality-based review of RCTs, Gerber et al. (2011) found PDT to be at least as efficacious as another active treatment in 34 of 39 studies (87%). In comparison with inactive conditions, PDT was superior in 18 of 24 adequate comparisons (75%).

In another quality-based review of RCTs, Thoma et al. (2012) examined the methodological quality of RCTs of cognitive-behavioral therapy (CBT) in depression. Contrary to their expectation, the authors found no significant differences in methodological quality between RCTs of CBT in depression and RCTs of PDT. Taking the frequently put forward criticism of the methodological quality of studies of PDT into account (e.g., Bhar & Beck, 2009), the result reported by Thoma et al. (2012) is of some importance. In another context, we showed that often double standards were applied when studies of PDT were criticized by representatives of other approaches (Leichsenring & Rabung, 2011).

Evidence-based medicine and empirically supported treatments

Several proposals have been made to grade the available evidence of both medical and psychotherapeutic treatments (Canadian Task Force on the Periodic Health Examination, 1979; Chambless & Hollon, 1998; Clarke & Oxman, 2003; Cook, Guyatt, Laupacis, Sacket, & Goldberg, 1995; Nathan & Gorman, 2002). Apart from other differences, all available proposals regard

RCTs (efficacy studies) as the "gold standard" for the demonstration that a treatment is effective. According to this view, only RCTs can provide level I evidence, which is the highest level of evidence. RCTs are conducted under controlled experimental conditions, allowing one to control for variables systematically influencing the outcome apart from the treatment. The defining feature of an RCT is the random assignment of subjects to the different conditions of treatment (Shadish, Cook, & Campbell, 2002). Randomization is regarded as indispensable in order to ensure that a priori existing differences between subjects are equally distributed. The goal of randomization is to attribute the observed effects exclusively to the applied therapy. Thus, randomization is used to ensure the internal validity of a study (Shadish et al., 2002). Gabbard, Gunderson, and Fonagy (2002) discuss different types of RCTs that provide different levels of evidence. The most stringent test of efficacy is achieved by comparison with rival treatments, thus controlling for specific and unspecific therapeutic factors (Chambless & Hollon, 1998, p. 8). Furthermore, such comparisons provide explicit information regarding the relative benefits of competing treatments. Treatments that are found to be superior to rival treatments are more highly valued.

As RCTs are carried out under controlled experimental conditions, their internal validity is usually high. However, for this very reason, their external validity may be limited, in that their results may not be fully representative of clinical practice. In contrast to RCTs, naturalistic studies (observational or effectiveness studies) are conducted under the conditions of clinical practice. Thus, their results are usually more representative for clinical practice with regard to patients, therapists, and treatments (external validity). RCTs and observational studies address different questions of research, i.e., efficacy under controlled experimental conditions versus effectiveness under the conditions of clinical practice (Leichsenring, 2004). For this reason, RCTs are not "bad" and observational studies are not "good" or vice versa. Their relationship is complementary rather than one of rival (Leichsenring, 2004).

Methods

Definition of Psychodynamic Therapy (PDT)

PDT operates on an interpretive–supportive continuum (Gunderson & Gabbard, 1999; Wallerstein, 1989). Interpretive interventions enhance the patient's insight about repetitive conflicts sustaining his or her problems (Gabbard, 2004; Luborsky, 1984). Supportive interventions aim to strengthen abilities ("ego-functions") that are temporarily not accessible to a patient due to acute stress (e.g., traumatic events) or that have not been sufficiently developed (e.g., impulse control in borderline personality disorder; BPD). Thus, supportive interventions maintain or build ego functions (Wallerstein, 1989). Supportive interventions include, for example, fostering a therapeutic alliance, setting goals, or strengthening ego functions such as reality testing or impulse control (Luborsky, 1984). The use of more supportive or more interpretive (insight-enhancing) interventions depends on the patient's needs. The more severely disturbed a patient is, or the more acute his or her problem is, the more supportive and less interpretive interventions are required and vice versa (Luborsky, 1984; Wallerstein, 1989). Borderline patients, as well as healthy subjects, in an acute crisis or after a traumatic event may need more supportive interventions (e.g., stabilization, providing a safe and supportive environment). Thus, a broad spectrum of psychiatric problems and disorders can be treated with PDT, ranging from milder adjustment disorders or stress reactions to severe personality disorders such as BPD or psychotic conditions.

Inclusion and exclusion criteria

The following inclusion and exclusion criteria were applied: (1) PDT according to the definition above was applied, (2) RCT, (3) reliable and valid measures for diagnosis and outcome, (4) use of treatment manuals, and (5) study of specific mental disorders. Studies examining the combination of psychodynamic therapy and medication were not included, however, concomitant medication in both treatment arms was allowed.

We collected studies of PDT that were published between 1970 and September 2013 by use of a computerized search of MEDLINE, PsycINFO, and Current Contents. The following search terms were used: (psychodynamic or dynamic or psychoanalytic★) and (therapy or psychotherapy or treatment) and (study or studies or trial★) and (outcome or result★ or effect★ or change★) and (psych★ or mental★) and (RCT★ or control★ or compare★). Manual searches in articles and textbooks were performed. In addition, we communicated with authors and experts in the field.

Efficacy studies of PDT in specific mental disorders

A total of 47 RCTs providing evidence for the efficacy of PDT in specific mental disorders were identified and included in this review. These studies are presented in Table 7.1.

Models of PDT

In the studies identified, different forms of PDT were applied (Table 7.1). The models developed by Luborsky (1984), Shapiro and Firth (1985), and Malan (1976) were used most frequently.

Table 7.1 Overview of RCTs providing evidence for the efficacy of PDT in specific mental disorders

Study	Disorder	N (PP)	Comparison group	Concept of PP	Treatment duration
Depressive disorders					
Barber et al. (2012)	Major depression	51	Pharmacotherapy: N = 55; Placebo: N = 50	Luborsky	20 sessions; 16 weeks
Barkham et al. (1996)	Major depression	18	CBT: N = 18	Shapiro and Firth	8 versus 16 sessions
Driessen et al. (2013)	Major depression	117	CBT: N = 164	de Jonghe	16 sessions
Gallagher-Thompson and Steffen (1994)	Major, minor or intermittent depression	30	CBT: N = 36	Mann, Rose and DelMaestro	16–20 sessions
Johannson et al. (2012)	Major depression	46	Structured support: N = 46	Internet-guided self-help; Silverberg	10 weeks
Maina et al. (2005)	Dysthymic disorder	10	Supportive therapy: N = 10; Waiting list: N = 25	Malan	15–30 sessions
Salminen et al. (2008)	Major depression	26	Fluoxetine: N = 25	Mann, Malan	16 sessions
Shapiro et al. (1994)	Major depression	58	CBT: N = 59	Shapiro and Firth	8 versus 16 sessions
Thompson et al. (1987)	Major depression	24	BT: N = 25; CBT: N = 27; Waiting list: N = 19	Horrowitz and Kaltreiter	16–20 sessions
Anxiety disorders					
Bögels et al. (2003)	Social phobia	22	CBT: N = 27	Malan	36 sessions
Crits-Christoph et al. (2005)	Generalized anxiety disorder	15	Supportive therapy: N = 16	Luborsky; Crits-Christoph et al.	16 sessions
Knijnik (2004)	Social phobia	15	Credible placebo control group: N = 15	Knijnik et al.	12 sessions
Leichsenring et al. (2009)	Generalized anxiety disorder	28	CBT: N = 29	Luborsky; Crits-Christoph et al.	30 sessions
Leichsenring et al. (2013a)	Social phobia	207	Cognitive therapy: N = 2009	Luborsky, Leichsenring, Beutel; Leibing	30 sessions

Study	Disorder	N (PP)	Comparison group	Concept of PP	Treatment duration
Milrod et al. (2007)	Panic disorder	26	Waiting list: N = 79 CBT (applied relaxation), N = 23	Milrod et al.	24 sessions
Mixed samples of depressive and anxiety disorders					
Bressi et al. (2010)	Depressive and anxiety disorders	30	TAU: N = 30	Malan	40 sessions
Knet et al. (2008a, b)	Depressive and anxiety disorders	128, 101	Solution-focused therapy: N = 97	Malan; Sifneos; Gabbard	235 sessions; 49.9 sessions; 29.9 sessions
Brom et al. (1989)	PTSD	29	Desensitization: N = 31 Hypnotherapy: N = 29	Horowitz	18.8 sessions
Somatoform disorders					
Creed et al. (2003)	Irritable bowel	59	Paroxetine: N = 43 TAU: N = 86	Hobson; Shapiro and Firth	8 sessions
Faramasrzi et al. (2013)	Functional dyspepsia	24	Medical treatment: N = 25	Luborsky, Book	16 sessions
Guthrie et al. (1991)	Irritable bowel	50	Supportive listening: N = 46	Hobson; Shapiro and Firth	8 sessions
Hamilton et al. (2000)	Functional dyspepsia	37	Supportive therapy: N = 36	Spapiro and Firth	7 sessions
Monsen and Monson (2000)	Somatoform Pain disorder	20	TAU/no therapy: N = 20	Monson and Monson	33 sessions
Sattel et al. (2012)	Multi-somatoform disorder	107	Enhanced medical care: N = 104	Hardy; Barkham et al.	12 sessions
Eating disorders					
Bachar et al. (1999)	Anorexia nervosa, bulimia nervosa	17	Cognitive therapy: N = 17 Nutritional counseling: N = 10	Barth; Goodsitt; Geist	46 sessions
Dare et al. (2001)	Anorexia nervosa	21	Cognitive-analytic therapy (Ryle): N = 22 Family therapy: N = 22 Routine treatment: N = 19	Malan; Dare et al.	M = 24.9 sessions

continued

Table 7.1 continued

Study	Disorder	N (PP)	Comparison group	Concept of PP	Treatment duration
Zipfel et al. (2013)	Anorexia nervosa	80	Enhanced CBT: N = 80 Enhanced CBT: 44.8 sessions Optimized TAU: 50.8 sessions	Schauenburg et al.	LTPP: 39.9 sessions
Fairburn et al. (1986)	Bulimia nervosa	11	CBT: N = 11	Rosen; Stunkard; Bruch	19 sessions
Garner et al. (1993)	Bulimia nervosa	25	CBT: N = 25	Luborsky	19 sessions
Gowers et al. (1994)	Anorexia nervosa	20	TAU: N = 20	Crisp	12 sessions
Tasca et al. (2006)	Binge eating disorder	48	Group CBT: N = 47 Waiting list: N = 40	Tasca et al.	16 sessions
Substance related disorders					
Crits-Christoph et al. (1999, 2001)	Cocaine dependence	124	CBT + group DC: N = 97 Individual DC: N = 92 Individual DC + group DC: N = 96	Mark and Luborsky + group DC	Up to 36 individual and group sessions; 4 month
Sandahl et al. (1998)	Alcohol dependence	25	CBT: N = 24	Foulkes	15 sessions (M = 8.9)
Woody et al. (1983, 1990)	Opiate dependence	31	DC: N = 35 CBT + DC: N = 34	Luborsky + DC	12 sessions
Woody et al. 1995	Opiate dependence	57	DC: N = 27	Luborsky + DC	26 sessions
Borderline personality disorder					
Bateman and Fonagy (1999, 2001)	BPD	19	TAU: N = 19	Bateman and Fonagy	18 month
Bateman and Fonagy (2009)	BPD	71	Structured clinical management: N = 63	Bateman and Fonagy	18 month

Study	Disorder	N (PP)	Comparison group	Concept of PP	Treatment duration
Clarkin et al. (2007)	BPD	30	Dialectical behavioral therapy: N = 30 Supportive therapy: N = 30	Kernberg; Clarkin et al.	12 month
Doering et al. (2010)	BPD	43	Treatment by experienced community therapist: N = 29	Clarkin et al.	Assessment after 1 year
Giesen-Bloo et al. (2006)	BPD	42	CBT: N = 44	Kernberg; Clarkin et al.	3 years with sessions twice a week
Gregory et al. (2008)	BPD	15	TAU: N = 15	Gregory and Remen	24.9 sessions
Munroe-Blum and Marziali (1995)	BPD	31	Interpersonal group: N = 25	Kernberg	17 sessions
Cluster C personality disorders					
Muran et al. (2005)	Cluster C personality disorders	22	Brief relational therapy: N = 33	Pollack et al.	30 sessions
			CBT: N = 29		
Svartberg et al. (2004)	Cluster C personality disorders	25	CBT: N = 25	Malan; McCullough Vaillant	40 sessions
			Waiting list: N =18		
Avoidant personality disorder					
Emmelkamp et al. (2006)	Avoidant personality disorder	23	CBT: N = 21	Malan; Luborsky; Luborsky and Mark; Pinsker et al.	20 sessions
Samples of mixed personality disorders					
Abbass et al. (2008)	Heterogeneous personality disorders	14	Minimal contact: N = 14	Davenloo	27.7 sessions (mean)
Hellerstein et al. (1998)	Primarily Cluster C personality disorders	25	Brief supportive psychotherapy: N = 24	Davenloo	40 sessions

Evidence for the efficacy of PDT in specific mental disorders

The studies of PDT included in this review will be presented for different mental disorders. However, from a psychodynamic perspective, the results of a therapy for a specific psychiatric disorder (e.g., depression, agoraphobia) are influenced by the underlying psychodynamic features (e.g., conflicts, defenses, personality organization), which may vary considerably within one category of psychiatric disorder (Kernberg, 1996). These psychodynamic factors may affect treatment outcome and may have a greater impact on outcome than the phenomenological DSM categories (Piper, McCallum, Joyce, Rosie, & Ogrodniczuk, 2001).

Depressive disorders

At present, several RCTs are available that provide evidence for the efficacy of PDT compared to CBT in major depressive disorder (Barkham et al., 1996; Driessen et al., 2013; Gallagher-Thompson & Steffen, 1994; Shapiro et al., 1994; Thompson, Gallagher, & Breckenridge, 1987). It is of note that due to the large sample size the RCT by Driessen et al. (2013) was sufficiently powered for an equivalence trial. Different models of PDT were applied (Table 7.1). Thase (2013) concluded from this RCT: "On the basis of these findings, there is no reason to believe that psychodynamic psychotherapy is a less effective treatment of major depressive disorder than CBT." (p. 954)

In another RCT by Salminen et al. (2008), PDT was found to be equally efficacious as fluoxetine in reducing symptoms of depression and improving functional ability. However, with sample sizes of N1 ¼ 26 and N2 ¼ 25, statistical power may have not been sufficient to detect possible differences between treatments. In a small RCT, Maina, Forner, and Bogetto (2005) examined the efficacy of PDT and brief supportive therapy in the treatment of minor depressive disorders (dysthymic disorder, depressive disorder not otherwise specified, or adjustment disorder with depressed mood). Both treatments were superior to a waiting-list condition at the end of treatment. At six-month follow-up, PDT was superior to brief supportive therapy. In a recent study by Barber, Barrett, Gallop, Rynn, and Rickels (2012), PDT and pharmacotherapy were equally effective in the treatment of depression. However, neither PDT nor pharmacotherapy was superior to placebo.

An earlier meta-analysis (Leichsenring, 2001) found PDT and CBT to be equally effective with regard to depressive symptoms, general psychiatric symptoms, and social functioning. These results are consistent with the findings of more recent meta-analyses by Barth et al. (2013) and Driessen et al. (2010; Abbass & Driessen, 2010). Barth et al. (2013) did not find significant differences in outcome between different forms of psychotherapy of depression. Driessen et al. (2010) found PDT significantly superior to control conditions.

If group therapy was included, PDT was less efficacious compared to other treatments at the end of therapy. If only individual therapy was included, there were no significant differences between PDT and other treatments (Abbass & Driessen, 2010). In three-month and nine month follow-ups, no significant differences between treatments were found.

Meanwhile, internet-guided self-help is also available for PDT. In an RCT, Johansson et al. (2012) found internet-guided self-help based on PDT significantly more efficacious than a structured support intervention (psychoeducation and scheduled weekly contacts online) in patients with major depressive disorder. Treatment effects were maintained at ten-month follow-up. Psychodynamically oriented self-help was based on the concept by Silverberg (2005). Silverberg's internet-guided self-help based on PDT is a promising approach, especially for patients who do not receive psychotherapy. Further studies should be carried out.

In summary, several RCTs provide evidence for the efficacy of PDT in depressive disorders.

Pathological grief

In two RCTs by McCallum and Piper (1990) and Piper et al. (2001), the treatment of prolonged or complicated grief by short-term psychodynamic group therapy was studied. In the first study, short-term psychodynamic group therapy was significantly superior to a waiting list (McCallum & Piper, 1990). In the second study, a significant interaction was found. With regard to grief symptoms, patients with high quality of object relations improved more in interpretive therapy, and patients with low quality of object relations improved more in supportive therapy. For general symptoms, clinical significance favored interpretive therapy over supportive therapy (Piper et al., 2001).

Anxiety disorders

For anxiety disorders, several RCTs are presently available (Table 7.1). With regard to panic disorder (with or without agoraphobia), Milrod et al. (2007) showed in an RCT that PDT was more successful than applied relaxation. For social phobia, three RCTs of psychodynamic therapy exist. In the first study, short-term psychodynamic group treatment for generalized social phobia was superior to a credible placebo control (Knijnik, Kapczinski, Chachamovich, Margis, & Eizirik, 2004).

In a study by Bögels, Wijts, and Sallerts (2003), PDT proved to be as effective as CBT in the treatment of (generalized) social phobia. However, with sample sizes of N ¼ 22 and N ¼ 24, statistical power may have not been sufficient to detect possible differences between treatments.

In a large-scale multicenter RCT, the efficacy of PDT and cognitive therapy (CT) in the treatment of social phobia was studied (Leichsenring et al., 2013a).

In an outpatient setting, 495 patients with a primary diagnosis of social phobia were randomly assigned to CT, PDT, or the waiting list.

Treatments were carried out according to manuals and treatment fidelity was carefully controlled for. Both treatments were significantly superior to the waiting list. Thus, this trial provides evidence that PDT is effective in the treatment of social phobia according to the criteria proposed by Chambless and Hollon (1998). There were no differences between PDT and CT with regard to response rates for social phobia (52% vs. 60%) and reduction of depression. There were significant differences between CT and PDT in favor of CT, however, with regard to remission rates (36% vs. 26%), self-reported symptoms of social phobia, and reduction of interpersonal problems. Differences in terms of between-group effect sizes, however, were small and below the priori set threshold for clinical significance (Leichsenring, Salzer, & Leibing, 2013; Leichsenring et al., 2013a). Taking these results referring to clinically significant differences into account, recommending CBT over PDT in social anxiety disorders is not warranted. As Kraemer (2011) puts it: "Only if the ES [effect size] is greater than some value d⋆ [threshold of clinical significance] is a strong clinical recommendation of one treatment over the other warranted." (p. 1350) For the comparison of PDT with CBT, this was not the case. Furthermore, in the follow-up study 6, 12, and 24 months after end of therapy, neither statistically significant nor clinically significant differences were found between CT and PDT in any outcome measure (Leichsenring et al., 2013b). In general, the differentiation between statistical and clinical significance has not yet been sufficiently taken into account in psychotherapy research. From small, but statistically significant differences, the conclusion is drawn that one treatment is superior to another (Leichsenring et al., 2014).

In a randomized controlled feasibility study of generalized anxiety disorder, PDT was equally effective as a supportive therapy with regard to continuous measures of anxiety, but significantly superior on symptomatic remission rates (Crits-Christoph, Connolly Gibbons, Narducci, Schamberger, & Gallop, 2005). However, the sample sizes of that study were relatively small (N ¼ 15 vs. N ¼ 16), and the study was not sufficiently powered to detect more possible differences between treatments. In another RCT of generalized anxiety disorder, PDT was compared to CBT (Leichsenring et al., 2009). PDT and CBT were equally effective with regard to the primary outcome measure. However, in some secondary outcome measures, CBT was found to be superior, both at the end of therapy and at the six-month follow-up. Other differences may exist that were not detected due to the limited sample size and power (CBT: N ¼ 29; PDT: N ¼ 28). In the one-year follow-up, results proved to be stable (Salzer, Winkelbach, Leweke, Leibing, & Leichsenring, 2011). Contrary to short-term PDT (STPP), a core element in the applied method of CBT consisted of a modification of worrying. This specific difference between the treatments may explain the superiority of CBT in the Penn State Worry Questionnaire (Meyer, Miller, Metzger, & Borkovec, 1990) and, in part, also in the State-Trait Anxiety Inventory (trait measure) (Spielberger, Gorsuch, & Lushene, 1970)—the latter also contains several items related to worrying. The results of that study may suggest that the outcome of STPP in generalized anxiety disorder may be further optimized by employing a stronger focus on the process of worrying. In PDT, worrying can be conceptualized as a mechanism of defense that protects the subject from fantasies or feelings that are even more threatening than the contents of his or her worries (Crits-Christoph, Wolf-Palacio, Ficher, & Rudick, 1995).

According to the available RCTs, PDT is efficacious in anxiety disorders. If differences between PDT and CBT were found, they showed up in secondary outcome measures or corresponded to small differences in effect size. This is consistent with a recent meta-analysis by Baardseth et al. (2013) who did not find significant differences in favor of CBT compared to bona fide treatments.

For CBT, a recent historical review showed that the efficacy of treatments for anxiety disorders has not increased but rather decreased from the 1980s to the present (Öst, 2008). Furthermore, a substantial proportion of patients do not sufficiently benefit from the treatments and the proportion of non-responders does not appear to have decreased over time (Öst, 2008). For these reasons, there is a need to further improve the treatment of anxiety disorders (Schmidt, 2012). This is true not just for CBT, but also for PDT as well (Leichsenring, Klein, Salzer, 2014). In one of the most promising approaches to address this problem, psychotherapy research is moving from single-disorder-focused manualized approaches toward "transdiagnostic" and modular treatments (e.g., Barlow, Allen, & Choate, 2004; McHugh, Murray, & Barlow, 2009). The rationale for transdiagnostic treatments focuses on similarities among disorders, particularly in a similar class of diagnoses (e.g., anxiety disorders), including high rates of comorbidity and improvements in comorbid conditions when treating a principal disorder (Barlow et al., 2004; McHugh et al., 2009). For these reasons, researchers in the field of CBT have developed transdiagnostic treatment protocols (e.g., Barlow et al., 2004; McHugh et al., 2009; Norton & Phillip, 2008). It is an advantage that PDT is traditionally less tailored to single mental disorders, but focuses on core underlying processes of mental disorders. A recent review has shown that the empirically supported methods of PDT for specific anxiety disorders have core treatment components in common (Leichsenring & Salzer, 2014). These components have been distilled and integrated into an evidence-based Unified Psychodynamic Protocol for ANXiety disorders (UPPAnx; Leichsenring & Salzer, 2014).

Integrating treatment elements of empirically supported methods of PDT for specific anxiety disorders, the manualized UPP-Anx has the potential to: (1) be more effective than single-disorder psychotherapy, (2) be more effective than routine PDT, (3) improve comorbid symptoms, (4) enhance patients' quality of life, (5) facilitate translation of research into clinical practice of mental health professionals, (6) facilitate training for practitioners and dissemination of the approach relative to training in several distinct single-disorder treatments,

(7) be more cost efficient (e.g., by additionally improving comorbid symptoms), and (8) have an impact on both the health-care system and public health. As a next step, we are planning to evaluate the UPP-Anx in a RCT.

Mixed samples of depressive and anxiety disorders

Knekt et al. (2008a, 2008b) compared STPP, long-term psychodynamic psychotherapy (LTPP), and solution-focused therapy (SFT) in patients with depressive or anxiety disorders. STPP was more effective than LTPP during the first year. During the second year of follow-up, no significant differences were found between long-term and short-term treatments. In the three-year follow-up, LTPP was more effective; no significant differences were found between the short-term treatments. With regard to specific mental disorders, it is of note that after three years significantly more patients recovered from anxiety disorders in LTPP (90%) compared to STPP (67%) and SFT (65%). For depressive disorders, no such differences occurred. In an RCT by Bressi, Porcellana, Marinaccio, Nocito, and Magri (2010), PDT was superior to Treatment as Usual (TAU) in a sample of patients with depressive or anxiety disorders.

Posttraumatic stress disorder

In an RCT by Brom, Kleber, and Defares (1989), the effects of PDT, behavioral therapy, and hypnotherapy in patients with posttraumatic stress disorder (PTSD) were studied. All of the treatments proved to be equally effective. The results reported by Brom et al. (1989) are consistent with that of a more recent metaanalysis by Benish, Imel, and Wampold (2008), which found no significant differences between bona fide treatments of PTSD. In a response to the metaanalysis by Benish et al. (2008), Ehlers et al. (2010) critically reviewed the study by Brom et al. (1989). A comprehensive discussion with a convincing reply to the critique by Ehlers et al. (2010) was given by Wampold et al. (2010). In the present context, we shall only address the critique put forward by Ehlers et al. (2010) against the study by Brom et al. (1989). Ehlers et al. (2010) reviewed the study by Brom et al. (1989) in the following way (p. 273, italics by the authors): "In this study, neither hypnotherapy nor psychodynamic therapy was consistently more effective than the waiting-list control condition across the analyses used [...]." In addition, Brom et al. (1989) pointed out that "Patients in psychodynamic therapy showed slower overall change than those in the other two treatment conditions, and did not improve in intrusive symptoms significantly [...]."

Results are different for different outcome measures. For the avoidance scale and the total score of the Impact of Event Scale (Horowitz, Wilner, & Alvarez, 1979), PDT was significantly superior to the waiting-list condition, both after therapy and at follow-up (Brom et al., 1989, p. 610, Table 7.1). While effect sizes for PDT were somewhat smaller at posttreatment (avoidance: 0.66, total: 1.10),

PDT achieved the largest effect sizes at follow-up (avoidance: 0.92, total: 1.56) as compared to CBT (avoidance: 0.73, total: 1.30) and hypnotherapy (avoidance: 0.88, total: 1.54).

For the intrusion scale of the Impact of Event Scale, the primary outcome measure, it is true that PDT was not superior to waiting list both at posttest and at three-month follow-up. Intrusion is one of the core symptoms of PTSD. Pre-post differences of PDT, however, were significant and the pre-post and pre-follow-up effect sizes were large (0.95 and 1.55, respectively). In contrast, the pre-post effect size for the waiting list was small (0.34). For the CBT condition (trauma desensitization), the pre-post and pre-follow-up effect sizes were 1.66 and 1.43, respectively. Thus, at follow-up, PDT achieved a larger effect size than CBT. While the effect size of CBT tended to decrease at follow-up, it tended to increase for PDT; as will be shown below, this is true for the avoidance scale and the total score of the Impact of Event Scale. For this reason, it is strange that the difference between PDT and the control condition was reported by Brom et al. (1989) to be not significant at follow-up. For intrusion, PDT achieved the lowest score of all conditions at follow-up. These results, however, were not reported by Ehlers et al. (2010). The figure presented by Ehlers et al. (2010, p. 273, Figure 2) only included the pre-post effect sizes, but not the pre-follow-up effect sizes, for which PDT achieved larger effect sizes, as shown above. In a critical review, results of all analyses should be presented, not only the results that support one's own perspective. Furthermore, for general symptoms, Brom et al. (1989) wrote that PDT "seems to withstand the comparison [with waiting list] best" (p. 610). Thus, after all, it seems to take (a little bit, i.e., three months!) longer for PDT to achieve its effects, but these effects are at least as large as those of CBT.

Further studies of PDT in PTSD are required. At present, only one RCT of PDT in PTSD is presently available.

Somatoform disorders

At present, five RCTs of PDT in somatoform disorders that fulfill the inclusion criteria are available (Table 7.1). In the RCT by Guthrie, Creed, Dawson, and Tomenson (1991), patients with irritable bowel syndrome, who had not responded to standard medical treatment over the previous six months, were treated with PDT in addition to standard medical treatment. This treatment was compared to standard medical treatment alone. According to the results, PDT was effective in two-thirds of the patients. In another RCT, PDT was significantly more effective than routine care, and as effective as medication (paroxetine) in, the treatment of severe irritable bowel syndrome (Creed et al., 2003). During the follow-up period, however, PDT, but not paroxetine, was associated with a significant reduction in health-care costs compared with TAU. In an RCT by Hamilton et al. (2000), PDT was compared to supportive therapy in the treatment of patients with chronic intractable functional dyspepsia, who had failed to respond to conventional pharmacological treatments. At the end of treatment, PDT was significantly superior to the control condition. The effects were stable in the 12-month follow-up.

An RCT by Faramarzi et al. (2013) corroborated these results with PDT combined with medical treatment being superior to medical treatment alone, with regard to gastrointestinal symptoms, defense mechanisms, and alexithymia, both at the end of therapy and at the 1- and 12-month follow-up. Monsen and Monsen (2000) compared PDT of 33 sessions with a control condition (no treatment or TAU) in the treatment of patients with chronic pain. PDT was significantly superior to the control group on measures of pain, psychiatric symptoms, interpersonal problems, and affect consciousness. The results remained stable or even improved in the 12-month follow-up. In a recent study, Sattel et al. (2012) compared PDT with enhanced medical care in patients with multi-somatoform disorders. At follow-up, PDT was superior to enhanced medical care with regard to improvements in patients' physical quality of life.

Abbass, Kisely, and Kroenke (2009) carried out a review and meta-analysis on the effects of PDT in somatoform disorders. They included both RCTs and controlled before and after studies. Meta-analysis was possible for 14 studies. It revealed significant effects on physical symptoms, psychiatric symptoms, and social adjustment, which were maintained in long-term follow-up. Thus, specific forms of PDT can be recommended for the treatment of somatoform disorders.

Bulimia nervosa

For the treatment of bulimia nervosa, three RCTs of PDT are available (Table 7.1). Significant and stable improvements in bulimia nervosa after PDT were demonstrated in the RCTs by Fairburn, Kirk, O'Connor, and Cooper (1986), Fairburn et al. (1995), and Garner et al. (1993). In the primary disorder-specific measures (bulimic episodes, self-induced vomiting), PDT was as effective as CBT (Fairburn et al., 1986, 1995; Garner et al., 1993). Again, however, the studies were not sufficiently powered to detect possible differences (see Table 7.1 for sample sizes). Apart from this, CBT was superior to PDT in some specific measures of psychopathology (Fairburn et al., 1986). However, in a follow-up (Fairburn et al., 1995) of the Fairburn et al. (1986) study using a longer follow-up period, both forms of therapy proved to be equally effective and were partly superior to a behavioral form of therapy. Accordingly, for a valid evaluation of the efficacy of PDT in bulimia nervosa, longer-term follow-up studies are necessary. In another RCT, PDT was significantly superior to both a nutritional counseling group and CT (Bachar, Latzer, Kreitler, & Berry, 1999). This was true of patients with

bulimia nervosa and a mixed sample of patients with bulimia nervosa or anorexia nervosa.

Anorexia nervosa

For the treatment of anorexia nervosa, however, evidence-based treatments
are barely available (Fairburn, 2005). This applies to both PDT and CBT. In
an RCT by Gowers, Norton, Halek, and Crisp (1994), PDT combined with
four sessions of nutritional advice yielded significant improvements in patients
with anorexia nervosa (Table 7.1). Weight and body mass index (BMI)
changes were significantly more improved than in a control condition
(TAU). Dare, Eisler, Russell, Treasure, and Dodge (2001) compared PDT
with a mean duration of 24.9 sessions to cognitive-analytic therapy, family
therapy, and routine treatment in the treatment of anorexia nervosa (Table
7.1). PDT yielded significant symptomatic improvements and PDT and
family therapy were significantly superior to the routine treatment with
regard to weight gain. However, the improvements were modest—several
patients were undernourished at the follow-up.

A recent RCT compared manual-guided psychodynamic therapy,
enhanced CBT, and optimized TAU in the treatment of anorexia nervosa
(Zipfel et al., 2013). After ten months of treatment, significant improvements
were found in all treatments, with differences in the primary outcome
measure (BMI). At the 12-months follow-up, however, psychodynamic
therapy was significantly superior to optimized TAU, whereas enhanced
CBT was not (Zipfel et al., 2013). Recovery rates were 35% versus 19%
versus 13% for psychodynamic therapy enhanced CBT and optimized TAU.
Thus, the method of psychodynamic therapy specifically tailored to the treatment of anorexia nervosa yielded promising effects.

Binge eating disorder

In an RCT by Tasca et al. (2006), a psychodynamic group treatment was as
efficacious as CBT and superior to a waiting-list condition in binge eating
disorder (e.g., days binged, interpersonal problems). For the comparison of
PDT with CBT, again the question of statistical power arises (N1 ¼ 48, N2
¼ 47, N3 ¼ 40).

Substance-related disorders

Woody et al. (1983; Woody, Luborsky, McLellan, & O'Brien, 1990) studied
the effects of PDT and CBT, both of which were given in addition to drug
counseling, in the treatment of opiate dependence (Table 7.1). PDT plus
drug counseling yielded significant improvements on measures of drug-
related symptoms and general psychiatric symptoms. At the seven-month

follow-up, PDT and CBT, plus drug counseling, were equally effective, and both conditions were superior to drug counseling alone. In another RCT, PDT of 26 sessions given in addition to drug counseling was also superior to drug counseling alone in the treatment of opiate dependence (Woody, McLellan, Luborsky, & O'Brien, 1995). At the six-month follow-up, most of the gains made by the patients who had received psychodynamic therapy remained.

In an RCT conducted by Crits-Christoph et al. (1999, 2001), PDT of up to 36 individual sessions was combined with 24 sessions of group drug counseling in the treatment of cocaine dependence. The combined treatment yielded significant improvements and was as effective as CBT, which was combined with group drug counseling as well. However, CBT and PDT plus group drug counseling were not more effective than group drug counseling alone. Furthermore, individual drug counseling was significantly superior to both forms of therapy concerning measures of drug abuse. With regard to psychological and social outcome variables, all treatments were equally effective (Crits-Christoph et al., 1999, 2001).

In an RCT by Sandahl, Herlitz, Ahlin, and Ronnberg (1998), PDT and CBT were compared concerning their efficacy in the treatment of alcohol abuse. PDT yielded significant improvements on measures of alcohol abuse, which were stable at a 15-month follow-up. PDT was significantly superior to CBT in the number of abstinent days and in the improvement of general psychiatric symptoms.

Borderline personality disorder

At present, seven RCTs are available for PDT in BPD (Bateman & Fonagy, 1999, 2009; Clarkin, Levy, Lenzenweger, & Kernberg, 2007; Doering et al., 2010; Giesen-Bloo et al., 2006; Gregory et al., 2008; Munroe-Blum & Marziali, 1995). Of these studies, several showed that PDT was superior to TAU (Bateman & Fonagy, 1999; Doering et al., 2010; Gregory et al., 2008). Bateman and Fonagy (1999, 2001) studied psychoanalytically oriented partial hospitalization treatment for patients with BPD. The major difference between the treatment group and the control group was the provision of individual and group psychotherapy in the former. The treatment lasted a maximum of 18 months. PDT was significantly superior to standard psychiatric care, both at the end of therapy and at the 18-month follow-up.

In a recent RCT, Transference-Focused Psychotherapy (TFP) based on Kernberg's model (Clarkin, Yeomans, & Kernberg, 1999) was compared to a treatment carried out by experienced community psychotherapists in borderline outpatients (Doering et al., 2010). TFP was superior with regard to borderline psychopathology, psychosocial functioning, personality organization, inpatient admission, and dropouts.

Another RCT compared PDT ('dynamic deconstructive psychotherapy') with TAU in the treatment of patients with BPD and co-occurring alcohol use disorder (Gregory et al., 2008). In this study, PDT, but not TAU, achieved significant improvements in outcome measures of parasuicide, alcohol misuse, and institutional care (Gregory et al., 2008). Furthermore, PDT was superior with regard to improvements in borderline psychopathology, depression, and social support. No difference was found in dissociation. This was true although TAU participants received higher average treatment intensity.

Another recent RCT found mentalization-based treatment (MBT) to be superior to manual-driven structured clinical management with regard to the primary (suicidal and self-injurious behaviors, hospitalization) and secondary outcome measures (e.g., depression, general symptom distress, interpersonal functioning) (Bateman & Fonagy, 2009).

With regard to the comparison of PDT to specific forms of psychotherapy, one RCT reported PDT as equally effective as an interpersonal group therapy (Munroe-Blum & Marziali, 1995). PDT yielded significant improvements on measures of borderline-related symptoms, general psychiatric symptoms, and depression, and was as effective as an interpersonal group therapy. Power, however, may have been insufficient to detect differences between treatments (N1 ¼ 22, N2 ¼ 26).

Giesen-Bloo et al. (2006) compared PDT (TFP) with schema-focused therapy (SFT), a form of CBT. Treatment duration was three years with two sessions a week. The authors reported statistically and clinically significant improvements for both treatments. However, SFT was found to be superior to TFP in several outcome measures. Furthermore, a significantly higher dropout risk for TFP was reported. This study, however, had serious methodological flaws. The authors used scales for adherence and competence for both treatments, for which they adopted an identical cutoff score of 60 indicating competent application. According to the data published by the authors (Giesen-Bloo et al., 2006, p. 651), the median competence level for applying SFT methods was 85.67. For TFP, a value of 65.6 was reported. While the competence level for SFT clearly exceeded the cutoff, the competence level for TFP just surpassed it. Furthermore, the competence level for SFT is clearly higher than that for TFP. Accordingly, both treatments were not equally applied in terms of therapist competence. Thus, the results of that study are questionable. The difference in competence was not taken into account by the authors, neither with regard to the analysis of resulting data nor in the discussion of the results. Thus, this study raises serious concerns about an investigator allegiance effect (Luborsky et al., 1999).

Another RCT compared PDT (TFP), dialectical behavior therapy (DBT), and psychodynamic supportive psychotherapy (Clarkin et al., 2007). Patients treated with all three modalities showed general improvement in the study. However, TFP was shown to produce improvements not demonstrated by either DBT or supportive therapy. Those participants who received TFP were more likely to move from an insecure attachment classification to a secure one. They also showed significantly greater changes in mentalizing capacity and narrative coherence compared to the other two groups. TFP was associated with significant improvement in 10 of the 12 variables across the six symptomatic domains, compared to six in supportive therapy and five in DBT. Only TFP made significant changes in impulsivity, irritability, verbal assault, and direct assault. TFP and DBT reduced suicidality to the same extent. Here as well, power may have been insufficient to detect further possible differences (N1 ¼ 23, N2 ¼ 17, N3 ¼ 22).

In summary, there is clear evidence that specific forms of manual-guided PDT are efficacious in BPD (Leichsenring, Leibing, Kruse, New, & Leweke, 2011). For TFP and MBT, two RCTs carried out in independent research settings are available which provide evidence that both MBT and TFP are efficacious and specific treatments of BPD, according to the criteria of empirically supported treatments proposed by Chambless and Hollon (1998). Studies of both psychotherapy and pharmacotherapy in BPD were recently reviewed by Leichsenring, Leibing et al. (2011). For bona fide treatments, including MBT, TFP, DBT, and schema-focused therapy there is no evidence that one form of psychotherapy is superior to another (Leichsenring, Leibing et al., 2011).

Cluster C personality disorders

There is also evidence for the efficacy of PDT in the treatment of Cluster C personality disorders (i.e., avoidant, compulsive, or dependent personality disorder). In an RCT conducted by Svartberg, Stiles, and Seltzer (2004), PDT of 40 sessions in length was compared to CBT (Table 7.1). Both PDT and CBT yielded significant improvements in patients with DSM-IV Cluster C personality disorders. The improvements refer to symptoms, interpersonal problems, and core personality pathology. The results were stable at 24-months follow-up. Nonsignificant differences were found between PDT and CBT with regard to efficacy. However, this study was also not sufficiently powered to detect possible differences (N1 ¼ 25, N2 ¼ 25).

Muran, Safran, Samstag, and Winston (2005) compared the efficacy of psychodynamic therapy, brief relational therapy, and CBT in the treatment of Cluster C personality disorders and personality disorders not otherwise specified. Treatments lasted for 30 sessions. With regard to mean changes in outcome measures, no significant differences were found between the treatment conditions, neither at termination nor at follow-up. Furthermore, there were no significant differences between the treatments with regard to the patients achieving clinically significant change in symptoms, interpersonal problems, features of personality disorders, or therapist ratings of target complaints. At termination, CBT and brief relational therapy were superior to

PDT in one outcome measure (patient ratings of target complaints). However, this difference did not persist at follow-up. With regard to the percentage of patients showing change, no significant differences were found, either at termination or at the follow-up, except in one comparison: at termination, CBT was superior to PDT on the Inventory of Interpersonal Problems (Horowitz, Alden, Wiggins, & Pincus, 2000). Again, this difference did not persist at follow-up. The conclusion is that only a few significant differences were found between the treatments but these differences did not persist at follow-up.

Avoidant personality disorder

Avoidant personality disorder (AVPD) is among the above-mentioned Cluster C personality disorders. In a recent RCT, Emmelkamp et al. (2006) compared CBT to PDT and a waiting-list condition in the treatment of AVPD. The authors reported CBT as more effective than waiting-list control and PDT. However, the study suffers from several methodological shortcomings (Leichsenring & Leibing, 2007). In contrast to CBT, for example, no disorder-specific manual was used for PDT. Some outcome measures applied by Emmelkamp et al. (2006) were specifically tailored to effects for CBT (e.g., to beliefs). Furthermore, an arbitrary level of significance (p ¼ 0.10) was set by the authors so that a usually not significant difference (p ¼ 0.09) achieved significance in favor of CBT. At follow-up, no differences between CBT and PDT were found in primary outcome measures. In addition, Emmelkamp et al. (2006) reported that PDT was not superior to the waiting-list group. This was true, but may be attributed to the small sample size and low power of the study. Furthermore, CBT was superior to the waiting-list group in only two of six measures (Leichsenring & Leibing, 2007). Thus, design, statistical analyses and reporting of results raise serious concerns about an investigator allegiance effect (Luborsky et al., 1999).

Heterogeneous samples of patients with personality disorders

Winston et al. (1994) compared PDT with brief adaptive psychotherapy or waiting-list patients in a heterogeneous group of patients with personality disorders. Most of the patients showed a Cluster C personality disorder. Patients with paranoid, schizoid, schizotypal, borderline, and narcissistic personality disorders were excluded. Mean treatment duration was 40 weeks. In both treatment groups, patients showed significantly more improvements than the patients on the waiting list. No differences in outcome were found between the two forms of psychotherapy.

Hellerstein et al. (1998) compared PDT to brief supportive therapy in a heterogeneous sample of patients with personality disorders. Again, most of the patients showed a Cluster C personality disorder. The authors reported similar degrees of improvement both at termination and at six-month follow-up. However, the studies by Winston et al. (1994) and Hellerstein et al. (1998) were not sufficiently powered to detect possible differences (see Table 7.1 for sample sizes).

Abbass, Sheldon, Gyra, and Kalpin (2008) compared PDT (intensive short term dynamic psychotherapy, ISTDP) with a minimal contact group in a heterogeneous group of patients with personality disorders. The most common Axis II diagnoses were borderline (44%), obsessive compulsive (37%), and AVPD (33%). Average treatment duration was 27.7 sessions. PDT was significantly superior to the control condition in all primary outcome measures. When control patients were treated, they experienced benefits similar to the initial treatment group. In the long-term follow-up, two years after the end of treatment, the whole group maintained their gains and had an 83% reduction of personality disorder diagnoses. In addition, treatment costs were thrice offset by reductions in medication and disability payments. This preliminary study of ISTDP suggests that it is efficacious and cost-effective in the treatment of personality disorders.

At present, two meta-analyses on the effects of PDT in personality disorders are available (Leichsenring & Leibing, 2003; Town, Abbass, & Hardy, 2011). A meta-analysis addressing the effects of PDT and CBT in personality disorders reported that PDT yielded large effects sizes not only for comorbid symptoms, but also for core personality pathology (Leichsenring & Leibing, 2003). This was true especially for BPD. A more recent meta-analysis by Town et al. (2011) included seven RCTs on STPP in personality disorders. The authors drew the preliminary conclusion that PDT may be considered an efficacious empirically supported treatment option for a wide range of personality disorders, producing significant and medium to long-term improvements for a large percentage of patients.

Discussion

Under the requirements of the criteria proposed by the Task Force modified by Chambless and Hollon (1998), several RCTs are presently available that provide evidence for the efficacy of PDT in specific mental disorders (Leichsenring et al., 2014). There is evidence for the efficacy of PDT in depressive disorders, prolonged or complicated grief, anxiety disorders, PTSD, eating disorders, somatoform disorders, substance-related disorders, and personality disorders, including both less severe (Cluster C) and severe personality disorders (BPD). For PTSD, only one RCT exists (Brom et al., 1989). Thus, we urgently need further studies showing that PDT is effective in complex PTSDs, i.e., in patients suffering from childhood abuse. With regard to personality disorders, no RCTs exist for Cluster A personality disorders (e.g., paranoid, schizoid) and for some relevant Cluster B personality disorders (e.g., narcissistic). This is true, however, for CBT as well. In addition, further RCTs of PDT-LTPP, especially in complex mental disorders, are required.

In the studies reviewed here, PDT was either more effective than placebo therapy, supportive therapy or TAU, or no differences between PDT and CBT, or between PDT and pharmacotherapy, were found.

In a few studies, PDT was superior to a method of CBT (Milrod et al., 2007); in another study, PDT was superior to CBT in some outcome measures (Clarkin et al., 2007). However, most of the studies that found no differences in efficacy between PDT and another bona fide treatment were not sufficiently powered. As reported above, testing for non-inferiority (i.e., equivalence) requires $N1 = N2 = 86$ patients to detect an at least medium differences (effect size $d = 0.5$) between two treatments with a sufficient power (a $= 0.05$, two-tailed test, $1-b = 0.90$) (Cohen, 1988). At present, only four RCT comparing PDT with a bona fide treatment fulfill this criterion (Crits-Christoph et al., 1999; Driessen et al., 2013; Knekt et al., 2008a; Leichsenring et al., 2013a). The issue of small sample size studies, however, is not specific to studies of PDT, since many studies of CBT are also not sufficiently powered (Leichsenring & Rabung, 2011).

For comparisons of PDT with bona fide therapies, the between-group effect sizes were found to be small (Driessen et al., 2013; Leichsenring, 2001; Leichsenring, Salzer et al., 2011; Leichsenring et al., 2013a). Thus, it is an open question of research whether more highly powered studies would find significant differences. Furthermore, the question has to be addressed whether these (possibly small) differences are clinically relevant or significant (Jacobson & Truax, 1991).

It is important, however, to realize which mental disorders lack any RCTs of PDT. This is true, for example, for dissociative disorders and for some specific forms of personality disorders (e.g., narcissistic). For PTSD, only one RCT is presently available (Brom et al., 1989).

Some studies reported differences, at least in some measures, in favor of CBT. This is true, for example, for the studies on bulimia nervosa by Fairburn et al. (1986) and Garner et al. (1993), and for the studies on generalized anxiety disorder (Leichsenring et al., 2009) and social phobia (Leichsenring et al., 2013a). For the study on generalized anxiety disorder (Leichsenring et al., 2009), we discussed above whether a stronger focus on the process of worrying would possibly improve the results of PDT.

In general, future research should address the question whether the efficacy of PDT can be improved by putting a stronger focus on the specific mechanisms that maintain the psychopathology of the respective disorder. Mentalization-based therapy or TFP may serve as good examples for psychodynamic treatments that focus on the assumed processes or deficits maintaining a disorder.

According to the results of this review, further research of PDT in specific mental disorders is necessary, including studies of both the outcome and the active ingredients of PDT in these disorders. Not only measures of symptoms and DSM criteria of a disorder should be applied, but also measures more specific to PDT. Future studies should also examine if there are specific gains achieved only by PDT, i.e., the question of "added value." Furthermore, those methods of therapy that have proved to work under experimental conditions of RCTs need to be studied for their effectiveness in the field (effectiveness studies). The perception that PDT lacks empirical support is not consistent with available empirical evidence and may reflect selective dissemination of research findings (Shedler, 2010).

Note

1 This is a reprint of our chapter in Leuzinger-Bohleber, M.; Kächele, H. (2015) (Eds.). *An open door review of outcome and process studies in psychoanalysis*, 3rd Edition. London: IPA.

References

Abbass, A., & Driessen, E. (2010). The efficacy of short-term psychodynamic psycho- therapy for depression: A summary of recent findings. *Acta Psychiatrica Scandinavica, 121,* 398 (author reply, 398–399).

Abbass, A., Kisely, S., & Kroenke, K. (2009). Short-term psychodynamic psychother- apy for somatic disorders: Systematic review and meta-analysis of clinical trials. *Psy- chotherapy and Psychosomatics, 78,* 265–274.

Abbass, A., Sheldon, A., Gyra, J., & Kalpin, A. (2008). Intensive short-term dynamic psychotherapy for DSM-IV personality disorders: A randomized controlled trial. *Journal of Nervous and Mental Disorders, 196,* 211–216.

Baardseth, T., Godberg, S.B., Pace, B.T., Minami, T., Wislocki, A.P., Frost, N.D., … Wampold, B.E. (2013). Cognitive-behavioural therapy versus other therapies: Redux. *Clinical Psychology Review, 33,* 395–405.

Bachar, E., Latzer, Y., Kreitler, S., & Berry, E.M. (1999). Empirical comparison of two psychological therapies: Self psychology and cognitive orientation in the treatment of anorexia and bulimia. *Journal of Psychotherapy Practice and Research, 8,* 115–128.

Barber, J.P., Barrett, M.S., Gallop, R., Rynn, M.A., & Rickels, K. (2012). Short- term dynamic psychotherapy versus pharmacotherapy for major depressive disor- der: A randomized, placebo controlled trial. *Journal of Clinical Psychiatry, 73,* 66–73.

Barkham, M., Rees, A., Shapiro, D.A., Stiles, W.B., Agnew, R.M., Halstead, J., … Harrington, V.M. (1996). Outcomes of time-limited psychotherapy in applied set- tings: Replicating the Second Sheffield Psychotherapy Project. *Journal of Consulting and Clinical Psychology, 64,* 1079–1085.

Barlow, D.H., Allen, L.B., & Choate, M.L. (2004). Toward a unified treatment for emotional disorders. *Behavior Therapy, 35,* 205–230.

Barth, J., Munder, T., Gerger, H., Nüesch, E., Trelle, S., Znoj, H., … Cuijpers, P. (2013). Comparative efficacy of seven psychotherapeutic interventions for patients with depression: A network meta-analysis. *PLoS Medicine, 10,* e1001454. doi:10.1371/ journal.pmed.1001454.

Bateman, A., & Fonagy, P. (1999). Effectiveness of partial hospitalization in the treatment of borderline personality disorder: A randomized controlled trial. *American Journal of Psychiatry, 156*, 1563–1569.

Bateman, A., & Fonagy, P. (2001). Treatment of borderline personality disorder with psychoanalytically oriented partial hospitalization: An 18-month follow-up. *American Journal of Psychiatry, 158*, 36–42.

Bateman, A., & Fonagy, P. (2009). Randomized controlled trial of outpatient mentalization-based treatment versus structured clinical management for borderline personality disorder. *American Journal of Psychiatry, 166*, 1355–1364.

Benish, S.G., Imel, Z.E., & Wampold, B.E. (2008). The relative efficacy of bona fide psychotherapies for treating post-traumatic stress disorder: A meta-analysis of direct comparisons. *Clinical Psychology Review, 28*, 746–758.

Bhar, S.S., & Beck, A.T. (2009). Treatment integrity of studies that compare short-term psychodynamic psychotherapy with cognitive-behaviour therapy. *Clinical Psychology: Science and Practice, 16*, 370–378.

Bögels, S., Wijts, P., & Sallerts, S. (2003, September). Analytic psychotherapy versus cognitive-behavioural therapy for social phobia. Paper presented at the European Congress for Cognitive and Behavioural Therapies, Prague.

Bressi, C., Porcellana, M., Marinaccio, P.M., Nocito, E.P., & Magri, L. (2010). Shortterm psychodynamic psychotherapy versus treatment as usual for depressive and anxiety disorders: A randomized clinical trial of efficacy. *Journal of Nervous and Mental Disorders, 198*, 647–652. doi:10.1097/NMD.0b013e3181ef3ebb.

Brom, D., Kleber, R.J., & Defares, P.B. (1989). Brief psychotherapy for posttraumatic stress disorders. *Journal of Consulting and Clinical Psychology, 57*, 607–612.

Canadian Task Force on the Periodic Health Examination. (1979). The periodic health examination. *Canadian Medical Association, 121*, 1193–1254.

Chambless, D.L., & Hollon, S.D. (1998). Defining empirically supported therapies. *Journal of Consulting and Clinical Psychology, 66*, 7–18.

Clarke, M., & Oxman, A.D. (Eds.). (2003). Cochrane reviewer's handbook 4.2.0 (updated March 2003). *The Cochrane Library Database*, Issue 2. Oxford: Update Software.

Clarkin, J.F., Levy, K.N., Lenzenweger, M.F., & Kernberg, O.F. (2007). Evaluating three treatments for borderline personality disorder: A multiwave study. *American Journal of Psychiatry, 164*, 922–928. doi:10.1176/appi.ajp.164.6.922.

Clarkin, J.F., Yeomans, F.E., & Kernberg, O.F. (1999). *Psychotherapy of borderline personality*. New York: Wiley.

Cohen, J. (1988). *Statistical power analysis for the behavioural sciences*. Hillsdale, NJ: Lawrence Erlbaum.

Cook, D., Guyatt, G.H., Laupacis, A., Sacket, D.L., & Goldberg, R.J. (1995). Clinical recommendations using levels of evidence for antithrombotic agents. *Chest, 108*, 227–230.

Creed, F., Fernandes, L., Guthrie, E., Palmer, S., Ratcliffe, J., Read, N., ... Tomenson, B. (2003). The cost-effectiveness of psychotherapy and paroxetine for severe irritable bowel syndrome. *Gastroenterology, 124*, 303–317.

Crits-Christoph, P., Connolly Gibbons, M.B., Narducci, J., Schamberger, M., & Gallop, R. (2005). Interpersonal problems and the outcome of interpersonally oriented psychodynamic treatment of GAD. *Psychotherapy: Theory, Research, Practice, Training, 42*, 211–224. doi:10.1037/0033-3204.42.2.211.

Crits-Christoph, P., Siqueland, L., Blaine, J., Frank, A., Luborsky, L., Onken, L.S., … Beck, A.T. (1999). Psychosocial treatments for cocaine dependence: National Institute on Drug Abuse Collaborative Cocaine Treatment Study. *Archives of General Psychiatry, 56*, 493–502.

Crits-Christoph, P., Siqueland, L., McCalmont, E., Weiss, R.D., Gastfriend, D.R., Frank, A., … Thase, M.E. (2001). Impact of psychosocial treatments on associated problems of cocaine-dependent patients. *Journal of Consulting and Clinical Psychology, 69*, 825–830. doi:10.1037/0022-006X.69.5.825.

Crits-Christoph, P., Wolf-Palacio, D., Ficher, M., & Rudick, D. (1995). Brief supportive-expressive psychodynamic therapy for generalized anxiety disorder. In J. Barber & P. Crits-Christoph (Eds.), *Dynamic therapies for psychiatric disorders (Axis I)* (pp. 13–42). New York: Basic Books.

Dare, C., Eisler, I., Russell, G., Treasure, J., & Dodge, L. (2001). Psychological therapies for adults with anorexia nervosa: Randomised controlled trial of out-patient treatments. *British Journal of Psychiatry, 178*, 216–221. doi:10.1192/bjp.178.3.216.

Doering, S., Horz, S., Rentrop, M., Fischer-Kern, M., Schuster, P., Benecke, C., … Buchheim, P. (2010). Transference-focused psychotherapy v. treatment by community psychotherapists for borderline personality disorder: Randomised controlled trial. *British Journal of Psychiatry, 196*, 389–395. doi:10.1192/bjp.bp.109.070177.

Driessen, E., Cuijpers, P., deMaat, S.C., Abbass, A.A., de Jonghe, F., & Dekker, J.J. (2010). The efficacy of short-term psychodynamic psychotherapy for depression: A meta-analysis. *Clinical Psychology Review, 30*, 25–36. doi:10.1016/j.cpr.2009.08.010.

Driessen, E., Van, H.L., Don, F.J., Peen, J., Kool, S., Westra, D., … Dekker, J.J. (2013). The efficacy of cognitive-behavioural therapy and psychodynamic therapy in the outpatient treatment of major depression: A randomized clinical trial. *American Journal of Psychiatry, 170*, 1041–1050. doi:10.1176/appi.ajp.2013.12070899.

Ehlers, A., Bisson, J., Clark, D.M., Creamer, M., Pilling, S., Richards, D., … Yule, W. (2010). Do all psychological treatments really work the same in posttraumatic stress disorder? *Clinical Psychology Review, 30*, 269–276. doi:10.1016/j.cpr.2009.12.001.

Emmelkamp, P.M., Benner, A., Kuipers, A., Feiertag, G.A., Koster, H.C., & van Apeldoorn, F.J. (2006). Comparison of brief dynamic and cognitive-behavioural therapies in avoidant personality disorder. *British Journal of Psychiatry, 189*, 60–64.

Fairburn, C.G. (2005). Evidence-based treatment of anorexia nervosa. *International Journal of Eating Disorders, 37*, 26–30. doi:10.1002/eat.20112.

Fairburn, C.G., Kirk, J., O'Connor, M., & Cooper, P.J. (1986). A comparison of two psychological treatments for bulimia nervosa. *Behavioural Research Therapy, 24*, 629–643.

Fairburn, C.G., Norman, P.A., Welch, S.L., O'Connor, M.E., Doll, H.A., & Peveler, R.C. (1995). A prospective study of outcome in bulimia nervosa and the long-term psychoanalytic psychotherapy effects of three psychological treatments. *Archives of General Psychiatry, 52*, 304–312. doi:10.1001/archpsyc.1995.03950160054010.

Faramarzi, M., Azadfallah, P., Book, H.E., Tabatabaei, K.R., Taheri, H., & Shokrishirvani, J. (2013). A randomized controlled trial of brief psychoanalytic psychotherapy in patients with functional dyspepsia. *Asian Journal of Psychiatry*, *6*, 228–234. doi:10.1016/j.ajp.2012.12.012.

Fonagy, P., Roth, A., & Higgitt, A. (2005). Psychodynamic psychotherapies: Evidence-based practice and clinical wisdom. *Bulletin of the Menninger Clinic*, *69*(1), 1–58. doi:10.1521/bumc.69.1.1.62267.

Gabbard, G.O. (2004). *Long-term psychodynamic psychotherapy: A basic text*. Washington, DC: American Psychiatric Publishing.

Gabbard, G., Gunderson, J.G., & Fonagy, P. (2002). The place of psychoanalytic treatments within psychiatry. *Archives of General Psychiatry*, *59*, 505–510.

Gallagher-Thompson, D., & Steffen, A.M. (1994). Comparative effects of cognitive-behavioural and brief psychodynamic psychotherapies for depressed family caregivers. *Journal of Consulting and Clinical Psychology*, *62*, 543–549.

Garner, D.M., Rockert, W., Davis, R., Garner, M.V., Olmsted, M.P., & Eagle, M. (1993). Comparison of cognitive-behavioural and supportive-expressive therapy for bulimia nervosa. *American Journal of Psychiatry*, *150*, 37–46.

Gerber, A.J., Kocsis, J.H., Milrod, B.L., Roose, S.P., Barber, J.P., Thase, M.E., … Leon, A.C. (2011). A quality-based review of randomized controlled trials of psychodynamic psychotherapy. *American Journal of Psychiatry*, *168*, 19–28. doi:10.1176/appi.ajp.2010.08060843.

Giesen-Bloo, J., van Dyck, R., Spinhoven, P., van Tilburg, W., Dirksen, C., van Asselt, T., … Arntz, A. (2006). Outpatient psychotherapy for borderline personality disorder: Randomized trial of schema-focused therapy vs. transference-focused psychotherapy. *Archives of General Psychiatry*, *63*, 649–658. doi:10.1001/archpsyc.63.6.649.

Gowers, S., Norton, K., Halek, C., & Crisp, A.H. (1994). Outcome of outpatient psychotherapy in a random allocation treatment study of anorexia nervosa. *International Journal of Eating Disorders*, *15*, 165–177. doi:10.1002/1098-108X.

Gregory, R.J., Chlebowski, S., Kang, D., Remen, A.L., Soderberg, M.G., Stepkovitch, J., & Virk, S. (2008). A controlled trial of psychodynamic psychotherapy for co-occurring borderline personality disorder and alcohol use disorder. *Psychotherapy: Theory, Research, Practice, Training*, *45*, 28–41. doi:10.1037/0033-3204.45.1.28.

Gunderson, J.G., & Gabbard, G.O. (1999). Making the case for psychoanalytic therapies in the current psychiatric environment. *Journal of the American Psychoanalytic Association*, *47*, 679–704.

Guthrie, E., Creed, F., Dawson, D., & Tomenson, B. (1991). A controlled trial of psychological treatment for the irritable bowel syndrome. *Gastroenterology*, *100*, 450–457.

Hamilton, J., Guthrie, E., Creed, F., Thompson, D., Tomenson, B., Bennett, R., & Liston, R. (2000). A randomized controlled trial of psychotherapy in patients with chronic functional dyspepsia. *Gastroenterology*, *119*, 661–669.

Hellerstein, D.J., Rosenthal, R.N., Pinsker, H., Samstag, L.W., Muran, J.C., & Winston, A. (1998). A randomized prospective study comparing supportive and dynamic therapies: Outcome and alliance. *Journal of Psychotherapy Practice and Research*, *7*, 261–271.

Horowitz, L.M., Alden, L.E., Wiggins, J.S., & Pincus, A.L. (2000). *Inventory of interpersonal problems: Manual*. Odessa, FL: The Psychological Corporation.

Horowitz, M.J., Wilner, N., & Alvarez, W. (1979). Impact of event scale: A measure of subjective stress. *Psychosomatic Medicine*, *41*, 209–218.

Jacobson, N.S., & Truax, P. (1991). Clinical significance: A statistical approach to defining meaningful change in psychotherapy research. *Journal of Consulting and Clinical Psychology*, *59*, 12–19. doi:10.1037//0022-006X.59.1.12.

Johansson, R., Ekbladh, S., Hebert, A., Lindstrom, M., Moller, S., Petitt, E., … Andersson, G. (2012). Psychodynamic guided self-help for adult depression through the internet: A randomised controlled trial. *PLoS One*, *7*, e38021. doi:10.1371/journal.pone.0038021.

Kernberg, O.F. (1996). A psychoanalytic model for the classification of personality disorders. In M. Achenheil, B. Bondy, R. Engel, M. Ermann, & N. Nedopil (Eds.), *Implications of psychopharmacology to psychiatry* (pp. 66–78). New York: Springer.

Knekt, P., Lindfors, O., Harkanen, T., Valikoski, M., Virtala, E., Laaksonen, M.A., … Renlund, C. (2008a). Randomized trial on the effectiveness of long- and short-term psychodynamic psychotherapy and solution-focused therapy on psychiatric symptoms during a 3-year follow-up. *Psychological Medicine*, *38*, 689–703. doi:10.1017/S003329170700164X.

Knekt, P., Lindfors, O., Laaksonen, M.A., Raitasalo, R., Haaramo, P., & Jarvikoski, A. (2008b). Effectiveness of short-term and long-term psychotherapy on work ability and functional capacity: A randomized clinical trial on depressive and anxiety disorders. *Journal of Affective Disorders*, *107*, 95–106. doi:10.1016/j.jad.2007.08.005.

Knijnik, D.Z., Kapczinski, F., Chachamovich, E., Margis, R., & Eizirik, C.L. (2004). Psychodynamic group treatment for generalized social phobia. *Revista Brasileira de Psiquiatria*, *26*, 77–81. doi:10.1590/S1516-44462004000200003.

Kraemer, H.C. (2011). Another point of view: Superiority, noninferiorty, and the role of an active comparator. *Journal of Clinical Psychiatry*, *72*, 1350–1352.

Leichsenring, F. (2001). Comparative effects of short-term psychodynamic psychotherapy and cognitive-behavioural therapy in depression: A meta-analytic approach. *Clinical Psychology Review*, *21*, 401–419.

Leichsenring, F. (2004). Randomized controlled versus naturalistic studies: A new research agenda. *Bulletin of the Menninger Clinic*, *68*, 137–151. doi:10.1521/bumc.68.2.137.35952.

Leichsenring, F., Klein, S., & Salzer, S. (2014). The efficacy of psychodynamic psychotherapy in specific mental disorders: A 2013 update of empirical evidence. *Contemporary Psychoanalysis*, *50*(1–2), pp. 89–130.

Leichsenring, F., Klein, S., & Salzer, S. (2014). Evidence for psychodynamic therapy in anxiety disorders. In P. Emmelkamp & T. Ehring (Eds.), *Wiley handbook of anxiety disorders: Theory, research, practice* (Vol. II; pp. 852–864). New York: Wiley-Blackwell.

Leichsenring, F., & Leibing, E. (2003). The effectiveness of psychodynamic therapy and cognitive behaviour therapy in the treatment of personality disorders: A meta-analysis. *American Journal of Psychiatry*, *160*, 1223–1232. doi:10.1176/appi.ajp.160.7.1223.

Leichsenring, F., & Leibing, E. (2007). Cognitive-behavioural therapy for avoidant personality disorder. *British Journal of Psychiatry*, *190*, 80; (author reply, 80–81). doi:10.1192/bjp.190.1.80.

Leichsenring, F., Leibing, E., Kruse, J., New, A., & Leweke, F. (2011). Borderline personality disorder. *Lancet*, *377*, 74–84. doi:10.1016/S0140-6736(10)61422-5.

Leichsenring, F., & Rabung, S. (2011). Double standards in psychotherapy research. *Psychotherapy and Psychosomatics*, *80*, 48–51; (author reply, 53–44). doi:10.1159/000315365.

Leichsenring, F., & Salzer, S. (2014). A unified protocol for the transdiagnostic psychodynamic treatment of anxiety disorders: An evidence-based approach. *Psychotherapy*, *51*(2), 224–245. doi: 10.1037/a0033815. Epub 2013 Dec 30.

Leichsenring, F., Salzer, S., Beutel, M.E., Herpertz, S., Hiller, W., Hoyer, J., Huesing, J., … Leibing, E. (2013a). Psychodynamic therapy and cognitive therapy in social anxiety disorder: A multi-center randomized controlled trial. *American Journal of Psychiatry*, *170*, 759–767. doi:10.1176/appi.ajp.2013.12081125.

Leichsenring, F., Salzer, S., Beutel, M.E., Herpertz, S., Hiller, W., Hoyer, J., Huesing, J., … Leibing, E. (2013b). Long-term effects of psychodynamic therapy and cognitive therapy in social anxiety disorder. Unpublished manuscript.

Leichsenring, F., Salzer, S., Hilsenroth, M., Leibing, E., Leweke, F., & Rabung, S. (2011). Treatment integrity: An unresolved issue in psychotherapy research. *Current Psychiatry Reviews*, *7*, 313–321. doi:10.2174/157340011797928259.

Leichsenring, F., Salzer, S., Jaeger, U., Kächele, H., Kreische, R., Leweke, F., … Leibing, E. (2009). Short-term psychodynamic psychotherapy and cognitive-behavioural therapy in generalized anxiety disorder: A randomized, controlled trial. *American Journal of Psychiatry*, *166*, 875–881. doi:10.1176/appi.ajp.2009.09030441.

Leichsenring, F., Salzer, S., & Leibing, E. (2013). Response to Dr. Clark. *American Journal of Psychiatry*, *170*, 1365–1366.

Luborsky, L. (1984). *Principles of psychoanalytic psychotherapy: Manual for supportive-expressive treatment*. New York: Basic Books.

Luborsky, L., Diguer, L., Seligman, D., Rosenthal, R., Krause, E.D., Johnson, S., … Schweizer, E. (1999). The researcher's own therapy allegiances: A "wild card" in comparisons of treatment efficacy. *Clinical Psychology: Science and Practice*, *6*, 95–106. doi:10.1093/clipsy.6.1.95.

Maina, G., Forner, F., & Bogetto, F. (2005). Randomized controlled trial comparing brief dynamic and supportive therapy with waiting list condition in minor depressive disorders. *Psychotherapy and Psychosomatics*, *74*, 43–50. doi:10.1159/000082026.

Malan, D.H. (1976). *Toward the validation of dynamic psychotherapy*. New York: Plenum.

McCallum, M., & Piper, W.E. (1990). A controlled study of effectiveness and patient suitability for short-term group psychotherapy. *International Journal of Group Psychotherapy*, *40*, 431–452.

McHugh, R.K., Murray, H.W., & Barlow, D.H. (2009). Balancing fidelity and adaptation in the dissemination of empirically-supported treatments: The promise of transdiagnostic interventions. *Behaviour Research and Therapy*, *47*, 946–953.

Meyer, T.J., Miller, M.L., Metzger, R.L., & Borkovec, T.D. (1990). Development and validation of the Penn State Worry Questionnaire. *Behaviour Research and Therapy*, *28*, 487–495.

Milrod, B., Leon, A.C., Busch, F., Rudden, M., Schwalberg, M., Clarkin, J., … Shear, M.K. (2007). A randomized controlled clinical trial of psychoanalytic psychotherapy for panic disorder. *American Journal of Psychiatry*, *164*, 265–272.

Monsen, K., & Monsen, T.J. (2000). Chronic pain and psychodynamic body therapy. *Psychotherapy: Theory, Research, Practice, Training*, *37*, 257–269.

Munroe-Blum, H., & Marziali, E. (1995). A controlled trial of short-term group treatment for borderline personality disorder. *Journal of Personality Disorders*, *9*, 190–198. doi:10.1521/pedi.1995.9.3.190.

Muran, J.C., Safran, J.D., Samstag, L.W., & Winston, A. (2005). Evaluating an alliance-focused treatment for personality disorders. *Psychotherapy: Theory, Research, Practice, Training, 42*, 532–545. doi:10.1037/0033-3204.42.4.532.

Nathan, P.E., & Gorman, J.M. (2002). *A guide to treatments that work* (2nd ed.). London: Oxford University Press.

Norton, P.J., & Phillip, L.M. (2008). Transdiagnostic approaches to the treatment of anxiety disorders: A quantitative review. *Psychotherapy Theory, Research, Practice, Training, 45*, 214–226.

Öst, L.G. (2008). Cognitive behavior therapy for anxiety disorders: 40 years of progress. *Nordic Journal of Psychiatry, 47*, 5–10.

Piper, W.E., McCallum, M., Joyce, A.S., Rosie, J.S., & Ogrodniczuk, J.S. (2001). Patient personality and time-limited group psychotherapy for complicated grief. *International Journal of Group Psychotherapy, 51*, 525–552. doi:10.1521/ijgp.51.4.525.51307.

Salminen, J.K., Karlsson, H., Hietala, J., Kajander, J., Aalto, S., Markkula, J., … Toikka, T. (2008). Short-term psychodynamic psychotherapy and fluoxetine in major depressive disorder: A randomized comparative study. *Psychotherapy and Psychosomatics, 77*, 351–357. doi:10.1159/000151388.

Salzer, S., Winkelbach, C., Leweke, F., Leibing, E., & Leichsenring, F. (2011). Long-term effects of short-term psychodynamic psychotherapy and cognitive-behavioural therapy in generalized anxiety disorder: 12-month follow-up. *Canadian Journal of Psychiatry, 56*, 503–508.

Sandahl, C., Herlitz, K., Ahlin, G., & Rönnberg, S. (1998). Time-limited group psychotherapy for moderately alcohol dependent patients: A randomized controlled clinical trial. *Psychotherapy Research, 8*, 361–378.

Sattel, H., Lahmann, C., Gundel, H., Guthrie, E., Kruse, J., Noll-Hussong, M., … Henningsen, P. (2012). Brief psychodynamic interpersonal psychotherapy for patients with multisomatoform disorder: Randomised controlled trial. *British Journal of Psychiatry, 200*, 60–67. doi:10.1192/bjp.bp.111.093526.

Schmidt, N.B. (2012). Innovations in the treatment of anxiety psychopathology: Introduction. *Behavior Therapy, 43*, 465–467.

Shadish, W.R., Cook, T.D., & Campbell, D.T. (2002). *Experimental and quasi-experimental designs for generalized causal inference.* Boston, MA: Houghton Mifflin.

Shapiro, D.A., Barkham, M., Rees, A., Hardy, G.E., Reynolds, S., & Startup, M. (1994). Effects of treatment duration and severity of depression on the effectiveness of cognitive-behavioural and psychodynamic interpersonal psychotherapy. *Journal of Consulting and Clinical Psychology, 62*, 522–534. doi:10.1037/0022-006X.62.3.522.

Shapiro, D.A., & Firth, J.A. (1985). *Exploratory therapy manual for the Sheffield Psychotherapy Project* (SAPU Memo 733). Sheffield: University of Sheffield.

Shedler, J. (2010). The efficacy of psychodynamic psychotherapy. *American Journal of Psychology, 65*, 98–109. doi:10.1037/a0018378.

Silverberg, F. (2005). *Make the leap: A practical guide to breaking the patterns that hold you back.* New York: Marlowe.

Spielberger, C.D., Gorsuch, R.C., & Lushene, R.E. (1970). *Manual for the State Trait Anxiety Inventory.* Palo Alto, CA: Consulting Psychologists Press.

Svartberg, M., Stiles, T.C., & Seltzer, M.H. (2004). Randomized, controlled trial of the effectiveness of short-term dynamic psychotherapy and cognitive therapy for cluster C personality disorders. *American Journal of Psychiatry*, *161*, 810–817.

Tasca, G.A., Ritchie, K., Conrad, G., Balfour, L., Gayton, J., Lybanon, V., ... Bissada, H. (2006). Attachment scales predict outcome in a randomized controlled trial of two group therapies for binge eating disorder: An aptitude by treatment interaction. *Psychotherapy Research*, *16*, 106–121. doi:10.1080/10503300500090928.

Thase, M.E. (2013). Comparative effectiveness of psychodynamic psychotherapy and cognitive behavioural therapy: It's about time, and what's next? *American Journal of Psychiatry*, *170*, 953–956. doi:10.1176/appi.ajp.2013.13060839.

Thoma, N.C., McKay, D., Gerber, A.J., Milrod, B.L., Edwards, A.R., & Kocsis, J.H. (2012). A quality-based review of randomized controlled trials of cognitive-behavioural therapy for depression: An assessment and meta-regression. *American Journal of Psychiatry*, *169*, 22–30. doi:10.1176/appi.ajp.2011.11030433.

Thompson, L.W., Gallagher, D., & Breckenridge, J.S. (1987). Comparative effectiveness of psychotherapies for depressed elders. *Journal of Consulting and Clinical Psychology*, *55*, 385–390.

Town, J.M., Abbass, A., & Hardy, G. (2011). Short-term psychodynamic psychotherapy for personality disorders: A critical review of randomized controlled trials. *Journal of Personality Disorders*, *25*, 723–740. doi:10.1521/pedi.2011.25.6.723.

Wallerstein, R.S. (1989). The psychotherapy research project of the Menninger Foundation: An overview. *Journal of Consulting and Clinical Psychology*, *57*, 195–205.

Wampold, B.E., Imel, Z.E., Laska, K.M., Benish, S., Miller, S.D., Fluckiger, C., ... Budge, S. (2010). Determining what works in the treatment of PTSD. *Clinical Psychology Review*, *30*, 923–933. doi:10.1016/j.cpr.2010.06.005.

Winston, A., Laikin, M., Pollack, J., Samstag, L.W., McCullough, L., & Muran, J.C. (1994). Short-term psychotherapy of personality disorders. *American Journal of Psychiatry*, *151*, 190–194.

Woody, G., Luborsky, L., McLellan, A.T., & O'Brien, C.P. (1990). Corrections and revised analyses for psychotherapy in methadone maintenance patients. *Archives of General Psychiatry*, *47*, 788–789.

Woody, G.E., Luborsky, L., McLellan, A.T., O'Brien, C.P., Beck, A.T., Blaine, J., ... Hole, A. (1983). Psychotherapy for opiate addicts. Does it help? *Archives of General Psychiatry*, *40*, 639–645.

Woody, G.E., McLellan, A.T., Luborsky, L., & O'Brien, C.P. (1995). Psychotherapy in community methadone programs: A validation study. *American Journal of Psychiatry*, *152*, 1302–1308.

Zeeck, A., von Wietersheim, J., Weiss, H., Beutel, M., & Hartmann, S. (2013). The INDDEP study: inpatient and day hospital treatment for depression-symptom course and predictor of change. *BMC Psychiatry*, *13*, 100.

Zipfel, S., Wild, B., Groß, G., Friederich, H.-C., Teufel, M., Schellberg, D., ... Herzog, W. (2013). Focal psychodynamic therapy, cognitive behaviour therapy, and optimized treatment as usual in outpatients with anorexia nervosa (Antop study): Randomised controlled trial. *The Lancet*. doi:10.1016/S0140-6736(13)61746-8.

Clinical discussion of *Psychodynamic Therapy: a Meta-Analysis Testing Equivalence of Outcome*

Harriet Wolfe

It is an honor to discuss Dr. Leichsenring's work. He and his colleagues, including the first author on the 2017 paper, Christiane Steinert, have achieved a new methodological standard for the meta-analysis of psychotherapy research and offer us encouraging results regarding the equivalence of psychodynamic therapy with other active treatments, namely CBT and pharmacotherapy with SSRI's (Steinert, Munder, Rabung, Hoyer, & Leichsenring, 2017).

I am not a researcher. I am a psychiatrist psychoanalyst who values psycho-therapy research greatly. I work as a clinician–administrator–educator, and my competence to fully understand the details of the authors' methodology is limited. But studying the study—its logic, its main methodological points and its extensive and impressive bibliography—has expanded my thinking signifi-cantly and has acquainted me with issues that I think would benefit my fellow clinicians' and our trainees' clinical acuity enormously. I am grateful to Dr. Leichsenring and to the Sandler Conference organizers for this inspiring introduction to essential learning for non-researcher colleagues.

First, and speaking as I said primarily as a clinician, I will highlight the facets of this meta-analysis that seem to me most valuable and some clinical questions that arise on considering them. Then I will move on to specific clinical and cultural perspectives that are highlighted by the meta-analysis and that suggest areas for further study.

The important features of the meta-analysis from my clinical point of view are:

1 the quality of the studies included;
2 the assessment of allegiance/bias—of researchers, therapists, trainers, supervisors;
3 the logic of equivalency testing—defining a margin, searching for studies with one or more established comparators, applying the two one-sided test procedure.

Quality of studies included

The 23 randomized controlled studies considered in the meta-analysis were all manualized or manual-guided studies and each had been subjected to two or more randomized controlled trials in independent research settings. The treatments compared (the comparators) were well-known methods of psychotherapy or psychopharmacology with established efficacy for the disorder being treated. Since the quantitative evidence-base for cognitive behavioral therapy (CBT)—the sheer volume of studies—far exceeds the evidence-base for psychodynamic psychotherapy (PDT), the meticulous demonstration of equivalence succeeds in putting PDT on the same evidence-based level (Milrod, 2017).

From a clinician's point of view, it becomes interesting to know what treatment was efficacious for what disorder and whether that is discernible from a meta-analysis. This analysis included six diagnostic categories under the rubric of "mental disorders": anxiety, mood, PTSD, eating disorders, personality disorders and substance abuse disorders. Not all disorders were included. For example, psychosis was not.

Psychosis brings to mind the clinical reality that all diagnostic categories may include various, including psychotic, symptoms, whether for moments or extended periods of time. When working with a patient it is often hard to commit to a single diagnosis. It is even harder to commit to a monosymptom disorder. It is possible to create a contract with a patient (or a research design) to focus on one or a few "target symptoms" but the exercise necessarily involves reductionist thinking about the patient's experience because human beings are complex.

Patients have variable genetic loadings, endure complex life experiences, and form relationships in variable, complex ways. This array of complexities drives some practitioners away from psychotherapy research. However, the rigor which a study such as this meta-analysis demonstrates can alert the clinician to the potential for an unwitting retreat behind the defensive claim of complexity. This study demonstrates that there are rigorous methods for assessing what we *do* know.

The assessment of allegiance

I found the careful attention to excluding the factor of allegiance to be the most impressive aspect of this meta-analysis. We can consider this a form of respect for operational effects; that is, how the very fact of doing research changes the field being observed. Some of the operational effects are predictable. If a researcher—or a clinician, supervisor, trainer or trainee—engages in "investigator bias," he/she loses the opportunity to discover what is objectively verifiable; i.e., what is true not only about outcomes but also about a patient's disorder and what a truly useful clinical intervention may be. Studies motivated by the goal of showing that an intervention works, rather than exploring if and how it might work, are not unfamiliar to us. They are, to the benefit of our profession, excluded from this meta-analysis.

The logic of equivalency testing

This is a difficult concept for a non-statistician. This aspect of the meta-analysis introduces the importance of defining "margins." That is, when comparing outcomes one needs to avoid comparing apples and oranges. There are disorders that have little margin for error and the study of outcome requires a small margin of difference between the interventions being compared. When disorders are not life-threatening, the margin between compared outcomes can be larger. The margin is the maximum difference in outcome considered to be clinically irrelevant. The design of this meta-analysis included an equivalence interval that corresponds to a small effect size. As the authors Steinert et al. (2017) note, they used one of the smallest margins ever suggested as compatible with equivalence, and they used treatments established in efficacy as comparators (p. 949).

Clinical perspectives

What does this sort of meta-analysis offer the therapist, the patient and the combination of the two? It offers a lot. In establishing that the psychotherapeutic interventions of psychodynamic therapy and cognitive behavioral therapy are equivalent, the meta-analysis alerts the clinician to the fact that choice of intervention is not a black and white matter. The choice of intervention is actually not the issue. It is the fit of the intervention with a particular patient that matters. If a clinician can accept the findings of the meta-analysis, he/she recognizes that it is necessary to have more than one therapeutic skill to offer.

I have been seeing a young person who was traumatically injured through an unexpected fall. It was very disfiguring and has required multiple surgeries. This usually upbeat person maintains a bright outlook through the defensive use of sarcasm and reports having been baseline anxious throughout life. My psychoanalytic frame of reference recognized dynamic themes related to sibling rivalry, self-esteem and body image problems, and identifications with competent, hard-working parents who were projectively seen as critical of the patient's slow return to work and erratic moods. The presence of nightmares, ruminative and scattered thinking, avoidance of fall-related heights, social avoidance because of appearance, and extreme self-criticism led me to the working diagnosis of acute post-traumatic stress disorder with an underlying generalized anxiety disorder.

John Markowitz and Barbara Milrod discuss the kind of problems I faced with my patient in their 2015 article in the *Lancet/Psychiatry* called "What to do when a psychotherapy fails" (Markowitz & Milrod, 2015). Although my patient was attached to meeting with me, it started to become clear that he was not improving and not engaging around what he would like to see change. His meeting with me took on the air of a ritual. I found thinking about our impasse from a transference and countertransference point of view unhelpful. I began to listen to his references to needing and liking lists as a way to structure his day as a potential affinity for cognitive behavioral therapy. I thought it could be a more effective treatment for his acute PTSD than my natural inclination toward psychodynamic therapy.

Two immediate roadblocks existed. I knew little about CBT, and my patient felt allergic to change and was paranoid about losing his friends because of his unusual neediness and irritability.

Unlike a psychopharmacologist who may switch a patient's medications through a series of trials but does so without switching her/his clinical attitude, the psychotherapist who switches therapies alters the balance or nuance of a relationship when adopting a different method. The interpersonal adjustment in a psychotherapy switch is more prominent, even though the relationship and alliance between psychopharmacologist and patient is critical to compliance if not outcome.

If a therapist (like me) has little experience and hence less conviction about the value, in their particular hands, of another form of psychotherapy, the patient is put in a difficult position whether a referral is suggested or the clinician changes approach. It was clear to me that the suggestion of a referral was likely to confirm my patient's fear of rejection due to his irritability and neediness. Also, as Markowitz and Milrod point out, the switch in me related to trying a CBT approach would have changed me in subtle and not so subtle ways and introduced questions about my authenticity (Markowitz & Milrod, 2015). The existing sense of safety, warmth, empathy and acceptance was not likely to survive no matter how diplomatic, educative and confident I managed to be in suggesting something different.

I describe this case in part to demonstrate that from a clinical perspective it would be helpful to have research on non-responders and to be able to predict with some level of certainty whether a patient's response to treatment might change with a different psychotherapy or an augmented therapy. Markowitz and Milrod suggest large-scale, randomized, crossover trials to study patients who are non-responsive to one particular treatment but responsive to another/others.

Cultural perspectives

The call for large-scale randomized crossover trials with patients who are non-responsive to treatment A in order to establish whether treatment B or C has a reasonable chance of succeeding serves as a segue to discussing cultural perspectives on the role of meta-analysis in psychotherapy research and the importance of psychotherapy research for clinical practice.

Outcome studies of psychodynamic psychotherapy are small and they are relatively few in number. The meta-analysis under discussion provides a powerful argument for the equivalent value of psychodynamic therapy in its meticulous aggregation and assessment of available data. We are similarly empowered by the meta-analysis and the appeal for clinician-accessible reporting that Jonathan Shedler offered us first in 2010 (Shedler, 2010) and in this book. In today's fast-moving, twitter-oriented culture, sitting still to discuss one's life problems has become an ambivalent choice. Some of our "candidates in training" and their young friends out in the world think that psychodynamic therapy has never been more needed. But many of them nevertheless have trouble imagining paying for it or making a lot of time for it. Our obligation is to make clear its value. The argument is supported by meta-analysis, but we also need to find ways of communicating value in plain terms. At the same time, we would do well to demonstrate whether, why and for whom multiple sessions per week are recommended to accomplish enduring change or—even better—health and longer life.

The clearest research problem from a cultural perspective is the lack of financial support for large-scale, randomized, controlled psychotherapy outcome research, the sort of thing Markowitz and Milrod suggest. It may be somewhat different in the European Union. But in the United States funding for clinical research is increasingly tied to biomarkers. So far there are no well-defined biomarkers for psychotherapy. Suggestions have been made but funding again becomes a problem. The interesting prospect of brain-imaging before and after comparable treatments is difficult to fund. But additional and simpler markers are possible and may be much more easily tolerated by subjects, by children as well as adults. They include such possibilities as changes in heart rate, hospital days for physical illness, decline in earnings, work- or school-day absences, changes in IQ, or changes in telomere length as studied in the leukocyte DNA easily obtained through a buccal swab.

The health- and longevity-promoting role of psychodynamic psychotherapies, including psychoanalysis, is something we rarely emphasize. In the 1990s there were studies reported in the U.S., and there were others going back to the 1950s in Germany, that indicated significant healthful effects of psychoanalysis. Doidge (2001) reported a social science study by Edward Jeffery (2001) that indicated male psychoanalysts had a 48% lower mortality rate than the male population at large based on 30 years of available data from 1953–1982. Their death rate was also significantly lower than that for general psychiatrists who had comparable years of education and similar or higher incomes. Jeffery wondered if what differentiated the physician psychoanalysts was the fact they had been psychoanalyzed as part of their professional training.

But, as Doidge reports, there are many reasons to think that psychoanalytic treatments are health-promoting. He cites reports by Dührssen in 1956, and again in 1972, of the follow-up of 845 patients treated with psychoanalytic psychotherapy or psychoanalysis through the German national health service (Dührssen, 1956, 1972). The patients' health was compared to that of the general population. For five years patients were followed through direct interviews, questionnaires, and home visits. The average number of hospital days in West Germany for patients not in psychotherapy was 2.5. The average number of days for psychoanalytic patients before they were in treatment was 5.3 days/year. Five years after treatment they averaged 0.78 days per year. Another German study by Dossman et al. in 1997 found that patients in psychoanalytic treatment had a one-third decline in medical visits, a two-fifths decline in lost work days, a two-thirds decline in hospitalization and a one-third decline in the use of all medications (Dossmann, Kutter, Heinzel, & Wurmser, 1997). These were declines that had continued two and one-half years after therapy ended.

A June 2017 report in Nature by a South Korean group, Kim et al., supports the notion that the salutary effect of psychoanalytic treatment on health and longevity can be studied at a cellular level (Kim et al., 2017). Kim et al. focused on telomere length and the effect on it of trauma and PTSD based on existing data that suggested telomere length was a cellular marker for age-related diseases as well as psychosocial stress. The subjects studied were male veterans of the Vietnam War with and without PTSD. Their results suggest that PTSD with severe trauma (as opposed to mild to moderate trauma) may accelerate decrease in telomere length and that SSRI treatment may protect against this decrease in telomere length.

I will not attempt to present the details of the Korean study or its statistical methods. I will just say that it is a recent addition to a line of research related to telomere length and the apparent relationship of decrease in length to severe perceived or actual stress and its health effects (Mathur et al., 2016). The telomere is easily retrieved via leukocytes that are harvested by a buccal swab. It is not painful. It is quick. The assay appears to be reliable. What is inferred is that decrease in telomere length reflects accelerated cellular aging. In the Korean study, which involved veterans in their 60s, it appeared that SSRI use in those with severe trauma was protective; i.e., their telomeres were longer than those who had experienced severe trauma but had not been treated with SSRIs.

This finding takes me back to the meta-analysis we heard about today. The efficacy of psychodynamic therapy, CBT and SSRI's was found to be equivalent. There seems to be an indication that studying each of those groups in terms of telomere length before and after a significant period of treatment (e.g., one year or more) could be enlightening.

In summary, there is a study of increased longevity among psychoanalyst psychiatrists as compared to the general population and to general psychiatrists and there is a study that indicates cellular growth in severely traumatized subjects treated with SSRI medication. Showing the health and longevity-promoting effects of psychotherapy and psychoanalysis may be easier than we think.

There is evidence that anxiety reduction at a psychological level results in psychosomatic health at the whole person level and also health at cellular and sub-cellular levels. Improved mortality of the whole person was suggested by Kliman to Jeffery in 1970 (Kliman, G. Personal communication, February 2018) and later studied by Jeffery (2001). The study showed a significant advantage for psychoanalysis. The cellular substrate for such advantage in comparative studies of psychotherapies appears to be well within reach.

A focus on the cost-effectiveness of psychodynamic psychotherapies that includes the decreased costs associated with health benefits may provide paths to outcome measures that are operationally independent of specific therapy techniques themselves. Clinical research has unavoidable operational effects. Assessing what we may we consider psychosocial data more extensively might not only be freer of operational effects, it might have more socially persuasive value than the behavioral measures we tend to favor as psychologically-oriented investigators and clinicians.

The execution of psychotherapy studies is not only expensive, it is time-consuming and requires a well-trained, well-oiled research team. Even though human society as well as our professional society will benefit from such work, we may have moments of despair and frustration with the lack of financial and cultural support for psychotherapy research. But Doidge starts his summary of psychosomatic research with these heartening words:

> Hope deferred maketh a sick heart
> But desire fulfilled is as the Tree of Life.
>
> (Proverbs 13:12)

References

Doidge, N. (2001). Introduction to Jeffery: Why psychoanalysts have low mortality rates. *J Am Psychoanal Assoc*, *49*(1), 97–102. doi:10.1177/00030651010490010701.

Dossmann, R., Kutter, P., Heinzel, R., & Wurmser, L. (1997). The long-term benefits of intensive psychotherapy: A view from Germany. *Psychoanalytic Inquiry, 1997 Suppl*, 74–86. doi:10.1080/07351699709534159.

Dührssen, A. (1956). Die Beurteilung des Behandlungserfolges in der Psychotherapie. *Zeitschrift für Psychosomatische Medizin*, *3*(3), 201–210.

Dührssen, A. (1972). Katamnestische Ergebnisse bei 1004 Patienten nach analytischer Psychotherapie. *Zeitschrift für Psychosomatische Medizin*, *7*(2), 74–86.

Jeffery, E.H. (2001). The mortality of psychoanalysts. *J Am Psychoanal Assoc*, *49*(1), 103–111. doi:10.1177/00030651010490011001.

Kim, T.Y., Kim, S.J., Choi, J.R., Lee, S.T., Kim, J., Hwang, I.S., … Kang, J.I. (2017). The effect of trauma and PTSD on telomere length: An exploratory study in people exposed to combat trauma. *Sci Rep*, *7*(1), 4375. doi:10.1038/s41598-017-04682-w.

Markowitz, J.C., & Milrod, B.L. (2015). What to do when a psychotherapy fails. *Lancet Psychiatry*, *2*(2), 186–190. doi:10.1016/s2215-0366(14)00119-9.

Mathur, M.B., Epel, E., Kind, S., Desai, M., Parks, C.G., Sandler, D.P., & Khazeni, N. (2016). Perceived stress and telomere length: A systematic review, meta-analysis, and methodologic considerations for advancing the field. *Brain Behav Immun*, *54*, 158–169. doi:10.1016/j.bbi.2016.02.002.

Milrod, B. (2017). The evolution of meta-analysis in psychotherapy research. *Am J Psychiatry*, *174*(10), 913–914. doi:10.1176/appi.ajp.2017.17050539.

Shedler, J. (2010). The efficacy of psychodynamic psychotherapy. *American Psychologist*, *65*(2), 98–109. doi:10.1037/a0018378.

Steinert, C., Munder, T., Rabung, S., Hoyer, J., & Leichsenring, F. (2017). Psychodynamic therapy: As efficacious as other empirically supported treatments? A meta-analysis testing equivalence of outcomes. *American Journal of Psychiatry*, *174*(10), 943–953. doi:10.1176/appi.ajp.2017.17010057.

Chapter 9

The LAC Study

A comparative outcome study of psychoanalytic and cognitive-behavioral long-term therapies of chronic depressive patients

Marianne Leuzinger-Bohleber, Lisa Kallenbach,
Ulrich Bahrke, Johannes Kaufhold, Alexa Negele,
Mareike Ernst, Wolfram Keller,[1] Georg Fiedler,
Martin Hautzinger, and Manfred E. Beutel

Introduction[2]

Today, depression is one of the most common mental illnesses worldwide. According to World Health Organization estimates in 2015, 322 million people worldwide suffer from depression. This are 4.4% of the current world population and 18% more than ten years ago. By 2020, depression will be the number two widespread disease. In Germany, 5.3 million are affected, which is 8.2% of the population. Many of them live with depression for years before it is diagnosed and treated accordingly. The consequences are severe mental suffering for those affected and their relatives as well as high (incalculable) costs for society (e.g., due to inability to work). Depressive parents, especially mothers, often pass the disease on to their children. Depression is therefore not only an individual fate, but also a problem for families and the entire society. The results of the large representative follow-up study conducted by the German Psychoanalytic Association (DPV) in the 1990s already showed that the combination of depression and personality disorders was one of the most frequent patient groups treated by DPV analysts in outpatient practices in the 1980s (cf. Leuzinger-Bohleber, Stuhr, Rüger, & Beutel, 2003). We assume that this is still true today (with a growing tendency) and also applies to the offices of analysts from other societies.

When we planned the LAC Depression Study in 2005, we were repeatedly confronted with polemics in the public discourse about the preservation of psychoanalytic procedures in the German care system, claiming there was a scientific proof of the effectiveness of psychoanalytic treatments. Already at that time it had been proven in various meta-analyses that this statement was not correct: There were enough studies on psychoanalytic short therapies that showed that their effectiveness did not differ from that of behavioral. Nevertheless, statements to the contrary were so frequently quoted by the health policy public that, for example, the Ärzteblatt (official paper of the medical doctors in Germany) claimed that the combination of cognitive behavioral therapy and psychopharmacotherapy was the only "scientifically proven" treatment for depressive patients. In addition, the Kompetenznetzwerk Depression (competence network depression), which is dominated by behavioral therapists, disseminated the claim that CBT is more or less the only form of treatment that cares for depressive patients in a highly effective way in the media. The objections to psychoanalytic long-term therapies and psychoanalyses were even more serious. In addition, there were hardly any empirical, and especially no RCT studies on the results of psychoanalytic long-term therapies available at that time. However, this also applied to other forms of long-term psychotherapy (cf. Leuzinger-Bohleber, 2010).

At the same time comparative outcome studies were met with great skepticism also within the psychoanalytic community, which is to some extent still true today. The question of whether and in what way psychoanalysis should take part in comparative outcome studies continues to be controversially discussed. Above all, psychoanalytic researchers at medical and psychological faculties strongly argued that psychoanalysis will fall victim to social marginalization if it eludes such comparative studies. In contrast: above all, psychoanalysts from the French-speaking world insist that methods and criteria of evidence-based medicine are not appropriate or even harmful for psychoanalysis as a science of the unconscious.

Despite these still ongoing controversies, the Open Door Review shows that a large number of process and outcome studies have now been carried out and that the acceptance of empirical research within the International Psychoanalytical Association has steadily increased (Leuzinger-Bohleber & Kaechele, 2019). Likewise Peter Lilliengren systematically collects all RCT studies in the field of psychoanalysis: there are currently 252 such studies.

As just mentioned, it was undisputed then and to an even greater extent today that RCT studies had proven the efficacy of both cognitive–behavioral and psychodynamic short-term therapies, but that such studies are still largely lacking for long-term treatments (cf. e.g., Leichsenring & Rabung, 2008). At the same time, the enormously high relapse rate of some patient groups— especially chronically depressed patients—in short-term therapy showed that these patients need long-term treatment in order to achieve a lasting improvement. But how can health insurance companies be persuaded to support long-term treatment of such patients? Can RCTs be expected from a group of severely ill patients, such as chronic depressives? Are they practical at all? And is the enormous cost of such studies even feasible?

The curiosity to find out more about the factors involved in psychoanalytic treatment compared to long-term CBT, the threat of social denial of psychoanalysis, but also the interest of some CBT researchers in getting longer treatments financed by the health insurance funds were the reasons why an interdisciplinary research group decided in 2005 to initiate a multi-center study on the outcome of cognitive and psychoanalytic long-term treatment in chronic depressive patients, the LAC Study (project chairs: M. Leuzinger-Bohleber, M. Hautzinger, M. Beutel, G. Fiedler, W. Keller).

The planning and implementation of the LAC Study took place against the background of these controversial discussions (see also introduction to this volume). For example, the research group opted for a design that combines a naturalistic study with an experimental one. In contrast to many studies of comparative psychotherapy research, in which for methodical and pragmatic reasons trained students or study therapists treated persons with precisely defined symptoms (often students) according to a manualized therapy method, in the LAC Study chronically depressive patients, as they are treated in private practices of psychotherapists in Germany today, were seen by experienced therapists in long-term psycho-therapies. We expected that many of them had already undergone several shorter therapies with only limited success, or even negative results, and therefore had a preference for a certain therapeutic procedure. They would therefore not be willing to be randomized for long-term treatment. There-fore, in the LAC Study, they could choose between the two therapies, cognitive behavioral therapy (CBT) and psychoanalytic long-term therapy (PAT). If they did not have a clear preference and were willing to do so, they were randomized.

Randomization of the patients, precisely described inclusion criteria, blind raters, reliable measuring instruments, manualized therapy procedures checked for their adherence, as well as the exact description of the samples, drop-outs and applied statistical procedures etc. belong to the criteria of the so-called "evidence-based medicine." These criteria must be met in order for the studies to be recognized both in the world of psychotherapy research and in health care systems. Therefore, the research group of the LAC Study tried to meet all these criteria.

In addition, the aforementioned epistemological and methodological con-cerns of the psychoanalytic community were taken seriously and a multi-perspective approach to the therapeutic outcome of these "difficult-to-treat" patients was chosen. Thus, in the second main publication of the LAC Study, one aspect of this complex problem was presented for discussion as an example: in the world of evidence-based medicine, it is well known that almost exclusively symptom changes are regarded as a success for psychother-apies, whereas psychodynamically, changes in the inner world of objects, so-called structural changes, characterize successful psychotherapies, because the goal of psychoanalytic treatments goes far beyond symptom changes and, as Freud postulated, is described as the ability to love, to work and to enjoy life (cf. e.g., Leuzinger-Bohleber, et al. 2019ab). Therefore, symptomatic and structural changes were compared and contrasted in the LAC Study (cf. Kaufhold et al. 2019).

In the meantime, the *Canadian Journal of Psychiatry* (Leuzinger-Bohleber et al. 2019a) has published the main results concerning symptomatic changes. In a second article in the *International Journal of Psychoanalysis*, the results of symptomatic and structural changes were compared (Leuzinger-Bohleber et al., 2019b). In addition, the modifications of the two English articles with comments by Peter Fonagy (psychoanalyst) and John Clarkin (behavioral therapist) were made available to a German readership in a special issue of PSYCHE in February 2019.

Therefore, in this chapter we can refer to already published work and limit ourselves to a summary of the methodological approach and the results both with regard to the symptom and the structural change.

Methods

Study design and overview

The LAC Study is a multicenter, controlled, single blind four-arm trial with a preference and a randomized section (see Figure 9.2). After being given a standardized general description of both forms of psychotherapy, patients were asked if they have a preference for one specific treatment (PAT or CBT). If they articulated a specific preference, patients were assigned accordingly. If they had no treatment preference, they were asked to give informed consent to random allocation.

Time points of measurement

Previous studies, e.g., the Stockholm Psychotherapy Study (Blomberg et al., 2001) or the Helsinki Study (Knekt et al. 2011), have repeatedly shown that sustained changes only become apparent in follow-up studies—after the therapies have been terminated. Therefore, the LAC Study was designed for five years.

Figure 9.1 gives an overview of the time points of measurement applied in our study. Figure 9.2 gives an overview of the applied instruments.

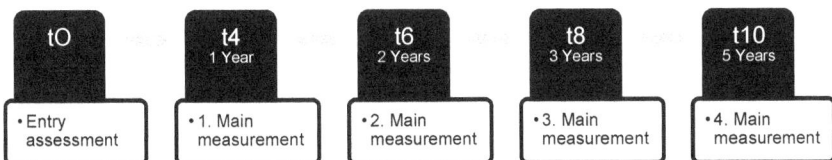

t0	t4 1 Year	t6 2 Years	t8 3 Years	t10 5 Years
• Entry assessment	• 1. Main measurement	• 2. Main measurement	• 3. Main measurement	• 4. Main measurement

Figure 9.1 Timeline of data assessment.

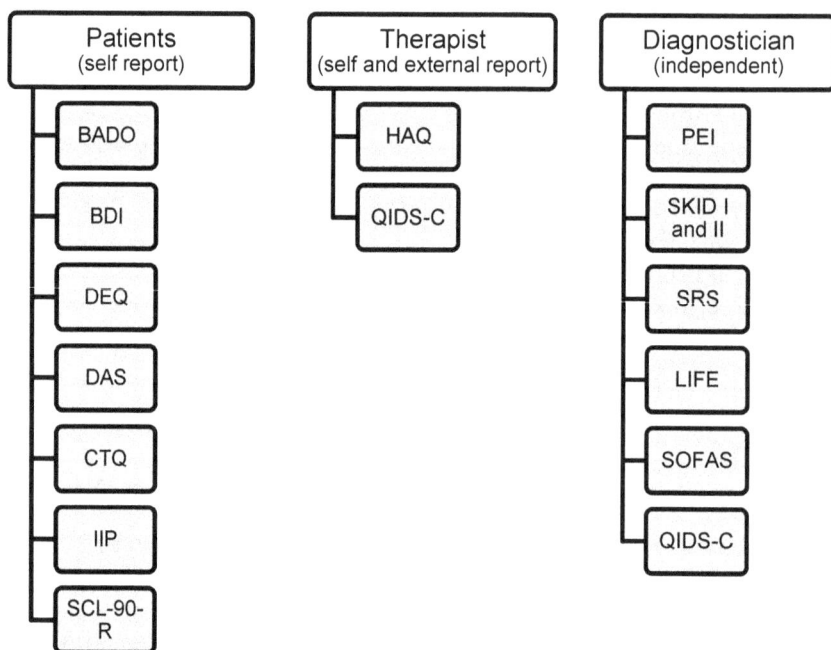

Figure 9.2 Scope of assessment.

Notes
BADO: Basic Documentation System. BDI: Beck Depression Inventory, DEQ: Depressive Experience Questionnaire, DAS: Dysfuntional Attitude Scale, CTQ: Child Trauma Questionnaire, IIP: Inventory of Interpersonal Problems, SCL-90-R: Symptom Checklist-90, QUIDS-C: Independent Clinical Rating; PEI: Psychoanalytic Interview; SKID I and II: Structural Clinical Interviews according to DSM-IV, SRS: Self-Reflective Functioning Scale; LIFE: Longitudinal Follow-Up Evaluation; SOFAS: Social Functioning Scale.

Patients

We included patients between 21 and 60 years of age suffering from chronic depression in four different study centers, Frankfurt a.M., Mainz, Berlin and Hamburg, who gave written informed consent to study participation. Patients had to be depressed for more than two years and meet diagnostic criteria of major depressive episode or dysthymia. Their current depression severity had to meet a Beck Depression Inventory (BDI) self-report score above 17 and a (blind, independent) clinician-rated Quick Inventory of Depressive Symptoms (QIDS-C) score of more than 9 points. Patients with antidepressant medication were included if they were on a stable dosage for more than four weeks.

As we have described in detail in our Consort diagram in the article in the *Canadian Journal of Psychiatry* (see Leuzinger-Bohleber, 2019a, figure 1) a total of 554 patients were interviewed. Of those 252 patients were included in the study. These patients were followed for three years receiving their preferred or their randomly assigned treatment. Typical for a naturalistic setting, treatment ended upon mutual agreement of therapist and patient. Originally 554 patients have been seen by our diagnosticians. Three-hundred-and-two patients did not fulfill the inclusion criteria. Fifty-five fell under the exclusion criteria. Based on the total sample of 252 study patients, at least one outcome criterion (BDI or QIDS) was available for 73.4% after one year, 63.9% after two, and 65.5% after three years.

As numbers of assessments differed between time points, we analyzed all patients who had completed at least one follow-up assessment. Those without any follow-up assessment were classified as drop-outs. Thus, 221 participants (87.7% of the total sample) could be included in the analyses, while 31 (12.3%) were classified as drop-outs.

Supplement table 2 (see Leuzinger-Bohleber et al., 2019a) summarizes baseline demographic and clinical characteristics of all, analyzed study subjects and drop-outs. The mean age of patients was about 41 years. Our patient sample suffered from chronic depression of high current symptom severity (mean BDI 32.1 points; QIDS-C 14.3 points). About two thirds were female. About two thirds were working, and 12% were unemployed. Two thirds had graduated from high school; 60% were married. Almost 60% reported work disability, the majority on a long-term basis, in the previous year. The majority suffered from recurring major depressive episodes, almost 30% from double depression and 12% from dysthymia. Over 72% had had previous outpatient psychotherapeutic treatments, of those the majority (63%) had had two or more previous treatments. At intake, about 47% were on antidepressant medication. Drop-outs did not differ from those analyzed regarding age, sex, severity of depression, diagnoses and antidepressant medication. However they had slightly lower education and more previous outpatient treatments (more details: Table A9.1).

In all our publications we have also illustrated characteristics of the patients of the LAC Study with case studies, so that we can refer to them in this context (see Leuzinger-Bohleber et al., 2019 a, b; Kaufhold et al., 2019; Leuzinger-Bohleber, 2015).

Treatments

Psychoanalytic therapy (PAT)

Psychoanalytic psychotherapy is well developed for severely and chronically depressed patients with comorbidity (see e.g., Bleichmar, 2010; Taylor, 2010; Leuzinger-Bohleber, 2015). Psychoanalytic authors have considered depression in the context of developmental processes, particularly pathological processes determined by unconscious fantasies and conflicts concerning (a) a differentiated, integrated, and realistic basic feeling of self and identity;

(b) the ability to engage in satisfying reciprocal interpersonal relationships; and (c) the ability to unfold one's own creativity in work, developmental tasks matching the patient's lifecycle, and satisfying management of everyday life situations. Discovering the unconscious determining factors due to failures in the development (archaic unconscious fantasies stimulated by traumatization, pathological relationships, burdened life situations, etc.) and working through idiosyncratic unconscious fantasies and conflicts due to developmental deficits and traumatization in the "here and now" of the therapeutic relationship is seen as indispensable for a long-lasting change of depressive symptoms. Thus, different forms of depression are not understood as clearly distinct entities due to specific genetic or neurobiological factors, but as products of complex interactions between genetic vulnerabilities and experiences in early relationships leading to pathological fantasies, developments, and adaptations. They constitute maladaptive attempts of the individual to cope with severe and lasting disruptions of his normal development. All psychoanalytic study therapists were trained in the Tavistock manual for treating chronically depressed patients in different workshops. This manual details psychoanalytic techniques to be applied with this group of patients, illustrated by clinical "anchor examples." Pretested in a British trial (Fonagy et al., 2015) with chronically depressed patients, it specifies a therapeutic approach, including establishing emotional contact, receptivity and openness, identification of fears, activity, and work in the "here and now" and in transference. A psychodynamic model of the evolvement of chronic depression provides a background of specific interventions. Psychoanalysts have had at least three years of clinical practice, participated in regular supervision groups, and were asked to record at least 40 therapy sessions, to permit independent control for adherence and competence.

Cognitive behavioral therapy (CBT)

Cognitive and behavioral therapy for depression followed a widely used and well-accepted CBT-manual (Hautzinger, 2013). Nearly all licensed behavior therapists are familiar with this manual and material, and have received formal training in using the manual. In general, CBT with depressed patients follows five phases within 25 to 45 sessions: *Phase 1*. Development, biographical information, problem analysis, goals, psycho-education, rationale for treatment, explanation of intervention steps. *Phase 2*: Behavior oriented interventions, activation, increasing pleasant activities, balance of negative and positive activities, situation analysis, structuring day and week. *Phase 3*: Cognitive interventions, thought control, focus on automatic thoughts and alternatives, influence basic assumptions and schemata. *Phase 4*: Skill training, social skills, problem-solving skills, communication skills, role play, stress management, etc. *Phase 5*: Maintenance, prepare for crisis and beginning depression, relapse prevention, transfer into everyday life.

This basic CBT for depression could be extended for chronic depressed patients by additional intervention elements (e.g., situational analysis, skill training, self-disclosure). All study CBT therapists were well trained and state licensed. They saw patients regularly, either in their own private practice or as therapists in cooperating outpatient units. Furthermore, they all participated in an initiating workshop about CBT of chronic depression and were supervised throughout the study. Supervision was offered at each site by experienced senior CBT therapists. At each site, workshops were offered regularly (one per year) to the study therapists. Each therapy session is taped and a selection of tapes of each therapy have been rated to control for adherence to cognitive behavioral therapy and for therapists' competence.

Adherence to treatment protocol

In a comparative study between different therapies, it is important to prove empirically that the study therapists actually practice the intervention they represent, i.e., to prove the so-called "adherence to treatment protocol." It was measured by the Comparative Psychotherapy Process Scale (CPPS, Hilsenroth et al., 2003) based on randomly selected audiotapes of therapies to distinguish between psychoanalytic and cognitive-behavioral treatments. A total of 137 therapy sessions (89 PAT, 48 CBT) were assessed by three independent raters. The average interrater-reliability was satisfactorily high (ICC > 0.85). According to CPPS the two psychotherapies could be distinguished very clearly, CBT therapists showing high scores on the CBT-subscale of the CPPS, PAT therapists high scores on the PAT-subscale of the CPPS, respectively.

Allegiance

Another crucial problem of comparative studies is the so-called allegiance. Many studies have shown that identification with a certain procedure has a significant influence on the results. In the LAC Study, part of the group of researchers had a psychoanalytic background, some had no clear preference, and some had a CBT background. Allegiance toward one of the two study psychotherapies was discussed openly before the study started and through treatment and follow-up phase. The study therapists were either psychoanalysts or cognitive behavioral therapists, but they had no influence on data collection, data management, or statistical analyses. The independent clinicians were blind to the treatment received, did not discuss treatment issues with the study patients, and were selected not having a bias toward PAT or CBT. An independent group of statisticians without allegiance to one or the other treatment was providing randomization lists and did the final analyses.

Outcome measures

Following evidence-based-medicine criteria, our outcome measures are evaluating mostly the change in symptoms in the view of the affected patients and independent observers (see introduction to this volume). Therefore, the *following primary outcome measures* were chosen to be: (1) the Beck Depression Inventory (BDI 2), a well-known self-rating scale for the patients and (2) the short form of the Inventory of Depressive Symptoms (QIDS-C), a rating scale for independent raters blind to treatments (see Figure 9.2, above). Connected to the symptom change was the remission rate, a particularly important measure for chronic depressed patients. Full remission rates were calculated by applying BDI and QIDS-C cut-off scores provided by representative samples (Hautzinger et al., 2006; Rush et al. 2003). All patients were diagnosed by the Structured Clinical Interview for DSM IV (SCID I and II) and followed over the three-year study period by the Longitudinal Follow-up Evaluation (LIFE). In addition, we assessed several secondary outcome measures and predictors (for details see Beutel et al., 2012). Intake interviews (SCIDs) and all ratings (QIDS-C) were conducted by independent, treatment blind, especially trained clinicians. Interrater reliability for the QIDS-C ratings was high (Pearson correlation $r = 0.95$ (CI: 0.889–0.999)).

Randomization

Randomization is one of the gold standards of evidence-based studies. Patients consenting to be randomized were coded by the respective study site and sent to the independent statistic department at LMU in Munich, which generated separate random allocation sequences for the study sites of the randomization arm.

Sample size calculation

Sample size calculation was based on meta-analyses with comparable interventions, patient groups and outcome measures (Spiker et al. 2013). A study comparing PAT and CBT directly was not available. Therefore, we used meta analysis data comparing psychotherapies and antidepressant medication in depressed outpatients to extrapolate a probable effect size of $d = 0.50$ between treatments (Thase et al., 1997). To detect this difference at $\alpha = 0.025$ (two-tailed) with a power of 0.80, a minimum number of 60 patients per cell or a total of 240 patients are required.

Statistical analysis

For a detailed description of statistical analyses we refer to our previous publication (Leuzinger-Bohleber et al., 2019a). The following section summarizes the statistical analyses of the independent methodological center at the University of Munich (Bernard Rüger, Joachim Küchenhoff, Felix Günther).

To analyze the time course of BDI and QIDS-C scores in the four treatment groups two Linear Mixed Models were estimated with the software package lme4 in R. In the main analysis missing data were assumed to be missing at random. The dependent variables of those models were the BDI-2 and QIDS-C scores of the patients one, two and three years after treatment start (time points T4, T6, T8). The time point of observation and the treatment group of the patient (CBT, PAT, randomized, preference) were included as categorical independent variables. To control for psychotropic medication at baseline, a three-categorical independent variable was included specifying whether or not a patient took antidepressant medication or if no information was available. Additionally a linear effect for the mean-centered baseline score of each patient (BDI/QIDS-C score before treatment start) and a patient-specific Gaussian random intercept were included into the models, to account for potentially differing disease levels before treatment and the repeated measurements of each patient. Effects of categorical independent variables were estimated using effect coding.

To test for differences between time points, between treatment groups, and for different time courses in the treatment groups three approximate F-tests based on the Kenward-Roger approach were performed for each of the two models with the R software package pbkrtest. To test for a general trend in expected score values over time and for overall differences in the expected scores of the four treatment groups, a linear mixed model was fitted with the respective covariate included (in addition to the baseline score, random intercept, and medication covariate) and tested against the (nested) baseline model without the respective covariate. To test for different time courses in the treatment groups the full model (including the interaction of time-point and treatment group) was tested against the model including only marginal time and treatment. Given the limitations of the sample sizes in detecting differences between treatments, we additionally computed 95% confidence intervals of the estimated group differences one and three years after treatment start to further illustrate the results and quantify uncertainty in estimation.

Results

Primary outcome measures: symptomatic changes in self- and independent (blind) ratings

Treatment outcomes

Table 9.1 presents the change scores of the main outcome criteria over the course of the trial, separately for the four treatment arms. Scores at one, two, and three years were subtracted from the baseline scores (change of BDI/

QIDS-C). Effect sizes (Cohen's d) were estimated based on mean change scores divided by the square-roots of scores' pooled variances (at the respective time point and baseline). Full remission rates (cut offs: BDI ≤ 12, QIDS-C ≤ 5) and numbers of participants with full data at each time point are also reported.

Table 9.1 Changes of patients' self-ratings (BDI) and expert (QIDS-C) ratings

BDI		PREF CBT	PREF PAT	RAND CBT	RAND PAT	TOTAL
Baseline	Score [mean (sd)]	32.0 (7.8)	31.2 (7.8)	32.6 (7.0)	33.9 (9.2)	32.1 (8.0)
	N	63	101	41	47	252
Year 1 (t4)	Diff [mean (sd)]	14.4 (12.1)	10.7 (11.1)	12.6 (13.3)	12.0 (12.7)	12.1 (12.0)
	Cohen's d	1.58	1.09	1.20	1.00	1.17
	Remission	38%	28%	47%	32%	34%
	N	37	76	34	38	185
Year 2 (t6)	Diff [mean (sd)]	15.2 (9.7)	13.9 (12.7)	11.9 (12.2)	15.2 (12.7)	14.1 (12.0)
	Cohen's d	1.77	1.38	1.03	1.39	1.38
	Remission	45%	38%	33%	33%	38%
	N	31	61	27	30	149
Year 3 (t8)	Diff [mean (sd)]	17.2 (10.7)	15.8 (10.9)	17.5 (12.4)	20.1 (11.9)	17.2 (11.4)
	Cohen's d	2.43	1.62	1.85	1.89	1.83
	Remission	43%	44%	50%	44%	45%
	N	28	64	30	27	149
QIDS-C		PREF CBT	PREF PAT	RAND CBT	RAND PAT	TOTAL
Baseline	Score [mean (sd)]	14.1 (3.0)	14.3 (3.0)	13.3 (2.6)	15.2 (3.4)	14.3 (3.1)
	N	63	101	41	47	252
Year 1 (t4)	Diff [mean (sd)]	7.1 (4.0)	5.7 (4.4)	6.6 (4.8)	6.8 (4.9)	6.4 (4,5)
	Cohen's d	1.90	1.46	1.92	1.39	1.56
	Remission	54%	33%	41%	33%	39%
	N	41	69	34	40	184
Year 2 (t6)	Diff [mean (sd)]	7.8 (4.5)	8.0 (4.4)	6.9 (5.9)	8.6 (4.9)	7.9 (4.8)
	Cohen's d	2.12	2.45	1.62	1.94	2.07
	Remission	57%	44%	46%	44%	47%
	N	35	64	28	34	161
Year 3 (t8)	Diff [mean (sd)]	7.0 (5.5)	8.0 (5.1)	9.7 (3.7)	10.1 (5.9)	8.5 (5.2)
	Cohen's d	1.69	1.85	3.43	2.38	2.08
	Remission	52%	55%	79%	68%	61%
	N	33	71	33	28	165

Note
Shown are mean baseline scores and standard deviations, means and standard deviations of differ- ence scores compared to baseline for participants one, two, and three years after baseline ("improvement" on BDI/QIDS-C scale). Effect sizes (Cohen's d) were estimated by subtracting patients' scores (1, 2, 3 years) from their baseline scores, divided by the square-root of pooled var- iance. Remission rates (BDI ≤ 12, QIDS-C ≤ 5) and number of participants with full data at each time point are also reported. PREF = preference arm; RAND = randomization arm.

The average BDI declined over the first year 12.1 points, and 17.2 points over three years. BDI overall mean effect sizes increased from $d = 1.17$ after one year to $d = 1.83$ after three years. Full remission rates for BDI increased from 34% after one year to 45% after three years. The average QIDS-C declined by 6.4 points, over the first year and by 8.5 points over three years. The QIDS-C overall effect sizes increased from $d = 1.56$ to $d = 2.08$, and full remission rates rose from 39% after one year to 61% after three years. (See also the estimated coefficients of the linear mixed models with BDI (A) and QIDS-C scores (B) as dependent variables in Leuzinger-Bohleber et al., 2019a, Table 9A.2.)

Shown are the estimated coefficients of the additive mixed models with the dependent variables BDI- and QIDS-C scores, the estimated standard errors, t-values and the significance of approximate F-tests of a model including the corresponding covariate/parameters against the smaller nested model.

As expected, a decrease (improvement) in BDI scores was observed over three years. The corresponding test of the time covariate rejects the null-hypotheses of no differences in expected BDI scores at the three different time points (1A; $p \leq 0.001$). We found no evidence for differences in BDI scores between the four study groups. The null-hypotheses of no differences in expected values for the treatment groups over all time points cannot be rejected (2A). This also applied to the test of the interaction between time points and treatment groups (3A). Medication at baseline was controlled as a covariate.

As expected, a decrease (improvement) of QIDS-C scores over three years was observed. For the QIDS-C scores the null-hypotheses of no time differences over all treatment groups could be rejected as well (1B, $p \leq 0.001$). There were no structural differences between the treatment groups over all time points (2B). However, a significant effect was found regarding the interaction between time points and treatment groups (3B, $p \leq 0.01$). Again, medication at baseline was controlled as a covariate. The course of change in the four treatment groups was based on expected values and 95% confidence intervals. Against the mean baseline scores, there were strong declines of expected BDI and QIDS-C scores to T4, which further declined to T8. As the figure indicates, the interaction between treatment group and time of QIDS-C is due to an increase of symptoms in the preference CBT arm and a further decrease of symptoms in the randomized CBT arm at T8. This corresponds to the difference of effect sizes calculated for CBT-preference ($d = 1.69$) and CBT-randomization ($d = 3.43$) at T8 (see Table 2 in Leuzinger-Bohleber et al., 2019a). 95% confidence intervals of score differences between treatment groups at time points T4 and T8 are presented in the supplement (supplementary Table 2 in Leuzinger-Bohleber et al., 2019a). The sensitivity analyses (supplementary Table 3, in Leuzinger-Bohleber et al., 2019a) showed similar results as the main analysis. In particular, based on the linear mixed models, there were no substantial differences between treatment groups. The interaction effect of treatment groups and time points is not significant for the models estimated on data with last available imputation.

Treatment intensity

PAT and CBT offer different treatment intensities and durations due to their divergent conceptualizations of chronic depression. One major aim of PAT is to achieve so called "structural changes," which is considered as presupposition for sustaining change in patients which often can only be observed in long follow-ups (see below). Our data showed that PAT had a mean of 80.4 session (SD 27.8) during the first year of treatment, CBT had a mean of 32.5 (SD 9.0) therapy sessions. Over three years, PAT had an average total of 234 sessions, while CBT had an average total of 57 sessions during the study period. PAT patients were in treatment for up to 36 months, while last CBT patients ended treatment after 15 months.

Short summary

In summary, the primary outcome measures showed a considerable reduction in the severity of symptoms in chronically depressed patients in psychoanalytic and cognitive-behavioral long-term therapies (with large effects sizes), which, however, did not differ significantly between the two therapeutic interventions (cf. Leuzinger-Bohleber et al., 2019ab). This result corresponds to the observation of other studies, especially on short therapies. Shedler comments on findings like this in his contribution to this volume, arguing that the mere absence of symptoms says nothing about the positive presence of inner abilities and resources. Does the dodo bird verdict therefore only apply to studies measuring outcomes of different therapies focusing on symptom changes? Can differences be found in the results of the LAC Study if the research microscope is adjusted differently and, for example, so-called "structural changes" are investigated? And do structural changes focus on different mechanisms of change in the psychoanalytic therapies compared to CBT? This question will be explored in the following section using one of the secondary outcome measures, the OPD, as an example.

Secondary outcome measures: the example of the operationalized psychodynamic diagnostics (OPD)

The structural change measures OPD and HSCS

As mentioned, we used a variety of instruments and defined a set of secondary outcome measures in the LAC Study (see Figure 9.2, above). The data is still being analyzed. In this context, we report exemplarily the results of an important secondary outcome criterion: structural change.

For many psychoanalytic psychotherapy researchers it has long been a central concern to identify sustainable psychological transformation processes in their psychotherapy studies. The focus is on structural changes and their operationalization in order to investigate them with the help of extra clinical empirical methods (cf. Fischmann, Russ, & Leuzinger-Bohleber, 2013; Fonagy, 2001; Josephs & Bornstein, 2011; Kantrowitz, 1986; Leuzinger-Bohleber, Stuhr, Ruger, & Beutel, 2003; R.S. Wallerstein, DeWitt, Hartley, Rosenberg, & Zilberg, 1989). By structural change we mean ongoing psychological transformations of the object and self-representations, the "inner world" of the patients, which are closely linked to the ability to mentalize. Clinically, they are regarded as a prerequisite for coming closer to the goals of psychoanalysis.

The OPD Task Force presented the most extensive work to date on the operationalization of such structural changes.[3] Therefore, in the LAC Study, we used this well validated instrument (see below) as one of the secondary outcome measures. The procedure and the results achieved are briefly described and quoted below.[4] For more details see Leuzinger-Bohleber et al. (2019b).

The primary objective behind the OPD manual was to provide a reliable and valid diagnostic instrument that complements the mere description or phenomenology of the psychiatric classification systems ICD-10 and DSM-IV with psychoanalytic dimensions, especially the identification of dysfunctional relationship patterns, strained internal conflict constellations as well as structural conditions of the patient. The basis is a video-recorded, semi-structured interview, conducted by a trained interviewer with appropriate theoretical background. In addition to the perception on the illness, it enquires about self- and object assessments in different areas of life. The questions are posed as open as possible, and no answer options are given. This interview is evaluated independently by at least two raters, then discussed together and rated on five axes. This approach allows for better objectivity, reliability, and validity of the diagnosis; comprehensive validity studies have demonstrated good psychometric properties of the OPD (Task force OPD 2008).

The OPD has a multi-axial structure and incorporates the international ICD-10 classification. In the LAC Study we used ratings of Axis III and IV:

Axis III: life-defining and unconscious conflicts of the patient.
Axis IV: structure (i.e., basal features of mental functioning).

Axis III corresponds to the classical psychoanalytic diagnostics and the central role of internal (neurotic) conflicts. In the OPD, life-determining, internalized conflicts can be juxtaposed with rather current, externally determined conflict situations. Axis IV represents qualities or deficits of psychological structural features. These include, for example, the self- and object perception, self-regulation, or different aspects of the quality of object relations.

Based on the OPD, a working group developed the *Heidelberg Structural Change Scale* (HSCS) (Rudolf et al., 2012; Leuzinger-Bohleber et al., 2019, p. 109). This instrument assesses different levels of awareness of one's unconscious conflicts and fantasies (foci)—and is thus connected with "structural change." Its formal setup is based on Stiles' APES scale (1992), but development stages of change are related to a specifically psychoanalytic process model. The starting point is a focus taken from the OPD rating, which includes a conflict or a structural feature. The seven-stage scale is used to estimate how aware the patient is of this focus. This is based on the assumption that an increasing awareness of this focus, an internal issue to be elaborated, leads to a more conscious approach to it in the concrete reality of life, thus also reducing the symptoms. While patients often begin psychoanalytic therapy at stage 2 (involuntary engagement with focus) or stage 3 (vague problem perception), after passing stages 4, they may proceed to stages 5 or 6. Higher levels of structural outcome have been shown as positive predictors of follow-ups of psychoanalytic treatments (Grande et al. 2009).

Findings on structural changes in the LAC Study

Since the evaluations of the OPD and the HSCS are very time consuming, 60 patients were selected for each of the therapy procedures. A total of 30 consecutive patients for each of the four arms were assessed by additional OPD interviews during the annual follow-up examinations one, three and five years after initiation of the therapy, with an emphasis on the detection of the degree of consciousness of the foci. After one year and after three years of treatment complete data were available for 102 patients. In consideration of the limited resources of the LAC Study, in addition to axis V, only axes III and IV were rated. The baseline data from patients with complete HSCS ratings (CBT: $N = 45$; PAT $N = 57$) were compared to the baseline of the LAC participants and showed no statistical differences. There was only one exception concerning the differential diagnoses: In the OPD sample we found more double depression in the PAT, and more dysthymia in CBT group. Yet, we considered participants of the OPD/HSCS subsamples as comparable as they did not differ regarding sociodemographic, medical history, symptom severity and structural data (see Table 9A.2, Appendix).

OVERVIEW OF FOCI IN THE HSCS AT BEGINNING OF TREATMENT T0

Following OPD-assessment, the five foci deemed most relevant for the individual patient were determined on the axes of conflict and structure. Foci or core problems of the patient were rated with regard to degree of consciousness. As mentioned above the HSCS defines seven steps of awareness. The interrater reliability ($ICC_{2,1}$) for all HSCS foci was 0.85, for the HSCI conflict foci 0.76

Frequencies of foci at the beginning of treatments

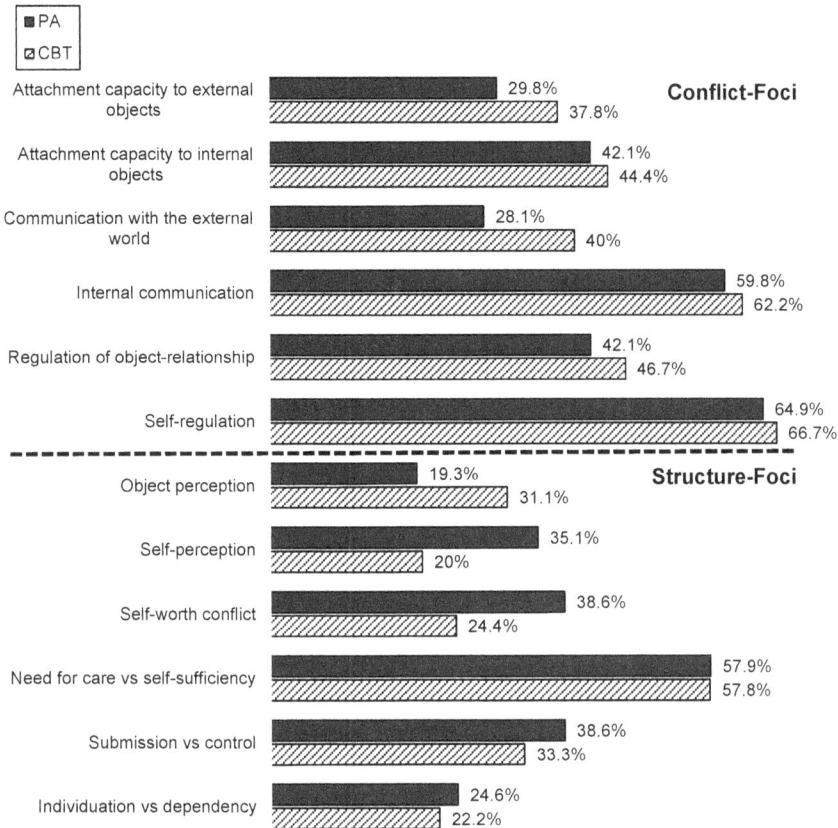

Legend:
- ■ PA
- ▨ CBT

Conflict-Foci

Focus	PA	CBT
Attachment capacity to external objects	29.8%	37.8%
Attachment capacity to internal objects	42.1%	44.4%
Communication with the external world	28.1%	40%
Internal communication	59.8%	62.2%
Regulation of object-relationship	42.1%	46.7%
Self-regulation	64.9%	66.7%

Structure-Foci

Focus	PA	CBT
Object perception	19.3%	31.1%
Self-perception	35.1%	20%
Self-worth conflict	38.6%	24.4%
Need for care vs self-sufficiency	57.9%	57.8%
Submission vs control	38.6%	33.3%
Individuation vs dependency	24.6%	22.2%

Figure 9.3 Frequencies of foci at the beginning of treatments.

and for the HSCS structure foci 0.71. These scores are in the same range of comparable studies (Rudolf & Grande, 2006).

Figure 9.3 shows the frequencies of the foci of the 102 patients at the beginning of treatment, separately for PAT and for CBT (cf. Kaufhold et al., 2017). The most frequent focus per patient was a structural focus of *Self-regulation* (rated in 13% of all focal ratings); as five ratings were made per patient, this applied to 67% of CBT, resp. 65% of PAT patients. Self-regulation is the ability to experience oneself as the agent of one's own competent actions, and to derive self-confidence and self-assurance from this experience of self-effectiveness. The second most frequent focus (12%) was *Internal communication*. The capability to have inner dialogues in order to understand oneself includes particularly the capability to experience one's own affects and one's bodily self as well as to use one's phantasies for understanding one's needs (present in 62% of CBT and 60% of PAT patients). The third most frequent focus (12%) was the conflict focus *Need for care versus self-sufficiency*, which refers to a conflict between a strong need for care vs. self-sufficiency or altruism (in 58% of all patients). There were no differences between CBT and PAT regarding the patterns of foci at baseline.

"STRUCTURAL CHANGE" ONE AND THREE YEARS AFTER BEGINNING OF THERAPY IN THE CBT- AND PAT-GROUP

According to Rudolf et al. (2012), the stages 4 and 5 of the HSCS are of central importance in terms of "structural changes": Stage 4 encompasses an active involvement with the focus; it is considered an indicator for a process of change taking place on a deeper level, which leads to a resolution of older structures at stage 5. As a consequence, Rudolf et al. (2012) defined positive "structural change" (SC positive) by two criteria: rating of at least two foci at a level of 4 and an increase of the HSCS total score of 1.5 levels compared to the beginning of treatment. The total score of HSCS (T0, T4, T8) is based on the mean of the five foci of each measurement time point. No "structural change" is observed when no focus reaches stage 4 and the difference between baseline and the follow-up assessment short of 1.5 stages.[5]

STATISTICAL ANALYSIS

Categorical variables were investigated by Chi^2-tests. Predictors for "structural change" were determined by linear regression analysis taking into account therapy group, baseline HSCS-score, age and gender, separately for one- and three-year assessments. In order to determine the influence of "structural change" (yes/no), treatment arm (PAT vs CBT) and their interaction on symptom severity, we computed a two-way ANOVA with baseline symptom score as a covariate and symptom score as dependent variable (for BDI-2, respectively QIDS) (full data analyses cf. Tables 1, 2, 3, 4 in Leuzinger-Bohleber et al., 2019a). In order to investigate possible changes during therapy these analyses were done separately at T4 and T8. Following the procedure of Rudolf we only included cases of "positive" versus "no structural change" (see supplement table 5 in Leuzinger-Bohleber et al., 2019a). Baseline symptom severity was controlled as covariate. Statistical analyses were performed with SPSS 23.0 for Macintosh.

As Figure 9.4 illustrates, after one year of treatment, positive "structural change" was observed in 24% of patients of CBT and 26% of the psychodynamic treatments. After three years, "structural change" increased to about 60% of patients in the psychodynamic group significantly exceeding CBT with 36%. In contrast to our expectation, we did not find a statistical difference in "structural change" between PAT and CBT after one year of treatment (CBT: 24.2%; PAT 26.3%). This is surprising. One possible explanation

Percentages of patients with "structural changes"

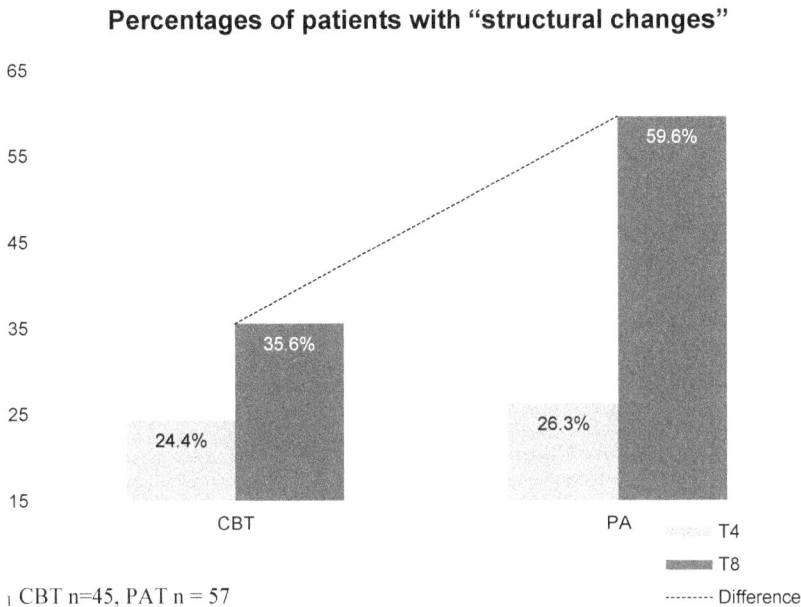

Figure 9.4 Percentages of patients with "structural changes" after one and three years of treatments by treatment approach (CBT vs. PAT[1]).

Note
1 CBT *n* = 45; PAT *n* = 57.

is offered by Lane et al. (2015).[6] These authors postulate that emotions play a central role in *all* kinds of therapies (e.g., also in CBT as well as in PAT) but are not conceptualized in many psychotherapies. In PAT irrational emotions in the transference are seen as one key to the unconscious. Understanding the unconscious meanings of the emotions and the (traumatic) memories connected with them is essential for any transformation in psychoanalysis—in contrast to CBT. However, according to Lane et al. (2015) we may expect that the intensive therapeutic work of empathic CBT therapists also leads to "structural changes" even if these kinds of changes are not conceptualized or intended in CBT. In contrast: discovering the unconscious mental functioning in the transference relationship and the working through in the psychoanalytic sessions is a central aim of PAT in order to achieve structural change. This may be one reason why the differences in "structural change" according to OPD/HSCS become more obvious and statistically significant after three years of treatment because PAT therapists are systematically working on structural changes with their patients—in contrast again to CBT therapists. Of course, we also have to consider that CBT are ending their therapies much earlier than psychoanalysts, another possible explanation for our findings.

Therefore we will have to test our findings further after all treatments have been terminated (see e.g., Blomberg et al., 2001; Huber, Zimmermann & Klug, 2016).

In order to determine the effect of treatment on "structural change" at T4 and T8, multiple regression was computed additionally entering sex, age and HSCS baseline score (see Table 9A.2, Appendix). One year after starting treatment (T4), neither the HSCS baseline score nor the type of therapy or demographic characteristics had a significant impact on "structural changes." However: after three years of treatment (T8), type of therapy was a predictor of "structural change": "structural change" occurred significantly more frequently in patients with psychoanalytical treatment.

In order to determine the relationship between structural change as defined by Rudolf et al. (2012) and symptom reduction, a two-way ANOVA with depressive symptoms as the dependent variable was calculated. Baseline symptom severity of our two primary outcomes was controlled as co-variable (see Table 9A.3, Appendix).

After one-year assessment (T4) for the BDI-II score, there were trends ($p < .10$) of treatment arm and structural change. Thus, the connection between structural change and symptom reduction at this time (one year after the beginning of treatment) turned out to be rather weak. There was no effect of baseline symptom severity, and no interaction effect between structural change and therapy group. After three years (T8), however, structural change was a statistically significant predictor of symptom severity. There was also a significant interaction between structural change at T8 and treatment arm, i.e., structural change had a stronger impact on outcome in PA compared to CBT (see Figure 9.4).

These findings show that indeed the two therapies, CBT and PAT, differ statistically with respect to "structural change" achieved as well as its influence on the reduction of depressive symptoms three years after start of treatment. To our knowledge, this is the first empirical study, which shows such a difference in the dimension of "structural change."

In this summarizing chapter we do not have the space to illustrate the symptomatic and structural changes with a detailed case study, but have to refer here to the other publications (cf. Kaufhold et al., 2019, p. 118ff.; Leuzinger-Bohleber, 2015; Leuzinger-Bohleber et al., 2019a, p. 113, 2019b, p. 93ff.)

Discussion

To the best of our knowledge, the LAC Study is the first controlled trial comparing the outcome of long-term psychodynamic and cognitive-behavioral treatments for chronically depressed patients either with randomized or with preferred allocation. As expected over one year both treatments led to similar positive effects (symptom reduction, remission rate). The full remission rates were increased over year two and three up to 45% (based on BDI), respectively

61% (based on QIDS-C). These remission rates exceeded previously reported rates for chronic depression. Thus, outcomes of our study point to the benefit of long-term treatment for this group of chronically depressed patients. Intensive, long-term psychoanalytic psychotherapies prove to be an efficient and long-lasting treatment for chronic depression that keeps up with well-established, evidence-based CBT.

Sustaining improvement of the depressive symptoms has a great relevance for these severely ill patients, who suffer from enormously high relapse rates. Preventing relapses of the chronic depressed is also significant for the families preventing the intergenerational transmission of depression. It also may reduce costs in the Mental Health Services, a topic of a future analysis of our data.

Contrary to our expectation, being treated by the preferred psychotherapy did not result in better outcome than randomly assigned psychotherapy. Clearly, patients were reluctant to be randomized. After being educated about both psychotherapies offered in this trial, about two-thirds of our sample had articulated treatment preference and were assigned, accordingly. Surprisingly, we even found that being randomized to CBT led to better outcome than receiving CBT by personal preference. We found this statistical effect only in the clinician rating scores (QIDS-C) and only for CBT. We consider the effect a statistical artefact produced by the underpowered CBT-randomization arm (see limitations below).

We took great care to conduct an outcome study relevant for clinical practice. Therefore, treatments were delivered under regular clinical conditions in out-patient settings and private practice, performed by experienced psychotherapists, and reimbursed by health insurance. Thus, our study achieved high external validity under the conditions of regular psychotherapeutic care. Another advantage of this trial is its long duration, following patients over three years after the beginning of out-patient treatment.

PAT and CBT offered different intensities and durations of treatment due to their divergent theoretical conceptualizations of chronic depression and of the treatment process. Future analyses also including the secondary outcome instruments need to scrutinize sub-groups of chronic depressed patients who improved more in PAT or in CBT and how they differ from patients with less favorable outcomes. This will offer important insights into moderator and mediator variables for successful outcome of PAT or CBT and for the relevant question who needs which kind and amount of treatment Analyses of direct and indirect costs of these treatments are investigated at the moment.

We have taken great care to characterize our patients according to different dimensions of mental functioning beyond symptoms. As we reported elsewhere, our baseline findings showed that around 80% of the patients of the LAC Study have suffered from severe and cumulative childhood trauma, particularly early emotional neglect (Negele et al., 2015). Following the psychoanalytical conceptualization of depression, chronic depressed patients suffer from pathological self- and object-representations connected to unbearable emotions (despair, helplessness, hopelessness) and chronic dissociative states of the mind. Modifying structural deficits in the self-object representations takes time and an intensive working through in the professional "corrective" emotional relationship to the psychotherapist. These sustained psychic transformations or so called "structural changes" are described in detail in other publications (Leuzinger-Bohleber et al., 2019a, 2019b; Kaufhold et al., 2019). In this chapter we summarized these results on structural changes as one of the secondary outcome measures based on the OPD/HSCS data. With these instruments, the increasing awareness of patients for their psychodynamically significant unconscious fantasies and conflicts was examined, which is regarded as an important prerequisite for structural changes in the sense of HSCS. Even if it is not yet possible to record lasting changes in therapy at this point, the results indicate differences between patients in psychoanalytic and long-term behavioral therapy already after three years of treatment.

The intrapsychic conflicts or structural deficits assessed at the beginning of treatment did not differ between CBT and PAT. The frequencies of the focuses identified by the raters blinded to the treatment condition in both treatment groups corresponded to psychodynamic conceptualizations of chronically depressed patients (cf. e.g., Bleichmar, 2010; Leuzinger-Bohleber, 2015): problems in connection with the structural dimensions of "self-regulation," "internal communication" and the conflict focus of "care versus self-sufficiency." According to the HSCS thesis, changes in the conscious perception of these focuses can lead to sustaining psychological transformations in depressive patients in the sense of structural changes. One year after the start of treatment, the proportions of structural changes between PAT (26%) and CBT (24%) were only insignificantly different. After three years, at 60%, more patients in PAT met the criteria for a structural change in comparison to CBT (36%)—analogous to the objective in these treatments. In the control of baseline HSCS, sex and age, the treatment arm remained a highly significant predictor of structural changes; in general, the therapy procedure was able to predict the structural changes. In PAT, these changes were significantly more frequent than in CBT three years after the start of treatment. Further analyses showed that the structural changes defined by OPD/HSCS are also a predictor of symptomatic changes. As the interaction of therapy form and structural change showed, after three years there was a stronger correlation between structural changes and reduction of depressive symptoms in PAT than in CBT.

Thus structural change, defined by increasing awareness of psychodynamically relevant unconscious intrapsychic conflicts and deficits in mental structure, proved to be particularly relevant for long-term psychoanalytic psychotherapies. In line with the model of Lane et al. (2015), a structural change requires a high emotional intensity in the therapeutic relationship and takes time. The psychoanalytic technique of working intensively with patients in the therapeutic relationship over a long period of time can create an extraordinary opportunity to activate emotions and associated "embodied memories" of unconscious, early traumatic experiences. They learn to endure them in the therapeutic relationship and—thanks to the analyst's containment and holding function—to relive them emotionally in their hitherto unbearable intensity. This makes these memories accessible to a common understanding. These activations and the therapeutic working through make it possible to observe in detail the specific influence of traumatic experiences on current conflicts and emotional experiences in transmission with an emotional intensity and liveliness that, according to Lane et al. (2015), is difficult to achieve with other psychotherapeutic methods. As illustrated in a detailed case study (Leuzinger-Bohleber et al., 2019, p. 113ff.), traumatization and the unconscious fantasies stimulated by the traumatic loss could be integrated into a more mature self and identity, which were no longer unconsciously determined by past traumatization and associated fantasies and conflicts (cf. e.g., Bohleber & Leuzinger-Bohleber, 2016; Negele, Kaufhold, Kallenbach, & Leuzinger-Bohleber, 2015).

These are possible explanations as to why structural changes were observed more frequently in patients in PAT after three years of treatment than in the CBT group. We expect structural changes to continue to consolidate in the upcoming analysis of the LAC Study data five years after treatment initiation. It is currently being examined whether these changes are associated with a reduction in incapacity to work, one of the sources of the enormous indirect health costs associated with chronic depression. Shedler (2010) summarized as follows:

> Especially noteworthy is the recurring finding that the benefits of psychodynamic therapy not only endure but increase with time, a finding that has now emerged from at least five independent meta-analyses [...]. In contrast, the benefits of other (non-psychodynamic) empirically supported therapies tend to decay overtime for the most common disorders.
>
> (pp. 101f.)

From a cognitive-behavioral perspective, we need to understand by what mechanisms deeply ingrained maladaptive behavior patterns are influenced by less intensive intervention. The mechanism of change should be different between CBT and PAT or structural changes can be achieved by more confronting, active, focused interventions. We have assessed study patients with identical batteries of tests and interviews. This should make it possible to take a step closer to answer such questions.

Therefore, we hope to gain further insights through the ongoing detailed data analysis as to who of the chronically depressed patients are more likely to be treated with psychoanalytic long-term therapy and which with cognitive-behavioral long-term therapy. We owe this to these seriously ill people and their years of suffering: the times of horse racing between different psychotherapy schools and the associated fantasy of omnipotence, that one certain approach is suitable for every patient, are over!

Limitations

Our naturalistic, but controlled trial with four arms, two very different active treatments and two kinds of allocation suffers from several shortcomings that limit our conclusions. First, we powered our design to detect treatment differences of an effect size of 0.5. Due to unavailable previous studies, we might have over-estimated this difference and therefore underpowered our design. Now, there is no doubt, that we would have needed a much larger sample overall and each design arm. Due to prevailing preferences of patients the randomized treatment arms ended with an even smaller cell size than expected. With only about 40 subjects in each cell, we cannot reliably detect the unexpectedly small differences between treatments. Not finding a significant difference between CBT and PAT as well as between preferential and randomized allocation may therefore be a matter of statistical power. Second, although, we could demonstrate that PAT therapists acted quite different from CBT therapists, and both groups showed great adherence to their kind of intervention, more control would have been needed. Third, the complexity of the design, recruitment of difficult-to treat patients under naturalistic conditions and the long duration of the trial led to a considerable proportion of missing data at single time points. However, by our statistical mixed model analysis approach we handled missing data by including all available assessments. The missing at random assumption could be problematic. Different imputation techniques could have led to slightly different results. Furthermore, we conducted a sensitivity analysis using the last available assessment for missing data. Fourth, we could not thoroughly control the effect of antidepressant medication taken over the duration of study time. We were only able to control statistically the influence of medication taken at intake.

In spite of all these limitations the conclusion of this study is that psychoanalytic long-term psychotherapy as well as cognitive behavioral *long-term* treatments help chronically depressed patients to achieve a sustaining reduction of their depressive symptoms and to improve substantially the remission rates.

Appendix

Table 9A.1 Baseline data from patients with complete HSCS ratings; CBT (*N* = 45) vs. PA (*N* = 57)

Variable	CBT		PA		Total		
	N	%	N	%	N	%	p
Sex							
Women	31	68.9	38	66.7	69	67.6	
Men	14	31.1	19	33.3	33	32.4	
Marital Status							
Single	26	60.5	32	57.1	58	58.6	
Married	7	16.3	18	32.1	25	25.3	
Divorced/separated	10	23.3	6	10.7	16	16.2	
Children							
No children	25	58.1	32	57.1	57	57.6	
1 child	7	16.3	8	14.3	15	15.2	
2 children	7	16.3	14	25.0	21	21.2	
3 children and more	4	9.3	2	3.6	6	6.1	
Education level							
CSE/primary school	2	4.7	1	1.8	3	3.1	
GCSE	9	20.9	10	18.2	19	19.4	
High school	32	74.4	44	80.0	76	77.6	
Job status							
Working full/part time	34	79.1	40	74.1	74	76.3	
Not working	2	4.7	6	11.1	8	8.2	
Education	1	2.3	4	7.4	5	5.2	
Unemployed	6	14.0	4	7.4	10	10.3	
Diagnosis							
Double depr.	10	22.2	17	29.8	27	26.5	0.005**
Dysthymia	13	28.9	3	5.3	16	15.7	
Depr. episode	22	48.9	37	64.9	59	57.8	
	Mean	SD	Mean	SD	Mean	SD	
Age	41.1	10.4	41.3	11.6	41.2	11.1	
HSCS							
T0	2.33	0.48	2.3	0.36	2.33	0.42	
T4	3.41	0.89	3.3	0.76	3.42	0.81	
T8	3.75	1.01	4.21	1.05	4.01	1.05	0.03*
BDI2							
T0	30.58	6.24	29,68	7.08	30.08	6.70	
T4	14.90	10.76	19.90	10.45	17.67	10.83	0.025*
T8	13.83	9.24	13.33	10.99	13.55	10.19	
QIDS-C							
T0	12.91	2.31	13.72	2.62	13.36	2.51	
T4	5.44	3.93	7.11	3.93	6.40	4.58	
T8	5.20	4.75	4.67	3.91	4.91	4.30	

Table 9A.2 Logistic regression with structural change (T4 & T8) and therapy-group, HSCS-total score T0, age and sex (N = 102)

	Regression-coefficient B	Standard error	Wald	df	Sig.	Exp(B)
T4						
Treatment arm	−0.074	0.465	0.025	1	0.873	0.929
Sex	0.599	0.474	1.593	1	0.207	1.819
Age	0.017	0.021	0.612	1	0.434	1.017
HSCS_T0	0.424	0.569	0.556	1	0.456	1.529
Constant	−2.948	1.727	2.915	1	0.088	0.052
T8						
Treatment arm	−0.985	0.414	5.668	1	0.017*	0.373
Sex	0.324	0.438	0.548	1	0.459	1.383
Age	−0.006	0.019	0.099	1	0.753	0.994
HSCS_T0	0.125	0.499	0.063	1	0.801	1.134
Constant	0.236	1.479	0.025	1	0.873	1.266

Note
* $p < 0.05$; Exp(B): Odds ratio

Table 9.A3 Two-way analyses of variance of symptom severity (BDI 2) after one year (T4) and after three years (T8) with HSCS and treatment arm as independent variables and baseline symptom severity as co-variable (separate analyses for T4 and T8)

BDI2 total score T4[a] Source	Type III sum of squares	df	Mean square	F	Sig.	Partial eta square[c]
Corrected model	1063.73[a]	4	265.93	2.44	0.056	0.134
Intercept	280.18	1	280.18	2.57	0.114	0.039
BDI2_T0 (co-variate)	229.32	1	229.32	2.10	0.152	0.032
Treatment arm	416.61	1	416.61	3.82	0.055	0.057
HSCS_T4 SC	308.27	1	308.27	2.82	0.098	0.043
Treatment arm * HSCS_T4 SC	43.21	1	43.21	0.40	0.532	0.006
Error	6877.04	63	109.16			
Total	28906.00	68				
Corrected total	7940.77	67				
BDI2 total score T8[b] Source	Type III sum of squares	df	Mean square	F	Sig.	Partial eta square[c]
Corrected model	3671.89[b]	4	917.97	13.92	0.000	0.498
Intercept	517.18	1	517.18	7.84	0.007	0.123
BDI2_T0 (co-variate)	1822.21	1	1822.21	27.62	0.000**	0.330
Treatment arm	14.11	1	14.11	0.21	0.646	0.004

BDI2 total score T4[a] Source	Type III sum of squares	df	Mean square	F	Sig.	Partial eta square[c]
HSCS_T8 SC	549.19	1	549.19	8.33	0.006**	0.129
Treatment arm * HSCS_T8 SC	289.52	1	289.52	4.38	0.041*	0.073
Error	3694.44	56	65.97			
Total	18282.00	61				
Corrected total	7366.33	60				

Notes
* $p < 0.05$;
** $p < 0.01$.

Prediction of symptom scores at T4/T8 by the total model:
a. $R^2 = 0.134$ (adjusted $R^2 = 0.079$);
b. $R^2 = .498$ (adjusted $R^2 = .463$);
c. Eta square effect sizes: 0.02 ~ small, 0.13 ~ medium, 0.26 ~large effect.

Table 9A.4 HSCS foci at T0, T4 and T8

Foci	HSCS at beginning of treatment T0	HSCS one year after starting treatment (T4)	HSCS tree years after starting treatment (T8)
Submission vs. control conflict	3+	6	6
Care vs. autarchy conflict	3	5	5+
Affect tolerance	3-	4+	5
Balance of interests	3	4	6
Accepting help	3+	5	5+

Note
Foci determined by the raters in the evaluation of the OPD interview and the results achieved in the HSCS up to three years after the beginning of the therapy.

Notes

1 Sadly Wolfram Keller died in May 2019.
2 This chapter is a longer, adapted version and based on results already published in two articles in English in the *International Journal of Psychoanalysis* and in German in the journal *PSYCHE* (Leuzinger-Bohleber et al., 2019c; Kaufhold et al., 2019).
3 The OPD research group, founded in 1990, included Manfred Cierpka, Reiner W. Dahlbender, Harald J. Freyberger, Tilman Grande, Gereon Heuft, Paul L. Janssen, Franz Resch, Gerd Rudolf, Henning Schauenburg, Wolfgang Schneider, Gerhard Schüssler, Michael Schulte-Markwort, Michael Stasch, Matthias von der Tann.
4 As we have discussed elsewhere, the definition of structural change in the OPD only partially corresponds to the aforementioned understanding in clinical psychoanalytical literature. Structural change in the OPD means a change on the structural axis. Since the gradations on the structural axis were relatively global at the time the design of the LAC Study was determined, we decided to dispense with its rating in the follow-up studies. In the meantime, S. Döring,

among others, is working on a differentiation of the structural axis of the OPD. When we speak of structural changes in the sense of transformations, we refer to our evaluations of HSCS and Rudolf's definition (Leuzinger-Bohleber et al., 2019b, p. 106ff.).

5 For understanding "structural changes" it is important to consider these criteria: Moving from stage 3 to stage 4 on the HCSC means, for example, a categorical change: the different stages have a specific meaning, which is evaluated by the raters. In contrast to other scales there is not simply a continuity in intensity: it is a fundamental difference in quality of the level of psychic functioning. 28 (15 CBT, 13 PAT) patients whose criteria for "structural change" are only partially fulfilled (less than two foci of 4 or a change score smaller than 1.5 stages) are not taken into account in the analyses of positive vs. no structural change, as described below.

6

> Time and cost considerations aside, the technique of meeting three, four or five times per week for several years creates a special opportunity to activate old memories and observe their influence on present-day construals and emotional experiences with an emotional intensity and vividness that is difficult or impossible with other methods.
>
> (Freud 1914/1958)

As such, this approach has the potential to offer something not available with other modalities that can have pervasive effects on a person's functioning in a wide variety of social, occupational, and avocational settings. New learning can involve improvement in function above and beyond symptom reduction, such as better self-esteem, greater ability to tolerate and manage stress, improved flexibility in social relations, a greater capacity for intimacy and the construction of a coherent life narrative that exceed what would be expected based on symptomatic improvement alone (Shedler 2010) (Lane et al., 2015, p. 16).

References

Beutel, M.E., Leuzinger-Bohleber, M., Rüger, B., Bahrke, U., Negele, A., Haselbacher, A., ... Hautzinger, M. (2012). Psychoanalytic and cognitive-behavior therapy of chronic depression: Study protocol for a randomized controlled trial. *Trials*, 13, 117. doi:10.1186/1745-6215-13-117.

Bleichmar, H. (2010). Pathological mourning: Subtypes and the need for specific therapeutic interventions. *International Forum of Psychoanalysis*, 19(4), 204–209. doi:10.1080/0803706X.2010.520734.

Blomberg, J., Lazar, A., & Sandell, R. (2001). Long-term outcome of long-term psychoanalytically oriented therapies: First findings of the Stockholm outcome of psychotherapy and psychoanalysis study. *Psychotherapy Research*, 11(4), 361–382. doi:10.1093/ptr/11.4.361.

Fischmann, T., Russ, M.O., & Leuzinger-Bohleber, M. (2013). Trauma, dream, and psychic change in psychoanalyses: A dialog between psychoanalysis and the neurosciences. *Front Hum Neurosci*, 7, 877. doi:10.3389/fnhum.2013.00877.

Fonagy, P. (2001). *The open door review* (1st ed.). London: The International Psychoanalytical Association.

Fonagy P., Rost F., Carlyle J., McPherson S., Thomas R., Pasco Fearon R. et al. (2015). Pragmatic randomized controlled trial of long-term psychoanalytic psychotherapy for treatment-resistant depression: the Tavistock Adult Depression Study (TADS). *World Psychiatry*, 14(3), 312–321.

Grande, T., Dilg, R., Jakobsen, T., Keller, W., Krawietz, B., Langer, M., ... Rudolf, G. (2009). Structural change as a predictor of long-term follow-up outcome. *Psychother Res*, 19(3), 344–357. doi:10.1080/10503300902914147.

Hautzinger, M. (2013). Kognitive Verhaltenstherapie bei Depressionen: Mit Online-Materialien. Beltz.

Hautzinger, M., Keller, F., & Kühner, C. (2006). *Beck Depressions Inventar* (BDI 2). Frankfurt: Harcourt Test Service.

Hilsenroth, M.J., Ackerman, S.J., Blagys, M.D., Baity, M.R., & Mooney, M.A. (2003). Short-term psychodynamic psychotherapy for depression: An examination of statistical, clinically significant, and technique-specific change. *J Nerv Ment Dis.* 191(6): 349–357.

Huber, D., Zimmermann, J., & Klug, G. (2016). Change in personality functioning during psychotherapy for depression predicts long-term outcome. *Psychoanalytic Psychology*, 34, 434–445 doi:10.1037/pap0000129.

Josephs, L., & Bornstein, R.F. (2011). Beyond the illusion of structural change: A process priming approach to psychotherapy outcome research. *Psychoanalytic Psychology*, 28(3), 420–434. doi:10.1037/a0023449.

Kantrowitz, J.L. (1986). The role of the patient-analyst "match" in the outcome of psychoanalysis. *Annual of Psychoanalysis*, 14, 273–297.

Kaufhold, H., Bahrke, U., Kallenbach, L., Negele, A., Ernst, M., Keller, W., Rachel, P., Fiedler, G., Hautzinger, M., Leuzinger-Bohleber, M., Beutel, M. (2019). Wie können nachhaltige Veränderungen in Langzeittherapien untersucht werden? Symptomatische versus strukturelle Veränderungen in der LAC-Depressionsstudie. *Psyche-Z Psychoanal*, 73, 2019, 106–133. doi:10.21706/ps-73-3-106.

Kaufhold, J., Negele, A., Leuzinger-Bohleber, M., Kallenbach, L., Ernst, M., & Bahrke, U. (2017). [Conflict dynamics in chronic depression – Results of the conflict and structure axis using the OPD in the LAC Study]. *Z Psychosom Med Psychother*, 63(2), 151–162. doi:10.13109/zptm.2017.63.2.151.

Knekt, P., Lindfors, O., Laaksonen, M.A., Renlund, C., Haaramo, P., Härkänen, T., Virtala, E., & the Helsinki Psychotherapy Study Group (2011). Quasi-experimental study on the effectiveness of psychoanalysis, long-term and short-term psychotherapy on psychiatric symptoms, work ability and functional capacity during a 5-year follow-up. *Journal of Affective Disorders*, 132, 37–47.

Lane, R.D., Ryan, L., Nadel, L., & Greenberg, L. (2015). Memory reconsolidation, emotional arousal, and the process of change in psychotherapy: New insights from brain science. *Behav Brain Sci*, 38, e1. doi:10.1017/S0140525X14000041.

Leuzinger-Bohleber, M. (2010). Psychoanalysis as "science of the unconscious" in the IPA centenary. *News of the International Psychoanalytical Association*, 18, Special Edition, 24–26.

Leuzinger-Bohleber, M. (2015). Working with severely traumatized, chronically depressed analysands. *Int J Psychoanal*, 96(3), 611–636. doi:10.1111/1745-8315.12238.

Leuzinger-Bohleber, M. & Kächele, H. (Eds.) (2015). *An open door review of outcome and process studies in psychoanalysis*, 3rd Edition. IPA website www.research-gate.

net/publication/317335876_Comprehensive_compilation_of_randomized_control-
led_trials_RCTs_involving_psychodynamic_treatments_and_interventions.

Leuzinger-Bohleber, M., Stuhr, U., Ruger, B., & Beutel, M. (2003). How to study
the 'quality of psychoanalytic treatments' and their long-term effects on patients'
well-being: A representative, multi-perspective follow-up study. *International Journal
of Psychoanalysis*, 84(2), 263–290.

Leuzinger-Bohleber, M., Hautzinger, M., Fiedler, G., Keller, W., Bahrke, U.,
Kallenbach, L., … Beutel, M. (2019a). Outcome of Psychoanalytic and cognitive-
behavioural long-term therapy with chronically depressed patients: A controlled trial
with preferential and randomized allocation. *Can J Psychiatry*, 64(1), 47–58.
doi:10.1177/0706743718780340.

Leuzinger-Bohleber, M., Kaufhold, J., Kallenbach, L., Negele, A., Ernst, M., Keller, W.,
… Beutel, M. (2019b). How to measure sustained psychic transformations in long-
term treatments of chronically depressed patients: Symptomatic and structural
changes in the LAC Depression Study of the outcome of cognitive-behavioural
and psychoanalytic long-term treatments. *The International Journal of Psychoanalysis*,
100(1), 99–127. doi:10.1080/00207578.2018.1533377.

Leuzinger-Bohleber, M., Hautzinger, M., Keller, W., Fiedler, G., Bahrke, U.,
Kallenbach-L., Kaufhold, J., Negele, A., Küchenhoff, H., Günther, F., Rüger, B.
Ernst, M., Rachel, P., Beutel, M. (2019c). Psychoanalytische und kognitiv-behaviorale
Langzeitbehandlung chronisch depressiver Patienten bei randomisierter oder präferierter
Zuweisung. Ergebnisse der LAC Studie. *Psyche- Z Psychoanal*, 73, 77–105. doi:
10.217067ps-73-2-77.

Leichsenring, F., & Rabung, S. (2008). Effectiveness of long-term psychodynamic
psychotherapy: A meta-analysis. *Jama*, 300(13), 1551–1565.

Negele, A., Kaufhold, J., Kallenbach, L., & Leuzinger-Bohleber, M. (2015). Childhood trauma and its relation to chronic depression in adulthood. *Depress Res Treat*,
2015, 650804. doi:10.1155/2015/650804.

Rudolf, G., & Grande, T. (2006). Fokusbezogene psychodynamische Psychotherapie.
Psychotherapeut, 51(4), 276–289.

Rudolf, G., Jakobsen, T., Keller, W., Krawietz, B., Langer, M., Oberbracht, C., …
Grande, T. (2012). [Structural change as an outcome paradigm in psychodynamic
psychotherapy—results of the PAL-Study (long-term psychoanalytic psychotherapy
study]. *Z Psychosom Med Psychother*, 58(1), 55–66. doi:10.13109/zptm.2012.58.1.55.

Rush, A.J., Trivedi, M.H., & Ibrahim, H.M. (2003). The 16-item Quick Inventory of
Depressive Symptomatology (QIDS). Clinical rating (QIDS-C) and self-report
(QIDS-SR). A psychometric evaluation in patients with chronic major depression.
Biological Psychiatry, 54: 573–583.

Sandell, R., Lazar, A., Grant, J., Carlsson, J., Schubert, J., & Broberg, J. (2006).
Therapist attitudes and patient outcomes. III. A latent class analysis of therapists.
Psychol Psychother, Dec; 79(Pt 4):629–47.

Spiker, J., van Straten, A., Bockting, C.L. et al. (2013). Psychotherapy, anti-depressants,
and their combination for chronic major depressive disorder: A systematic review.
Can J Psychiatry, 58: 386–392.

Taylor, D. (2010). Tavistock-Manual der Psychoanalytischen Psychotherapie. *Psyche –
Z Psychoanal*, 64, 833–861.

Thase, M.E., Greenhouse, J.B., Frank, E., & Reynolds, C.F. (1997). Treatment of major depression with psychotherapy or psychotherapy–pharmacotherapy combinations. *Arch Gen Psychiatry*, 54: 1009–1015.

Wallerstein, R.S., DeWitt, K.N., Hartley, D., Rosenberg, S.E., & Zilberg, N.J. (1989). *The scales of psychological capacities*. San Francisco: University of California.

Chapter 10

Discussion of *The LAC Depression Study: a Comparative Outcome Study* and a clinical case vignette

Esther Dreifuss-Kattan

Thank you Professor Marianne Leuzinger-Bohleber, for sharing this very interesting long-term outcome study with chronically depressed patients. This is a unique project that compares two therapeutic approaches, cognitive behavioral therapy (CBT) and psychoanalytic therapy (PAT), in both the short and long term.

I will not repeat the details of the study, but I want to point out a few unique aspects that I was particularly excited about. First, I was impressed with the large sample of patients included, who as individuals with chronic depression are particularly challenging to treat. Second, the analysis of outcomes over several years is a huge achievement, and gives us a more sophisticated understanding of the different kinds of change that can happen for patients treated with alternative therapy models. As a therapist for 40 years, I am thrilled that researchers are capturing the complexity of therapeutic processes and the structural changes that can take place in chronically depressed patients. Third, the multiple levels of evaluation and analysis, including interviews and self-report measures, was extremely well-thought out, comprehensive, and the result of a lot of effort on the part of the researchers.

Let me also share with you the aspects of the results that I found particularly enlightening. I was surprised that many patients showed improvement after just one year, but it is also helpful to know that most patients with chronic depression need longer-term treatment. We found out that while both CBT and psychodynamic psychotherapy resulted in some symptom relief and structural change in the short term, the longer, more intensive psychodynamic treatment resulted in more structural change and better long-term outcomes. It is important to remember that the difference in intensity of treatment between the two modalities was very significant. I found it especially useful to know that CBT, even with much less frequent sessions, leads initially to symptom relief and even some structural changes in patients' lives. What I take away from this research is that with an insightful and well-trained CBT psychotherapist or psychoanalyst, it is possible to successfully treat chronically depressed patients even in a shorter period of time. However, longer-term, intensive psychodynamic psychotherapy can lead to recovery for these patients and an increase in their ability to live a full life.

As a psychodynamic psychotherapist, many others and I have reached similar conclusions, but it is so important to have high-quality research backing them up. This research is particularly important for encouraging insurance companies to contribute to the cost of treatment, especially in the US where these companies rarely pay for longer-term, insight-oriented therapy even when it is recommended. I hope that this study and other, similar projects pave the way for patients to have better access to treatment for their depression, as well as more financial help paying for it, as the majority of US patients cannot afford to pay for treatment on their own.

I was also deeply moved by the clinical case vignette Professor Leuzinger-Bohleber shared with us of the very successful, long-term psychodynamic treatment of one of the chronically depressed woman in her study. This patient was fortunate to be treated by Professor Leuzinger-Bohleber, a highly skilled psychoanalyst who offered her a stable, reliable, and safe therapeutic relationship. What struck me about the treatment was the way in which analysis of the transference led directly to structural changes that the patient was able to make in her life. This patient experienced these changes on all levels, including in her professional life, her ability to regulate her emotions, and her willingness to care for herself physically, and thus was ready to embark on a stable romantic relationship.

A short clinical case from an art–psychotherapy group for long-term cancer patients at the University of California in Los Angeles (UCLA)

When I think about providing chronically depressed patients with the opportunity to address their mood and make structural changes in their lives, I consider the art–psychotherapy group that I have led at UCLA. This group is for adult cancer patients and survivors of cancer, and aims to address symptoms of depressed due to cancer. These groups are free, and allow patients to meet with others going through similar journeys and share their art, thoughts, feelings, and associations in a supportive environment. Many group members stay up to five years, therefore allowing for long-term structural changes, while others come and go. Group art–psychotherapy is another model for therapy that can reach many patients in an efficient and meaningful way. To illustrate the changes that are possible in this context, I will present one case vignette.

Henry was a 69-year-old married man with one son and two grandchildren. A few years before I met Henry, his adult son was diagnosed with lymphoma and nearly died as a result of being treated with the wrong dose of chemotherapy. Henry's son spent three months in the intensive care unit with two collapsed lungs, nursed by his father and his stepmother, Henry's second wife. His son recovered after two bouts of cancer and is now healthy.

After going through the trauma of his son's cancer and near-death experience, Henry was diagnosed with myeloma, the blood cancer with the poorest prognosis. Henry projected to the group members and to me an adaptive denial, using excessive humor and sexual references to defend against his strong feelings of impotence, loss and mourning. Henry's cancer was treated with chemotherapy and radiation that provided temporary relief, but a relapse eventually made a stem cell transplantation necessary. This transplant is in itself a traumatic experience, as the danger of infection prevents the patient from leaving his hospital room and visiting with friends other than his closest family members.

For three years, Henry was a member of two separate art–psychotherapy groups I facilitated for adult cancer patients, each for patients at different stages of illness and at two different cancer centers. I therefore often saw him twice a week for three years, with each group session lasting two hours. Because of our close bond, Henry developed a strong transference relationship with me. Using just a few of Henry's art works as an example, I would like to give a short pictorial illustration of some of the psychological issues, including depression, that arise when a patient is faced with the trauma of a life threatening disease.

The powerful imagery of Henry's work expresses the destructive process of cancer, along with the restorative and reparative processes that are part of all artistic and art-therapeutic expressions. It exemplifies how a cancer patient reaches a longed-for transitional space, a space characterized by emotional support, strong transference, exceptional creativity, play, and a sense of expanding, infinite time that can counteract depressive moods.

The Figure 10.1 illustrates the hospital in which Henry was being treated. On the one side we see the monitor with its chemotherapy infusion bags, drawn in black and white. On the other side we see a pretty, blonde nurse with very blue eyes and cute, perky, pink breasts. The title suggests that when Henry focuses on the nurse's breasts, the scary, dehumanizing chemotherapy ride is not as bad. The nurse looks very similar to his wife, who was a stable, dependable, and loving support to him. Distracted and buoyed by his sexual fantasies, Henry manages to soldier on despite his fears of chemotherapy treatment.

The colorful scene in Figure 10.2 depicts three naked adults. In the middle we see a woman who seems like Henry's wife, who is looking straight at us. On one side, we see Henry in a kind of self-portrait, wearing a white undershirt with his penis uncovered. On the other side we find a thin, vulnerable, completely naked bald man who looks down. The red fire hydrant looms in the background. Together we interpreted Henry's ambivalent awareness of his situation: he feels healthy and strong in one image, but vulnerable and sickly in the other. The two parallel realities surfaced unconsciously, but as they began to appear on paper, Henry was confronted by them and could discuss this paradox with other group members who related to its complexity.

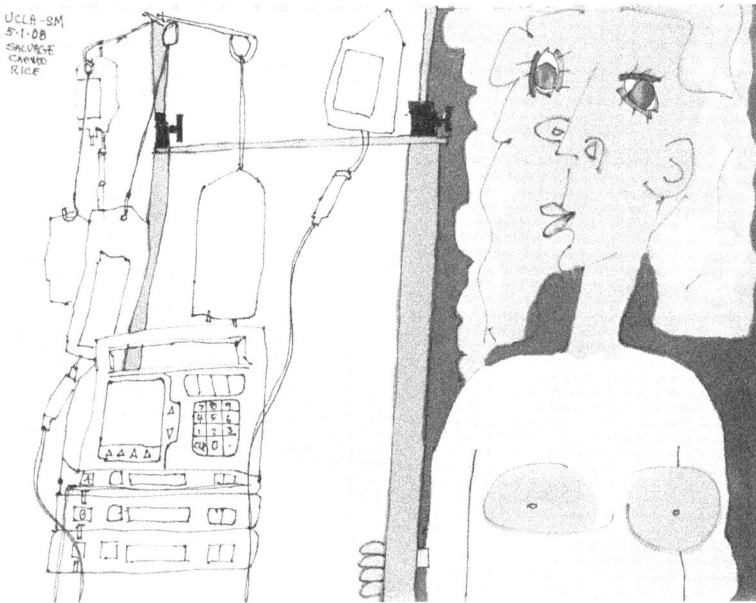

Figure 10.1 UCLA-SM, 2008, "Salvage Chemo Ride," pen and markers on paper.

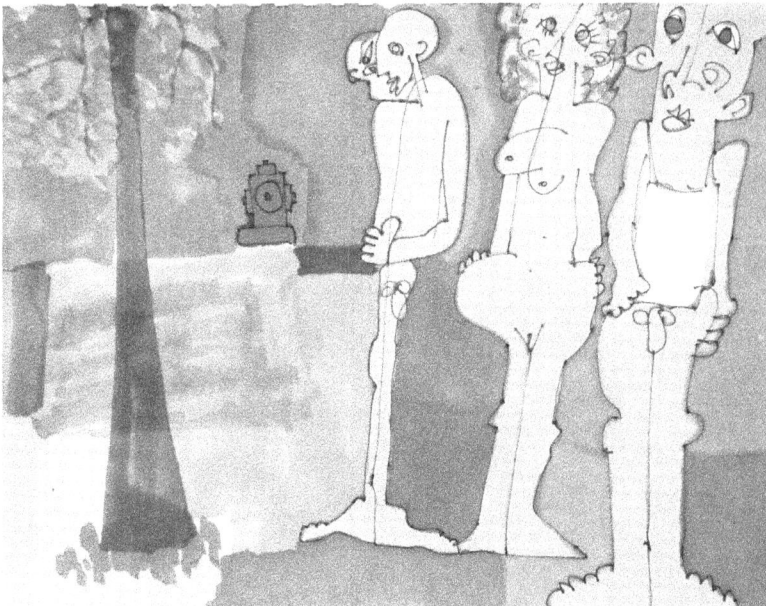

Figure 10.2 "Untitled," 2008, pen and markers on paper.

The red fire hydrant speaks to his wish to receive help in order to extinguish the "cancer fire" that seems to be spreading.

Henry portrays himself in the middle of a group of vulnerable, sick, naked adults. His use of a thin pen to draw makes this feeling of helplessness and weakness even more prominent. Henry identifies with all of his fellow cancer patients, like those in his art therapy group, who are very worried about their health. The support of his peers allows him to observe himself and others, and to acknowledge and express his sadness, fear of loss, and great physical and emotional defenselessness.

Figure 10.3 explains Henry's situation very well. He portrays himself in one corner with a woman, possibly representing his wife, as well as his therapist.

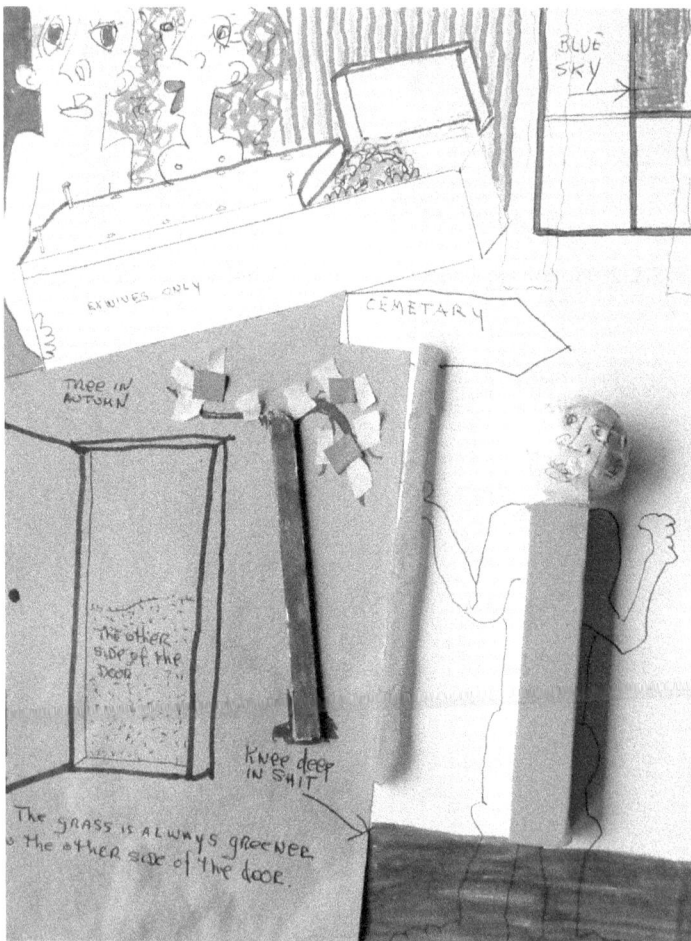

Figure 10.3 "Knee Deep in Shit" or "The Grass is Greener on the Other Side," 2009, mixed media, markers, masking tape, and wood.

Henry holds open the coffin lid, suggesting that it is not for him, but for his ex-wife, who is also the mother of his son. He still projects onto her their dissatisfying relationship, as well as his estranged relationship with his long-dead mother and most likely his ambivalent relationship to the art-therapist who cannot save him from death. The street sign directs us to the cemetery, and a desperate Henry is standing on the brown surface of "shit." There still seems to be a potential escape to the greener grass on the other side, or out of the window towards the blue sky. However, Henry realizes that time is running out for him, which he illustrates by drawing his legs already half inside the dirt, thus implying that he is being slowly buried.

The patient would like to shut the coffin on his bad internal objects—his aggressive father and unloving mother, who both still fill him with rage. With the help of the art therapist, Henry becomes aware that the rage that he directs towards his dead parents partly belongs to the destructive cancer that leaves him furious and impotent. He is sad that in spite of his good and caring oncologist, art-therapist, and devoted wife, he cannot stop the progression of his cancer.

I prompted the group members to first make a self-portrait and then make another portrait of somebody who came to mind. After Henry painted his self-portrait (Figure 10.4), he explained that the second portrait was of me, his art therapist (Figure 10.5). Shortly after our group, Henry had to be

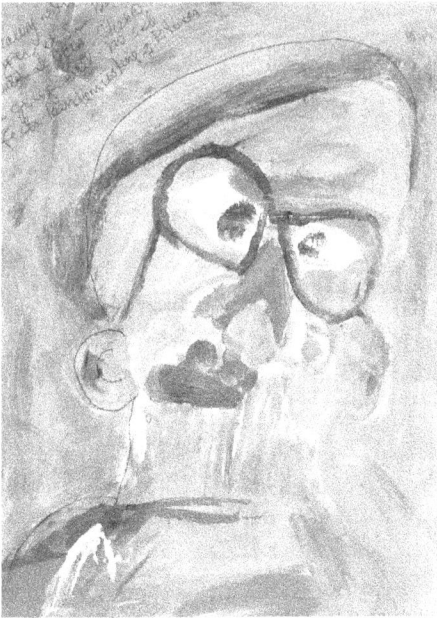

Figure 10.4 Two portraits: a dialog, acrylic on canvas.

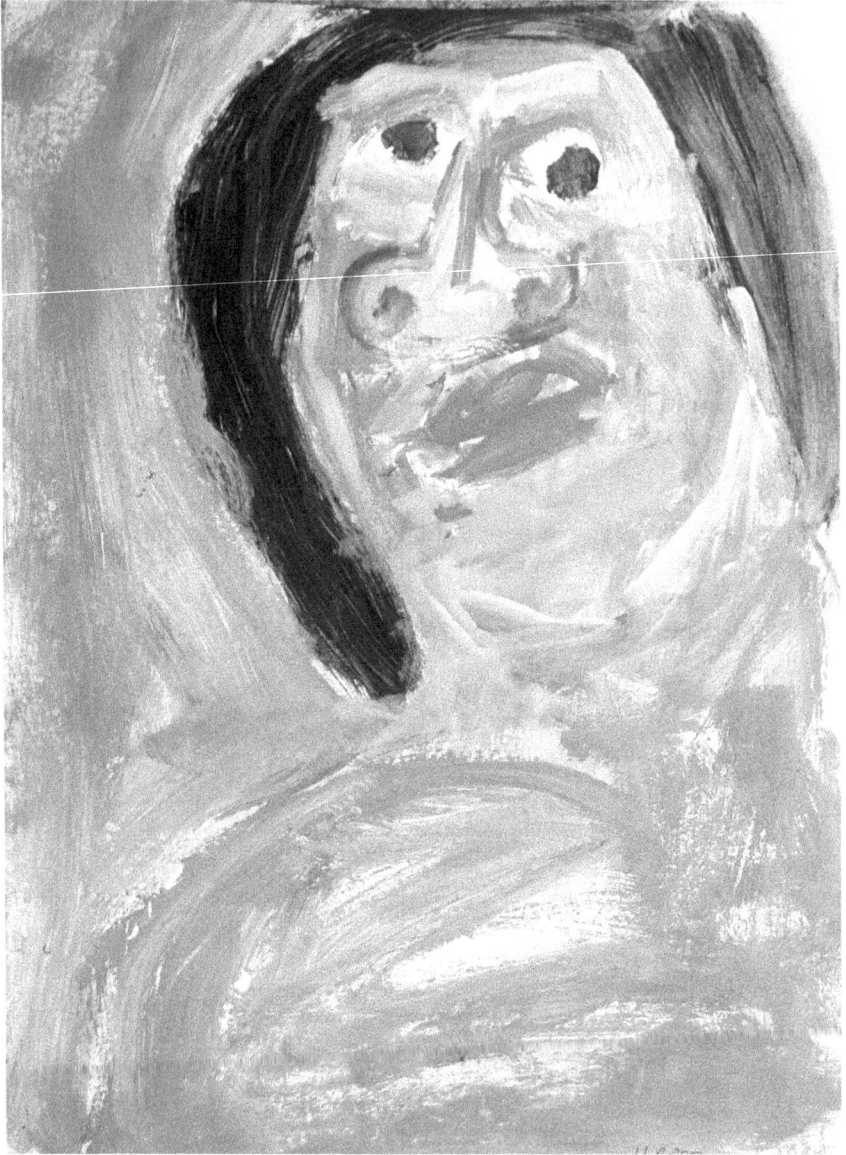

Figure 10.5 Two portraits: a dialog, acrylic on canvas.

admitted to the Intensive Care Unit in the hospital. Henry requested that I visit him, and when I walked into the room he was hooked up to many live-saving machines. He was too weak to talk, so he carefully and slowly wrote out a dialog with me on his laptop. He wrote that he did not want to die; he wanted to live longer because he was not yet done living. Even though his doctors suggested that he stay on the unit, he and his wife decided to go home the next day. On his way out of his hospital bed the following morning, Henry passed away in the presence of his beloved wife.

Without going into the details of this case, I wanted to illustrate that in certain life situations that foster depression, such as living with terminal cancer, depression can be addressed by different psychodynamic treatments. In this case, group art–psychotherapy allowed immediate access to the patient's unconscious, often without needing to express them with words. The group also provided a long-term supportive atmosphere, with patients going through similar cycles of illness, and a close transference relationship to the art-therapist. This example illustrates how long-term, intensive psychodynamic art–psychotherapy, in addition to long-term individual psychotherapy, may help treat depression that results from psychiatric or somatic diagnoses.

Reference

Dreifuss-Kattan, E. (2019): Art, death and mourning: the artist and art-psychotherapist perspective. *Cancer and Creativity: A Psychoanalytic Guide to therapeutic Transformation*, p. 147, Routledge 2019.

Comparative psychotherapy research focused on the treatment of borderline personality disorder

John F. Clarkin, Reed Maxwell, and
Julia F. Sowislo

Introduction

The psychoanalytic community has been extremely reluctant to empirically investigate the impact of their treatments on patient pathology (Kernberg, 2004). Some have argued that there is no need for superficial research methods, that the unconscious is beyond investigation, and that the art of psychotherapy with its intense, unique relationship between two individuals is beyond investigation. Placing the complexity of the individual into a psychiatric diagnosis is seen as too simplistic and lacking in specificity. In addition, the cognoscenti of psychotherapy research, dominated by those who are cognitive-behavioral in orientation, have ignored data from psychodynamic treatment studies falsely complaining at times that there is no data supporting dynamic treatments.

This state of affairs presents a challenge to those who see the need for research on psychoanalytic treatment approaches. If psychoanalytic treatment is to maintain a position of respect and influence in the field of psychotherapy, treatment outcome studies that are persuasive to the scientific community and the general public must be accomplished. In order to be persuasive, studies must meet methodological standards current in the field (Caligor, Roose, Hilsenroth, & Rutherford, 2015). Furthermore, to overcome the psychoanalytic critics who have justified concerns, research methods must be developed to measure complex psychodynamic concepts.

In this chapter, we survey the steps recommended to empirically develop a psychotherapeutic treatment. We have utilized these steps in developing a psychodynamic treatment for patients with borderline personality disorder (BPD) called transference-focused psychotherapy (TFP). This review is followed by a critique of the over-reliance on the randomized clinical trial (RCT) design, leading to our current efforts to go beyond the RCT to understand the complexity of the treatment of severe personality pathology.

Basic concepts and theoretical assumptions shared by all psychodynamic therapies, include a developmental perspective, recognition of unconscious motivation and intentionality, and a focus on the inner world and psychological causality (Caligor, Clarkin, Yeomans, & Kernberg, 2019). In addition, key features of the TFP treatment model for personality pathology include: (1) structuring the treatment with an oral contract, (2) a focus on disturbed interpersonal behaviors both in relationship to the therapist (transference) and in the patients' current daily interactions, (3) utilization of the process of interpretation to examine and modify internal representations of self and others, and (4) real world changes in interpersonal behavior particularly in the areas of work, friendships and intimate/love relations.

In order to participate in the empirical development of treatment for BPD, psychodynamic researchers must overcome a number of issues that provide the foundation for a proper evaluation of the complex approaches of psychodynamic thinking and treatment. This includes the development of instruments to measure the full range of borderline pathology including representations of self and others and related observable behaviors both before and after treatment. It also involves the generation of a treatment manual describing dynamic interventions, and measures of therapist adherence and competence in the treatment. These issues are described in later sections on the steps in treatment development.

Evolving conception of borderline personality pathology

The BPD diagnosis and comorbidities

BPD is one of 11 categorically defined personality disorders (American Psychiatric Association, 2013), identified by criteria focusing on identity and interpersonal dysfunction, impulsivity, and intense anger and other emotions. To complicate matters including the need for a homogeneous group of patients for research, however, there are three important issues that ensure that patients with a BPD diagnosis are a heterogeneous group of individuals. First, one meets the diagnosis on the basis of fulfilling any combination of five to nine criteria. This polythetic method provides many routes to obtain the diagnosis. Second, practically all BPD patients meet criteria for one or more additional personality disorders. For example, the combination of BPD, narcissistic personality disorder, and some antisocial traits is a poor prognostic sign for treatment (Lenzenweger, Clarkin, Cain, & Kernberg, 2018). Finally, there is the issue of BPD and comorbidity with symptom disorders such as depression, eating disorders, and substance abuse. There is a growing recognition that the coexistence of two or more psychiatric disorders is very high as approximately 50% of individuals with one psychiatric disorder meet criteria for a second disorder at the same time (Caspi et al., 2014).

For example, longitudinal studies of severe personality pathology and mood disorders (i.e., major depression and bipolar disorder) provide descriptions of the episodes of mood disturbance on the consistent platform of personality pathology. Patients with major depression relapse more frequently when co-morbid with BPD. Treatment of the personality pathology can lead to decrease in depression but not the other way around (Gunderson et al., 2014).

Emerging conception of core of personality pathology

There is an emerging consensus that the essential features of personality disorder involve difficulties with self-identity and interpersonal dysfunction (Bender & Skodol, 2007; Gunderson & Lyons-Ruth, 2008). This view, long espoused and central to object relations theory (Kernberg, 1984), is now reflected in *DSM-5*, section III (APA, 2013). Personality researchers and clinicians across diverse treatment orientations link self and interpersonal functioning to mental representations referred to by various theoreticians as cognitive affective units (Mischel & Shoda, 2008), schemas (Pretzer & Beck, 2004), internal working models (Bateman & Fonagy, 2006), and interpersonal copies (Benjamin, 2005). In contrast to this general agreement about the importance of mental representations in driving interpersonal behavior, the manner in which psychotherapeutic treatments address these cognitive/affective units varies in important ways.

For example, dialectical behavior therapy (DBT) (Linehan, 1993) uses an instructional approach to help the patient learn and utilize skills related to self-control and interpersonal behavior. Mentalization-based treatment (MBT) (Bateman & Fonagy, 2006) emphasizes the need to temper patient affect in therapy sessions, while also fostering the patients' mentalization or reflective capacities. In contrast, the TFP model of intervention provides a treatment framework that acknowledges the inevitability of affect arousal in a safe setting that provides the opportunity to modify extreme cognitions and related affects in the emotionally "hot" and immediate experience of the other; in this case, the therapist. This approach is consistent with current understandings of the processes in social cognition (Clarkin, Meehan, & Lenzenweger, 2015) and the contribution of brain systems related to the generation of primitive affects (Panksepp & Biven, 2012). The hypothesized mechanism of change in TFP is increased affect regulation achieved through the growing ability of the patient to reflect psychologically and place momentary affect arousal, especially in social interactions, into a more benign integration of emotion, thought and behavior (Levy et al., 2006; Yeomans, Clarkin, & Kernberg, 2015). Patients with personality disorders manifest a combination of both observable behavior that is interpersonally disruptive with internal symbolic representations of self and others that are dominated by sharp division of good and bad evaluations with extremes of affect (Lenzeweger, McClough, Clarkin, & Kernberg, 2012).

Empirical development of psychotherapies
for borderline personality disorder

Borderline patients were originally thought to be untreatable, but a number of specialized treatments such as MBT (Bateman & Fonagy, 2009) and DBT

(McMain et al., 2009), and our own transference-focused psychotherapy (TFP) (Clarkin, Levy, Lenzenweger, & Kernberg, 2007; Doering et al., 2010) have demonstrated significant reductions in symptomatology. A recent review of the meta-analyses of the different treatments for BPD by representatives of TFP, MBT, and DBT conclude that there are no detectable differences between the specialty treatments, and patients treated with these specialty treatments show more improvement than patients treated with treatment as usual (Levy, McMain, Bateman, & Clouthier, 2018). However, after treatment these borderline patients remain without work, on disability, and dysfunctional in friendships and intimate relations. This current state of the field raises two important questions that must be empirically addressed for the field to progress: (1) can psychotherapeutic treatment lead to improvements in social and intimate relations and work functioning, and (2) what are the biological and psychological predictors of potential response to the specific treatments?

Progressive steps in treatment development

The sequential steps in treatment development have been articulated as beginning with conceptualization of the pathology and the treatment approach with manualization of the treatment and training of therapists to adherence and competence (Kazdin, 2007). These initial steps are followed by preliminary data on the impact of the treatment followed by a randomized clinical trial demonstrating the effects of the treatment as compared to that of a control or comparison treatment. Final steps in the process include assessing the impact of moderators and mediators of change and generalization of the treatment to settings other than that of the initial demonstration site.

Object relations conceptualization of pathology and treatment

We have described previously the problems with the categorical diagnosis of BPD, resulting in a very heterogeneous group of individuals. In contrast to the DSM approach, object relations theory combines dimensions of severity of pathology and affiliation (introversion vs. extraversion) and allows for a categorical or prototypic classification of personality pathology across three levels of personality organization (Kernberg & Caligor, 2005). Each of the three levels of personality organization are characterized by different levels of identity, quality of object relations, defensive functioning, aggression, and moral values. Briefly, high level or neurotic personality organization is characterized by good identity formation but with compromised and conflicted quality of object relations. Borderline organization is marked by identity diffusion and compromised quality of object relations. Low level borderline organization is further invaded by aggression and variable moral functioning.

Patients with a DSM diagnosis of BPD can be found in the borderline organization range or in the low-level borderline organization. This approach has the advantage of utilizing both the severity of personality pathology and affiliation (interpersonal relatedness) while accommodating categories of personality organization extending from high (neurotic organization) to mid or borderline organization to severe or low-level borderline organization for treatment planning and application. This typology has received initial empirical support (Lenzenweger, Clarkin, Yeomans, Kernberg, & Levy, 2008) and replication (Yun, Stern, Lenzenweger, & Tiersky, 2013; Hallquist & Pilkonis, 2012), suggesting that the subtypes may be important to guide further efforts to understand underlying endophenotypes and genotypes and to guide treatment.

In order to assess these levels of personality organization, we developed a semi-structured interview, the Structured Interview for Personality Organization (STIPO) (Horz-Sagstetter, Caligor, Preti, Stern, & De Panfilis, 2017) and its recent revision, the STIPO-R (Clarkin, Caligor, Stern, & Kernberg, 2016). As described by current object relations theory, there are five domains of functioning assessed and rated in the STIPO-R: identity (capacity to invest in work and recreation, sense of self, sense of others), quality of object relations (interpersonal relations, intimate relations and sexuality, internal working models of relationships), defenses, aggression (self-directed and other-directed), and moral values. The STIPO has good psychometric properties including internal consistency (Stern et al., 2010; Doering et al., 2013) and construct validity (Doering et al., 2013; Preti, Punas, Sarno et al., 2012). Whereas there is a significant association between STIPO structural characteristics and *DSM* diagnoses, the STIPO domains were able to statistically identify treatment dropout among dual-diagnosis patients more effectively than personality disorder diagnoses (Preti, Rottoli, Dainese Di Pierro, Rancati, & Madeddu, 2015) suggesting that the levels of personality organization may be more clinically useful than DSM diagnoses.

In contrast to cognitive-behavioral treatments that design psychotherapy manuals specifying the same treatment modules for all patients, we have developed a principle-driven treatment manual in order to adapt the treatment principles to a heterogeneous group of patients with personality pathology. TFP was first described in manual form (Clarkin, Yeomans, & Kernberg, 1999), expanded and refined with extensive clinical experience (Clarkin, Yeomans, & Kernberg, 2006), and recently explicated with illustrative case examples (Yeomans et al., 2015). The treatment manuals were developed by studying in detail video-recordings of senior therapists treating borderline patients, distilling the treatment principles, and illustrating the application of the principles by clinical vignettes. After attending seminars on the treatment and its manual, the prospective TFP therapist is supervised on several video-recorded cases that are rated for adherence and competence by the instrument we have developed.

Impact of the treatment under development

Funded by a NIMH treatment development grant, we demonstrated significant impact of TFP on patients with a BPD diagnosis delivered in a one-year treatment episode with sessions two times a week (Clarkin, Foelsch, Levy, Hull, Delaney, & Kernberg, 2001). In comparison to the year prior to the year of TFP, borderline patients showed significant reduction in dangerousness of self-destructive behavior and lowering of health care costs by fewer emergency room visits and days of hospitalization.

The significant positive impact of TFP without harm to patients in this treatment development study led to two randomized controlled trials. An RCT conducted in New York City compared the impact of one year of TFP to DBT and a psychodynamic supportive treatment (Clarkin et al., 2007). Whereas significant symptom change was found in all three treatments, TFP was superior in the reduction of anger, verbal and direct assault, and irritability. This study was followed by an RCT comparing the impact of TFP to that of expert therapists in the community in a multi-site study in Munich, Germany, and Vienna, Austria (Doering et al., 2010). TFP was superior in terms of symptom change and changes in personality functioning, thus showing the impact of TFP and its generalization to settings other than the original site of development in New York.

Approaches to moderators and mediators

The fact that TFP is effective still leaves open the question of how does TFP have its impact, i.e., what are the mechanisms of change conceptualized as the relationship of techniques used by the TFP therapist with changes in patient functioning (Crits-Christoph, Gibbons, & Mukherjee, 2013). The TFP model of change can be conceptualized in five steps. **Step 1:** the BPD patient comes to treatment with serious difficulties in work and professional life and friendship/intimacy with others in her life. This dysfunctional state of development is directly related to the patient's internal representations of self and others infused with a preponderance of negative over positive affect and lack of effortful control in modulating affect in daily interpersonal interactions. **Step 2:** the focus of TFP is on the interaction, i.e., patient transference patterns with therapist. TFP provides a structured environment in which these transferences pattern, a window on the patient's internal representations of self and others, can be expressed, fully amplified in the relationship, and interpreted by the therapist. **Step 3:** the patient who is emotionally involved with the therapist and is open to the feedback from the therapist begins to change in her attitude and behavior toward the therapist. This is occurring as the transference pattern progresses from a paranoid mistrustful attitude toward a more positive and receptive attitude. **Step 4:** changes in the transference pattern toward the therapist are internalized by the patient, and the patient tries out new attitudes and behavior toward others in her daily environment. In the most beneficial situations, these changes in the patient's internal representations and interpersonal behavior are met with positive responses from others in the environment. **Step 5:** the patient's more positive interactions with others in the environment begins to result in more positive interactions in work and professional relationships. This is sometimes experienced by the patient with both pleasure in resuming development in life and sadness about time lost. More difficult is the step of engaging in intimate relations with selected others.

As described below, we have made a number of attempts to understand the process of change. This includes connecting pre-treatment patient characteristics and the process of change, examining disruptions in the alliance, increase in patients' reflective capacity, and changes in brain functioning connected to emotion regulation.

Pre-treatment patient characteristics and process of change

By utilizing the rates of change for each subject across multiple indicators of psychological and personality functioning in a randomized clinical trial of BPD patients, we explored the latent structure of these indicators and resolved three domains of change (aggressive dyscontrol, social adjustment/self-acceptance, and conflict tolerance/behavioral control) (Lenzenweger et al., 2012). Pre-treatment patient characteristics such as negative affectivity, identity diffusion, and social potency predicted the rates of change in these domains.

An examination of the patient–therapist interaction in psychotherapy for BPD patients reveals that patient executive attention is related to the quality of the therapeutic alliance, and this relationship is mediated by in-session mental state vacillations (i.e., rapid shifts in the perception of others, consistent with identity diffusion) made in the patient's discourse (Levy, Beeney, & Clarkin, 2010).

Our psychodynamic colleagues (Bateman & Fonagy, 2006) have postulated that the capacity for mentalization is a protective factor against developing severe personality pathology, and that the essence of treatment for BPD patients is an increase in mentalization. "Mentalization" in the general sense of the term overlaps with related concepts such as mindfulness, empathy, and affect consciousness and is difficult to measure (Choi-Kain & Gunderson, 2008). In a more precise definition the increase of the patient's ability to reflect and place momentary conceptions of self and others into perspective during "hot," emotional contexts is essential for smooth and satisfying relations with others. In this regard, an increase in mentalization through the use of interpretive techniques in TFP (Kernberg, 2018) is hypothesized as a mechanism of change in TFP. We have found in two RCTs that patients in

TFP demonstrate significant improvements in attachment representations and reflective functioning as compared to other treatments (Buchheim & Diamond, 2018).

Neurobiological changes in TFP

In a pilot study of ten BPD patients treated with TFP for one year, we hypothesized that as the patient experiences dominant object relations infused with negative and intense affect in the TFP sessions, the gradual analysis of the perception of self and others would modify extreme cognitive/affective perceptions (Perez et al., 2015). These changes would be consistent with enhanced modification of responses in the amygdala by the prefrontal cortex. These patients exhibited significant change in behavioral and psychological domains over the course of 1-year of TFP including a reduction in affective lability, interpersonal sensitivity, and paranoia. Importantly, at the end of the treatment, all patients in the study were employed in an occupation, displaying significant positive changes in work functioning.

In a comparison of pre-treatment and post-treatment fMRI scans, BPD patients manifested relative increased activation in cognitive control regions (right anterior-dorsal anterior cingulate cortex (ACC) and right dorsal-lateral prefrontal cortex (PFC) and relative decreased activation in the left inferior frontal gyrus and the left hippocampus. In addition, results showed that improvements in self-reported cognitive control over the course of one-year of TFP correlated positively with left anterior-dorsal ACC activation, while improvements in self-reported affective lability over one-year of TFP correlated positively with left posterior medial orbitofrontal cortex (OFC)/ventral striatum activation and correlated negatively with right amygdala/parahippocampal cortex activation. Finally, improvements in clinician-rated aggression over one year of TFP correlated positively with activation in the left inferior frontal gyrus. Taken together, these results suggest that treatment with TFP was associated with relative activation increases in emotional and cognitive control areas of the brain and relative activation decreases in areas of the brain associated with emotional reactivity and semantic-based memory retrieval.

Critique of existing empirical development of treatments for BPD

The empirical development of treatments for BPD has been dominated by the randomized clinical trial design. This focus has led to multiple trials that compare the treatment of interest to various levels of contrasting treatment including treatment as usual and some form of structured clinical management. Treatment outcome in these studies is usually limited to reduction in symptoms and/or BPD criteria. The randomized clinical trial (RCT) for psychotherapy research may be a method that provides some information about comparative effects of different treatments but is limited in its ability to provide more fine-grained information.

An effective RCT demands a homogeneous sample of patients. The field has used DSM diagnoses to choose a supposedly homogeneous sample of individuals. However, it has become clear that selecting a homogeneous sample using individual personality disorder diagnoses such as borderline personality disorder (BPD) does not have conceptual or practical usefulness. A second major factor in the RCT design is the requirement of a homogeneous intervention or therapy. Unlike a medication that is the same in every pill, therapists are not homogeneous and have varying abilities to relate to patients that are not captured in the treatment techniques as described in treatment manuals. It is known that therapist effects are a powerful predictor of outcome (Wampold, 2015). Different therapists not only relate differently, they also differ in their skill and ability to move patients along a trajectory of clinical improvement. Even if one were to successfully design a psychotherapy study in which a homogeneous sample of patients are exposed to a uniform treatment, a remaining issue is how the results would generalize to the more heterogeneous world of clinical practice. In ordinary clinical practice, patients present with multiple difficulties in the content of a wide range of personality functioning and environmental assets and liabilities. We are suggesting that the likelihood of the RCT model to produce useful knowledge varies from a specific symptom disorder matched with a standardized behavior treatment to the treatment of personality pathology that is not captured by a DSM diagnosis treated with a principle driven treatment such as TFP, MBT, or GPM.

Expanding the utilization of TFP principles

TFP was developed with the specific aim of treating patients with the diagnosis of BPD as described in *DSM-III* and its successors. However, given the self and interpersonal dysfunctions that extend across the personality disorder categories, we are currently applying the strategies and techniques of TFP to the entire range of personality pathology. The large general factor of personality pathology (Sharp et al , 2015) consistent with our clinical experience and the theoretical articulation of borderline personality organization has led us to articulate the strategies of object relations treatment across high, mid, and lower levels of personality organization (Caligor, Kernberg, Clarkin, & Yeomans, 2018).

In our current research efforts we are examining the impact of TFP delivered over 18 months duration on female borderline patients with careful diagnostic evaluation of their BPD diagnosis, co-morbid conditions, and level of personality organization. We are examining the trajectory of change in not only symptoms but most specifically functioning in work, friendships, and intimate relations. We are using an intensive design, with careful monitoring of patient pathology and functioning every three months during the treatment episode. We are using two novel methods of assessing patient change. In an effort to examine the generalization of patient changes in the transference patterns to changes in daily life, we are using an electronic diary method referred to as ecological momentary assessment (EMA; Trull, Ebner-Priemer, Brown, Tonko, & Scheiderer, 2012). The patient reports on daily interactions with others, including perceptions of self and others and related affects, in three waves of 14 days reporting. In addition, we are using fMRI assessment of affect regulation before and after the 18 months of treatment, further examining the results we found in our pilot study reported above.

There is a healthy tension between the clinical approach that focuses on the individual patient in his/her particular environment, and the psychotherapy research perspective that emphasizes treatment effects on a large group of individuals selected by diagnosis and treated by a defined and manualized intervention assumed to be uniform across different therapists and different patients. In this current study, as we did in our RCT (Clarkin et al., 2007), we are using statistical procedures that allow us to track changes specific to each individual in addition to changes in the sample as a whole.

TFP can be delivered in the individual treatment format with sessions two times a week during a treatment duration of one year or more as it has been empirically examined. However, there are local environmental conditions that may preclude this ideal delivery of TFP. Many national health care systems do not allow funding for treatment two times a week, and we are investigating the impact of TFP with once-a-week sessions in the United Kingdom, Spain, and Italy. In addition, TFP is being used in a group treatment format in hospital settings. The principles of TFP have been found to be useful in medical settings (Hersh, Caligor, & Yeomans, 2016) with patients who are resistant to the usual delivery of medical procedures.

Conclusion: what have we learned?

TFP is a theory-driven, manualized, intensive (sessions two times a week for a treatment duration of one year or more), and empirically supported treatment that was originally developed for patients with the diagnosis of borderline personality disorder (BPD). The aim of TFP is to effect change in both symptoms and interpersonal difficulties through structured psychological care that leads to the modification of patients' mental representations of self and other that guide behavior. The most recent development is to recognize the large general factor of personality pathology across the personality disorders (Sharp et al., 2015) and expand TFP to a transdiagnostic treatment for different levels of severity of personality pathology (Caligor et al., 2018).

Combining a clinical focus on patients with various levels of personality pathology with research aims and instruments has refined our thinking and forced us to attend to details of patient pathology and treatment nuances.

With the use of multiple pre-treatment assessment methods, we have refined our understanding of the heterogeneity of patients with the BPD diagnosis. There is considerable treatment relevant variation in the balance of positive and negative affect, level of narcissism, modulation of aggression, and moral functioning. Over time, our approach to the treatment has led to a balance between attention to the in-session transference and attention to the patients' current activities in daily interactions and work. We have also amplified our focus on patient motivation for and personal goals in treatment as a prerequisite for intense involvement in psychodynamic treatment of two times a week over a treatment duration of a year or more. We have become much more sophisticated in training therapists to both adherence and competence in TFP, as well as the application of the treatment tailored to the idiosyncrasies of the individual patient.

References

American Psychiatric Association. (2013). *Diagnostic and statistical manual of mental disorders* (5th ed.). Washington, DC: Author.

Bateman, A., & Fonagy, P. (2006). *Mentalization-based treatment for borderline personality disorder.* Oxford, UK: Oxford University Press.

Bateman, A., & Fonagy, P. (2009). Randomized controlled trial of outpatient mentalization-based treatment versus structured clinical management for borderline personality disorder. *American Journal of Psychiatry, 166*(12), 1355–1364.

Bender, D.S., & Skodol, A.E. (2007). Borderline personality as self-other representational disturbance, *Journal of Personality Disorders, 21*(5), 500–517.

Benjamin, L.S. (2005). Interpersonal theory of personality disorders: The structural analysis of social behavior and interpersonal reconstructive therapy. In M.F. Lenzenweger & J.F. Clarkin (Eds.), *Major theories of personality disorder* (2nd ed., pp. 157–230). New York, NY: Guilford.

Buchheim, A., & Diamond, D. (2018). Attachment and borderline personality disorder. *Psychiatric Clinics of North America, 41*(4), 651–668.

Caligor, E., Roose, S., Hilsenroth, M., & Rutherford, R. (2015). Developing a protocol design for an outcome study of psychoanalysis. *Psychoanalytic Inquiry, 35*(1), 150–168.

Caligor, E., Kernberg, O.F., Clarkin, J.F., & Yeomans, F.E. (2018). *Psychodynamic therapy for personality pathology: Treating self and interpersonal functioning.* Washington, DC: American Psychiatric Association Publishing.

Caligor, E., Clarkin, J.F., Yeomans, F.E., & Kernberg, O.F. (2019). Psychodynamic psychotherapy. In Laura Weiss Roberts (Ed.), *American Psychiatric Association textbook of psychiatry* (7th ed.). Washington, DC: American Psychiatric Association Publishing.

Caspi, A., Houts, R.M., Belsky, D.W., Goldman-Mellor, S.J., Harrington, H.L, Israel, S., Meier, M.H., Ramrakha, S., Shalev, I., Poulton, R., & Moffitt, T.E. (2014). The p factor: One general psychopathology factor in the structure of psychiatric disorders? *Clinical Psychological Science, 2*(2), 119–137.

Choi-Kain, L., & Gunderson, J.G. (2008). Mentalization: Ontogeny, assessment, and application in the treatment of borderline personality disorder. *American Journal of Psychiatry, 165(9),* 1127–1135.

Clarkin, J.F., Foelsch, P.A., Levy, K.N., Hull, J.W., Delaney, J.C., & Kernberg, O.F. (2001). The development of a psychodynamic treatment for patients with borderline personality disorder: A preliminary study of behavioral change. *Journal of Personality Disorder, 15(6),* 487–495.

Clarkin, J.F., Caligor, E., Stern, B., & Kernberg, O.F. (2016). *The Structured Interview for Personality Organization-Revised (STIPO-R).* Unpublished manuscript, Department of Psychiatry, Weill Cornell Medical College, NY, New York.

Clarkin, J.F., Levy, K.N., Lenzenweger, M.F., & Kernberg, O.F. (2007). Evaluating three treatments for borderline personality disorder: A multiwave study. *American Journal of Psychiatry, 164(6),* 922–928.

Clarkin, J.F., Yeomans, F.E., & Kernberg, O.F. (1999). *Psychotherapy for borderline personality.* New York, NY: Wiley.

Clarkin, J.F., Foelsch, P.A., Levy, K.N., Hull, J.W., Delaney, J.C., & Kernberg, O.F. (2001). The development of a psychodynamic treatment for patients with borderline personality disorder: A preliminary study of behavioral change. *Journal of Personality Disorders, 15(6),* 487–495.

Clarkin, J.F., Yeomans, F.E., & Kernberg, O.F. (2006). *Psychotherapy for borderline disorder: Focusing on object relations.* Washington, DC: American Psychiatric Publishing.

Clarkin, J.F., Meehan, K.B., & Lenzenweger, M.F. (2015). Emerging approaches to the conceptualization and treatment of personality disorder. *Canadian Psychology, 56(2),* 155–167.

Crits-Christoph, P., Connolly Gibbons, M.B., & Mukherjee, D. (2013). Psychotherapy process-outcome research. In: M.J. Lambert (Ed.), *Bergin and Garfield's handbook of psychotherapy and behavior change* (6th ed., pp. 298–340). Hoboken, NJ: Wiley & Sons, pp. 298–340.

Doering, S., Horz, S., Rentrop, M., Fischer-Kern, M., Schuster, P., Benecke, C., Buchheim, A., Martius, P., & Buchheim, P. (2010). Transference-focused psychotherapy versus treatment by community psychotherapists for borderline personality disorder: Randomized controlled trial. *British Journal of Psychiatry, 196(5),* 389–395.

Doering, S., Burgmer, M., Heuft, G., Menke, D., Baumer, B., Lubking, M., Feldmann, M., Horz, S., & Schneider, G. (2013). Reliability and validity of the German version of the Structured Interview of Personality Organization (STIPO). *BMC Psychiatry, 13,* 2010–223.

Gunderson, J.G., & Lyons-Ruth, K. (2008). BPD's interpersonal hypersensitivity phenotype. *Journal of Personality Disorders, 22(1),* 22–41.

Gunderson, J.G., Stout, R.L., Shea, M.T., Grilo, C.M., Markowitz, J.C., Morey, L.C., Sanislow, C., Yen, S., Zanarini, M.C., Keuroghlian, A.S., McGlashan, T.H., Skodol, A.E. (2014). Interactions of borderline personality disorder and mood disorders over 10 years. *Journal of Clinical Psychiatry, 75(8),* 829–834.

Hallquist, M.N., & Pilkonis, P.A. (2012). Refining the phenotype of borderline personality disorder: Diagnostic criteria and beyond. *Journal of Personality Disorders, 3(3),* 228–246.

Hersh, R.G., Caligor, E., & Yeomans, F.E. (2016). *Fundamentals of transference-focused psychotherapy: Applications in psychiatric and medical settings*. Cham, Switzerland: Springer International Publishing.

Horz-Sagstetter, S., Caligor, E., Preti, E., Stern, B., De Panfilis, C., & Clarkin, J.F. (2018). Clinician-guided assessment of personality using the structural interview and the Structured Interview of Personality Organization (STIPO). *Journal of Personality Assessment*, 100(1), 30–42.

Kazdin, A.E. (2007). Mediators and mechanisms of change in psychotherapy research. *Annual Review of Clinical Psychology*, 3, 1–27.

Kernberg, O.F. (1984). *Severe personality disorders: Psychotherapeutic strategies*. New Haven, CT: Yale University Press.

Kernberg, O.F (2004). *Contemporary controversies in psychoanalytic theory, technique, and their applications*. New Haven, CT: Yale University Press.

Kernberg, O.F. (2018). *Treatment of severe personality disorders: Resolution of aggression and recovery of eroticism*. Washington, DC: American Psychiatric Association Publishing.

Kernberg, O.F., & Caligor, E. (2005). A psychoanalytic theory of personality disorders. In M.F. Lenzenweger & J.F. Clarkin (Eds.), *Major theories of personality disorder* (2nd ed., pp. 114–156). New York, NY: Guilford Press.

Lenzenweger, M.F., Clarkin, J.F., Levy, K.N., Yeomans, F.E., & Kernberg, O.F. (2012). Predicting domains and rates of change in borderline personality disorder. *Personality Disorders: Theory, Research, and Treatment*, 3(2), 185–195.

Lenzenweger, M.F., Clarkin, J.F., Yeomans, F.E., Kernberg, O.F., & Levy, K.N. (2008). Refining the borderline personality disorder phenotype through finite mixture modeling: Implications for classification. *Journal of Personality Disorders*, 22(4), 313–331.

Lenzenweger, M.F., McClough, J.F., Clarkin, J.F., Kernberg, O.F. (2012). Exploring the interface of neurobehaviorally linked personality dimensions and personality organization in borderline personality disorder: The Multidimensional Personality Questionnaire and Inventory of Personality Organization. *Journal of Personality Disorders*, 26(6), 902–918.

Lenzenweger, M.F., Clarkin, J.F., Cain, N.M., & Kernberg, O.F. (2018). Malignant narcissism in relation to clinical change in borderline personality disorder. *Psychopathology*, 51(5), 318–325.

Levy, K.N., Beeney, J.E., & Clarkin, J.F. (2010). Conflict begets conflict: Executive control, mental state vacillations, and the therapeutic alliance in treatment of borderline personality disorder. *Psychotherapy Research*, 20(1), 413–422.

Levy, K.N., Meehan, K., Kelly, K., Reynoso, J., Weber, M., Clarkin, J.F., & Kernberg, O.F (2006). Change in attachment patterns and reflective function in a randomized control trial of transference-focused psychotherapy for borderline personality disorder. *Journal of Consulting and Clinical Psychology*, 74(6), 1027–1040.

Levy, K.N., McMain, S., Bateman, A., & Clouther, T. (2018). Treatment of borderline personality disorder. *Psychiatric Clinics of North America*, 41(4), 711–728.

Linehan, M.M. (1993). *Cognitive-behavioral treatment of borderline personality disorder*. New York, NY: Guilford.

McMain, S.F., Links, P.S., Gnam, W.H., Guimond, T., Cardish, R.J., Korman, L., & Streiner, D.L. (2009). A randomized trial of dialectical behavior therapy versus general psychiatric management for borderline personality disorder. *American Journal of Psychiatry*, *166*(*12*), 1365–1374.

Mischel, W., & Shoda, Y. (2008). Toward a unified theory of personality: Integrating dispositions and processing dynamics within the cognitive-affective processing system. In O.P. John, R.W. Robins, & L.A. Pervin (Eds.), *Handbook of personality: Theory and research* (3rd ed., pp. 208–241). New York, NY: Guilford.

Panksepp, J., & Biven, L. (2012). *The archaeology of mind: Neuroevolutionary origins of human emotions*. New York, NY: WW Norton.

Perez, D., Vago, D., Pan, H., Root, J., Tuescher, O., Fuchs, B., Leung, L., Epstein, J., Cain, N., Clarkin, J.F., Lenzenweger, M.F., Kernberg, O.F., Levy, K.N., Silbersweig, D.A., & Stern, E. (2015). Frontolimbic neural circuit changes in emotional processing and inhibitory control associated with clinical improvement following transference-focused psychotherapy in borderline personality disorder. *Psychiatry and Clinical Neurosciences*, *70*(*1*), 51–61.

Preti, E., Prunas, A., Sarno, I., & De Panfilis, C. (2012). Proprietà psicometriche della STIPO [Psychometric properties of the STIPO]. In: F. Madeddu & E. Preti (Eds.), *La diagnosi strutturale di personalità secondo il modello di O.F. Kernberg. La versione italiana della Structured Interview of Personality Organization* (pp. 59–84). Milan, Italy: Raffaello Cortina.

Preti, E., Rottoli, C., Dainese, S., Di Pierro, R., Rancati, F., Madeddu, F. (2015). Personality structure features associated with early dropout in patients with substance-related disorders and comorbid personality disorders. *International Journal of Mental Health and Addiction*, *13*(*4*), 536–547.

Pretzer, J.L., & Beck, A.T. (2004). A cognitive theory of personality disorders. In M.F. Lenzenweger & J.F. Clarkin (Eds.), *Major theories of personality disorder* (2nd ed, pp. 36–105). New York, NY: Guilford.

Sharp, C., Wright, A., Fowler, J., Frueh, B., Allen, J., Oldham, J., Clark, L. (2015). The structure of personality pathology: Both general ('g') and specific ('s') factors? *Journal of Abnormal Psychology*, *124*(*2*), 387–398.

Stern, B.L., Caligor, E., Clarkin, J.F., Critchfield, C., Horz, S., Maccornack, V., Lenzenweger, M.F., & Kernberg, O.F. (2010). Structured Interview of Personality Organization (STIPO): Preliminary psychometrics in a clinical sample. *Journal of Personality Assessment*, *92*(*1*), 35–44.

Trull, T.J., Ebner-Priemer, U.W., Brown, W.C., Tonko, R.I, & Scheiderer, E.M. (2012). Clinical psychology. In M.R. Mehl & T.S. Connor (Eds.), *Handbook of research methods for studying daily life* (pp. 620–635). New York, NY: Guilford Press.

Wampold, B.E. (2015). How important are the common factors in psychotherapy? An update. *World psychiatry*, *14*(*3*), 270–277.

Yeomans, F., Clarkin, J.F., Kernberg, O.F. (2015). *Transference-focused psychotherapy for borderline personality disorder: A clinician's guide*. Washington, DC: American Psychiatric Publishing.

Yun, R.J., Stern, B.L., Lenzenweger, M.F, Tiersky, L.A. (2013). Refining personality disorders subtypes and classification using finite mixture modeling. *Journal of Personality Disorders*, *4*(*2*), 121–128.

Chapter 12

Memory reconsolidation, emotional arousal and the process of change in psychoanalysis

Richard D. Lane

Introduction

It is an honor and privilege to contribute to this volume on outcome research and the future of psychoanalysis. For many years, and for understandable reasons, the field of psychoanalysis advanced primarily by linking careful clinical observations with sophisticated clinical theorizing. Relative to other psychotherapy modalities there was a strong preference for viewing "experience distant" objective clinical research as unnecessary or even unhelpful and, as such, the field stood as an outlier relative to other modalities in mainstream clinical psychology (Bornstein, 2001). More recently the need for such research has become evident if it is to survive in this era in which third party payers rely on outcome data to make decisions about reimbursement for care. Several excellent contributions by authors in this volume (e.g., Leichsenring & Rabung, 2008; Shedler, 2010) have demonstrated that psychodynamic psychotherapy and psychoanalysis (hereafter referred to as PDT) are indeed very effective. Within this context of competition and external scrutiny, it is important to be able to explain both how PDT fits into the wide range of modalities available and what PDT offers that distinguishes it from other approaches. To do so I will present a recent theory of change in psychotherapy based on advances in neuroscience that applies to all major psychotherapy modalities and will explain from that vantage point what PDT offers that may make it the treatment of choice under certain circumstances.

In a recent paper in Behavioral and Brain Sciences (BBS) (Lane et al., 2015a), my colleagues and I put forward the idea that enduring change in all psychotherapy modalities that bring about enduring change do so through reconsolidation of emotional memories. The fundamental advance that made this theory possible is the discovery that memories become labile or malleable whenever they are recalled and that information made available when the memories are in the labile state can be incorporated into the original memory in a process called memory reconsolidation (Nadel, Samsonovich, Ryan & Moscovitch, 2000; Elsey et al., 2018). We further proposed that emotion was the key ingredient in this updating process. As such, this theory was consistent with Freud's concept that patients "suffered from reminiscences" (Freud, 1910) as well as the central role that affect has played in psychoanalytic models of the mind and treatment since its inception (Freud, 1895; Spezzano, 1993).

Emotion is a particularly potent way to update memories because synaptic plasticity, which is the molecular basis for encoding memories, is enhanced by the neurotransmitters and hormones (e.g., norepinephrine, cortisol) that are activated by emotional arousal (Schwabe et al., 2012). As such, emotion makes otherwise neutral events more likely to be remembered, and, to the extent that emotional experiences were activated at the time of an event, those experiences constitute critical information that is incorporated into the memory of that episode. Any given event is encoded in memory in multiple ways corresponding to the modalities activated at the time (e.g., sight, sound, movement) (Schacter, Wagner and Buckner, 2000) and emotion is one such modality that can be updated. Moreover, memories are stored and retrieved in a mood congruent fashion (Bower, 1981). For example, when in a happy mood, happy memories are more likely to be recalled; when in a depressed mood, memories related to sadness and loss are more likely to be recalled. This intimate relation between emotion and memory may lie at the heart of the utility of the free association method.

In the BBS paper (Lane et al., 2015a) we proposed that the three essential ingredients for enduring change in psychotherapy, which apply to PDT as well as other modalities, are: (1) reactivating old memories whether through explicit recall or reminders, as well as activating the "old" (usually painful) affect associated with those old memories; (2) engaging in new emotional experiences during treatment that are incorporated into those reactivated memories via the process of reconsolidation; and (3) reinforcing the updated memory by practicing new ways of behaving and experiencing the world in a variety of contexts. These three ingredients have come to be known as the "LRNG Model" of change based on this first initials of the last names of the paper's authors (Lane, Ryan, Nadel, and Greenberg). This acronym also captures the notion that enduring change in psychotherapy involves a particular type of "learning" that involves interactions between emotion and memory as well as between different types of memory.

In the BBS paper we also introduced the "integrated memory model," which states that whenever episodic memory, semantic memory, or emotion are activated, the other two are activated as well. Our theory of change holds that what distinguishes between different psychotherapy modalities is how access is gained to the "integrated memory model." Thus, PDT preferentially enters this interactive matrix through episodic memories, whereas cognitive-behavioral therapy, for example, preferentially enters it through semantic memories and associated thoughts. The idea here is that new emotional experiences in psychotherapy contribute to the episodic memory of that episode, which interact with and potentially modify semantic memory or generalizable knowledge corresponding to the recurrent pattern that is the focus of treatment.

In the next sections I will review relevant advances in the neurosciences with regard to memory reconsolidation, the interaction between episodic and semantic memory, implicit emotion, emotion-memory interactions in the context of emotional trauma and the process of change. Following this I will then discuss how this model applies to PDT and how it helps to explain what PDT uniquely offers.

Memory reconsolidation

Memory consolidation refers to the transformation of memory from short (temporary) to long term (enduring). The traditional view of memory consolidation suggests that immediately after learning there is a period of time during which the memory is fragile and labile, but that after sufficient time has passed, the memory is more or less permanent. During this consolidation period, it is possible to disrupt the formation of the memory, but once the time window has passed, the memory may be modified or inhibited, but not eliminated. In contrast, multiple trace theory (MTT), a relatively new innovation in memory research, suggests that every time a memory is retrieved, the underlying memory trace once again enters into a fragile and labile state, and thus requires another consolidation period, referred to as "reconsolidation" (Nadel, Samsonovich, Ryan, & Moscovitch, 2000). The reconsolidation period provides an additional opportunity to amend or, under appropriate circumstances, even disrupt access to the memory.

MTT proposes that each time an episodic memory is recollected or retrieved, a new encoding is elicited, leading to an expanded representation or memory trace that makes the details of the event more accessible and more likely to be successfully retrieved in the future. This process is primarily initiated by active retrieval or recollection, although off-line reactivation that occurs during sleep and indirect reminder-induced reactivation can also trigger it (Hupbach, Gomez, Hardt & Nadel, 2007; Nadel, Campbell & Ryan, 2007; Wilson & McNaughton, 1994; Hardt, Einarsson & Nader, 2010). Critically, each time an event is recollected and re-encoded, an updated trace is created that incorporates information from the old trace, but now includes elements of the new retrieval episode itself the recollective experience—resulting in traces that are both strengthened and altered. This altered trace may incorporate additional components of the context of retrieval as well as new relevant information pertaining to the original memory. In this regard, MTT holds that memories are not a perfect record of the original event, but undergo revision and reshaping as memories age and, importantly, are recollected. The reconsolidation process, by this view, results in memories that are not just stabilized and strengthened, but are also qualitatively altered by the recollective experience.

This dynamic interplay between retrieval of the memory and reconsolidation has been demonstrated experimentally both in animals and humans. Animal studies have shown that well-established, supposedly consolidated, memories can be disrupted after reactivation (Nader, Schafe & Le Doux, 2000), even when that reactivation is nothing more than a reminder of the spatial context of the original event.

In discussing memory reconsolidation it is important to distinguish it from the behavioral phenomenon of extinction. Reconsolidation is assumed to actually change components of the reactivated memory, whereas extinction is assumed to merely create a new memory that over-rides the previously trained response (Milad & Quirk, 2002). Thus, an "extinguished" response is not really gone, since it can spontaneously recover over time, or be reinstated if the organism is exposed to a relevant cue in a new context. Recent work has shown that the cellular/molecular cascades in these two cases are different, and that whether reconsolidation or extinction is initiated depends upon the temporal dynamics of the test procedure, and how recently the memory in question was formed and/or reactivated (de la Fuente, Freudenthal & Romano, 2011; Inda, Muravieva & Alberini, 2011; Maren, 2011).

In humans, Hupbach and colleagues (2007; Hupbach, Hardt, Gomez & Nadel, 2008) have shown that when memories are reactivated through reminders, they are open to modification through the presentation of similar material that then becomes incorporated into the original event memory. Using a simple interference paradigm, Hupbach et al. (2007) had participants learn a set of objects during the first session. Forty-eight hours later, participants were either reminded of the first session or not and immediately afterward learned a second set of objects. Another 48 hours later, they were asked to recall the first set of objects only, that is, the objects they learned during the first session. Participants in the "reminder" condition showed a high number of intrusions from the subsequently learned object set, while those who had not been reminded showed almost no intrusions. The results demonstrated that updating of pre-existing memories can occur in humans, and that this updating is dependent upon reactivation of the original memory. Hupbach et al. (2008) subsequently showed that reminders of the spatial context of the original event were the most effective in triggering the incorporation of new information into the existing memory.

Episodic and semantic memory

Episodic and semantic memory seem, at least phenomenologically, quite different from one another. Episodic or autobiographical recollection involves thinking about a past event—it is personal, emotional, imbued with detail, temporally and spatially unique, and it often has great relevance to our sense of self and the meaning of our lives. Semantic memory, on the other hand, has to do with the knowledge and rules governing behavior that have been acquired through a lifetime of experiences—it is factual, and typically devoid of emotion or reference to the self, or specific times and places. While semantic knowledge conveys meanings, it is rarely the kind of personal meaning embodied in autobiographical and episodic memories. Instead, it provides us with expectations and allows us to predict the outcomes of new situations using the generic knowledge gained from similar situations in the past. This formulation suggests that episodic and semantic memory are representational systems that together capture both the regularities and irregularities of the world, allowing one to create concepts and categories (semantic memories), and also capture the time and place when one particular combination of entities was experienced, yielding an episode that may or may not be consistent with one's prior expectations (Ryan, Hoscheidt, & Nadel, 2008b).

It has long been assumed that these two types of memories are relatively independent of one another, both functionally and anatomically (Schacter & Tulving, 1994; Schacter et al., 2000; Tulving & Markowitsch, 1998; Aggleton & Brown, 1999). Recent research, however, has called this independence into question (see Ryan, Hoscheidt, & Nadel, 2008b, for review). In a series of functional MRI studies, Ryan and colleagues demonstrated that both semantic and episodic retrieval results in a similar pattern of hippocampal activation, particularly when the tasks were matched for spatial content (Ryan, Cox, Hayes & Nadel, 2008a; Ryan, Lin, Ketcham, & Nadel, 2010; Hoscheidt, Dongoankar, Payne & Nadel, 2013). Consistent with Tulving (2002), semantic memory and episodic memory are seen as interactive and complementary systems. Both semantic structures and singular episodic memories are important for identifying familiar circumstances, interpreting novel events and predicting outcomes, and choosing appropriate behaviors in response to situations and personal interactions.

Barsalou (1988) has long championed the idea that semantic knowledge is embedded within a network of autobiographical memories. Episodes are represented as single events that are connected to other related episodes. Semantic memory is essentially derived from similar event memories that can be convolved to emphasize common information that is experienced across contexts, giving rise to what we call semantic memory. This idea is the basis of latent semantic analysis models (Landauer & Dumais, 1997). By this view, semantic information may be indistinguishable from episodic memory at the level of the brain when it is first acquired, and only later becomes differentiated as similar experiences accumulate and structural regularities and rules are derived. This information can then be retrieved separately from a specific context if necessary.

Semantic memory is therefore not simply a stable record of past learning, but something that is generative, flexible, contextually bound, and subject to revision through personal experience. Semantic memory is generated anew each time it is required, in much the same way as Bartlett (1932) and others (Bergman & Roediger, 1999; Nadel et al., 2007) have noted that episodic memories are reconstructed and revised over time through multiple retrievals.

This stands in contrast to the classic distinction between episodic and semantic memories and the assumption that semantic memory, at least, is a faithful record of prior learning.

Implicit emotion

In contrast to a model of the unconscious as a cauldron of forbidden sexual and aggressive impulses and wishes, the "adaptive unconscious" (Bargh & Morsella, 2008) is conceptualized as an extensive set of processing resources that execute complex computations, evaluations and responses without requiring intention or effort. Much of this processing may be unavailable to conscious awareness, or at least, awareness is unnecessary for such processing to occur. More commonly, cognitive psychology refers to implicit processes to differentiate them from explicit processes that are engaged during intentionally-driven and goal-directed tasks. The distinction between implicit and explicit processing has been applied in some form to virtually all areas of cognition, including perception, problem solving, memory and, as we will discuss, emotion, leading Gazzaniga (1998) to suggest that 99% of cognition is implicit. Importantly, some psychoanalysts believe that this new way of understanding the unconscious as fundamentally adaptive calls for a revision of classic psychoanalytic models of the unconscious mind (Modell, 2010).

The distinction between implicit and explicit processes, a cornerstone of modern cognitive neuroscience, has also been applied to emotion (Kihlstrom, Mulvaney, Tobias, & Tobias, 2000; Lane, 2000). Emotions are automatic, evolutionarily older responses to certain familiar situations (Darwin, 1872). Emotion can be understood as an organism's or person's mechanism for evaluating the degree to which needs, values or goals are being met or not met in interaction with the environment and responding to the situation with an orchestrated set of changes in the visceral, somatomotor, cognitive, and experiential domains that enable the person to adapt to those changing circumstances (Levenson, 1994). Implicit processes apply to emotion in two important senses. First, the evaluation of the person's transaction with the environment often happens automatically, without conscious awareness, and is thus implicit. Importantly for this discussion, this implicit evaluation is based on an automatic construal of the meaning (implications for needs, values or goals) of the current situation to that person (Clore & Ortony, 2000). Second, the emotional response itself can be divided into bodily responses (visceral, somatomotor) and mental reactions (thoughts, experiences). The latter include an awareness that an emotional response is occurring and an appreciation of what that response is. A foundational concept of this chapter is that emotional responses can be implicit in the sense that the bodily response component of emotion can occur without concomitant feeling states or awareness of such feeling states.

There is now considerable evidence supporting an implicit view of emotion (Lambie and Marcel, 2002; Kihlstrom, Mulvaney, Tobias, & Tobias,

2000; Lane, 2008). Indeed, 25 years of research has demonstrated the occurrence of spontaneous affective reactions associated with changes in peripheral physiology and/or behavior that are not associated with conscious emotional experiences (Quirin et al., 2009; Winkielman & Berridge, 2004; Zajonc, 2000; Ledoux, 1996; Smith & Lane, 2016). For example, one can activate emotions with subliminal stimuli and demonstrate that the emotional content of the stimuli influences subsequent behavior, such as consummatory behavior, without the person being aware of such influences on behavior (Winkielman & Berridge, 2004).

The somatomotor component of implicit emotion refers to automatic motor expressions of emotion such as facial expressions and gestures but also involves more complex behavioral phenomena such as scripts, enactments and procedures. In 1991, Clyman wrote an important paper in a psychoanalytic journal on the procedural organization of emotion (Clyman, 1991). He put forward the idea that transference may be understood to be organized at the implicit, procedural level and that the processes of interaction in the transference reflect previously learned ways of enacting emotion. This is entirely consistent with what we now know about implicit emotion as the bodily expression of emotion at the visceromotor and somatomotor level that precedes the conscious *experience* of specific, differentiated emotion feeling that must be constructed, as opposed to uncovered (Lane et al., 2015b; Barrett, 2017). This procedural level can be thought of as "the doing of emotion"—rule-based schemas for how to express love, handle anger, get attention, joke around and obtain love and reassurance (Lane & Garfield, 2005). It is a key element of what the Boston Change Process Study Group (2007) meant by the "implicit level of relational knowing."

Emotional trauma

Trauma may consist of experiences that are emotionally overwhelming in the sense that the ability or resources needed to cognitively process the emotions (attend to, experience and know them) are exceeded. Trauma may consist of a single event but more commonly consists of a repeated pattern of abuse or mistreatment that is emotionally painful to the victim. In the context of growing up as a child in a family in which abuse repeatedly occurs, one makes cognitive and emotional adaptations to keep the subjective distress to a minimum. This helps to keep attention and other conscious resources available for other tasks (see Friston, 2010). The victim learns to accept certain kinds of mistreatments in order to continue in relationships, which appear to be (and often are) necessary for survival. The needed adjustments include tuning out awareness of one's own emotional responses or taking for granted certain things about the self (such as "you're no good and deserve to be punished"). Later in life, related situations are interpreted implicitly based on the implicit learning that occurred from these experiences (Edelman, 1989).

All too commonly, perhaps due to direct physical threats, shame or lack of available confidants, these experiences are never discussed with anyone. When a parent is the instigator of abuse it is often a "double whammy," first because of the violation or harm and second because the parent is not available to assist the victim in dealing with it (Newman, 2013). The lack of an available caregiver to provide comfort and support may be a critical ingredient in what makes the experience(s) overwhelming or traumatic. What this means emotionally is that the implicit emotional responses were never brought to the conscious level of discrete feeling through mental representation as in language. As a result, the traumatized individual knew the circumstances of the trauma but did not know how it affected them emotionally. This lack of awareness contributes to the tendency to experience traumatic threats in circumstances in an overly generalized manner that reflects the inability to distinguish circumstances that are safe from those that are not. It is often only in therapy when the experiences are put into words that the emotional responses are formulated for the first time (Stern, 1983; Lane & Garfield, 2005).

This perspective highlights the importance of becoming aware of the emotional impact of the experience(s) through symbolization and contextualization (narrative formation) (Liberzon & Sripada, 2008) and using this awareness in the promotion of more adaptive responses, i.e., converting implicit emotional responses to explicit emotional responses. When the trauma is first recalled, the description of experience likely includes strong emotions such as fear that were experienced at the time and contributed to strong encoding of the event (McGaugh, 2003). As the therapy process unfolds, the events are recalled in the context of a supportive therapist who also helps the patient to attend to contextual information that may not have been available to the patient at the time of the trauma (in part because of temporary hippocampal dysfunction; Nadel & Jacobs, 1998). This new information in therapy contributes to a construction of the events in a new way that leads to emotions that had not been formulated or experienced before, e.g., experiencing anger at abuse that could not be either expressed or experienced at the time because the threat may have been so severe. The anger is a signal that one needs to be protected. In that sense, the emotional response is adaptive to the circumstances. It likely was not permissible at the time of the trauma to experience or express it. This helps create a coherent narrative account of what occurred. This is not the same as catharsis (uncovering what was previously known and releasing pent up energy) but rather the creation of a more complete picture of what happened, how one responded, what one experienced and how it could have been different (Greenberg, 2010).

This suggests that distressing or traumatic event memories are incorporated into semantic structures that are used to predict the outcomes of subsequent experiences and to choose appropriate (or inappropriate) emotional and behavioral responses in novel situations. It is easy to see how highly emotional and accessible memories from the past become the dominant basis for maladaptive responses in novel circumstances that share some characteristics with the original distressing event.

MTT provides a way of understanding how distressing emotional memories can be both strengthened over time and also the potential for being altered therapeutically. Consider, for example, an emotionally distressing event such as a betrayal or abandonment. As we have seen, the emotional reaction is an integral component of the memory, connected via the spatial and temporal context to the event and bound to the self, forming an autobiographical memory. The more highly arousing the emotional reaction, the more likely the evoking situation will be remembered later on (McGaugh, 2003). When a memory is recalled, the emotional response is re-engaged and the sympathetic nervous system is reactivated via the amygdala. According to MTT, the recollected event and its newly experienced emotional response will be re-encoded into a new and expanded memory trace. Thus, memory for the original traumatic incident is strengthened, making it (and the now intensified emotional response) even more likely to be accessed in the future.

Process of change

MTT provides a mechanism for understanding how this same emotional memory might be revised. During therapy, patients are commonly asked to recall and re-experience a painful past event, often eliciting a strong emotional reaction, which is step 1 in the LRNG model of change. If the psychotherapy process leads to a re-evaluation of the original experience, a new, more adaptive and perhaps more positive, emotional response may ensue. The corrective experience occurs within a new context, the context of therapy itself, which can then be incorporated into the old memory through reconsolidation, which is step 2 in the LRNG model. Next, the new way of construing and responding to familiar problematic situations must be implemented in a variety of circumstances, which is step 3 and the "working through process." It is conceivable that once this transformation has taken place the original memory including the associated emotional response can no longer be retrieved in its previous form. By this view, psychotherapy is a process that not only provides new experiences, but also changes our understanding of past experience in fundamental ways through the interaction between memory and emotion and between different types of memory.

Applying these principles to relational psychoanalysis (Lane, 2018), the procedural or implicit aspects of emotion are in constant interchange between patient and analyst at the implicit level of relational knowing (Boston Change Process Study Group, 2007). A key phenomenon is that the analyst processes his or her own implicit (body based) and background (conscious but in the attentional background) feelings to make sense of the current interactive experience. This is accomplished by integrating an understanding of the patient's recurrent patterns with the analyst's current interoceptive and introspective experience in the present moment.

A key element of the work of psychoanalysis is for the analyst to construct his or own experience to inform how these recurrent patterns are being manifested in the present moment of interaction and how these influence the experience of all those with whom the patient interacts (Eagle, 2000). If this conscious processing is not done, the implicit emotion may be enacted. Indeed, while enactments are inevitable, explicit reflection upon and discussion of such enactments may be extremely useful therapeutically (Safran, Muran & Eubanks-Carter, 2011).

Wachtel (2009) has described how the recurrent patterns of the patient are maintained by virtue of the fact that the patient's actions induce emotions in the other person that lead to behavioral responses that maintain the patterns. These "cyclical relational patterns" typically operate at the implicit level— one action leads to actions by others in response via the emotions induced in the transaction. The analyst's job is twofold: to consciously construct and experience the emotion so induced, to understand its origin and meaning, and then to use this information to promote a corrective emotional experience in the patient, as opposed to repeating the pattern unknowingly.

The second step in the change process is corrective emotional experience. This is not the hokey, artificial, and manipulated corrective emotional experience attributed to Franz Alexander by his critics at the time that the concept was introduced (Alexander & French, 1946; Wallerstein, 1990) but rather the process of making use of the authentic emotional responses generated by the interaction to provide the patient with what she needs. For example, providing the experience of being understood, cared for and even loved when criticism, judgement, and shame are expected. Or, to be taken seriously and to be protected from harm when earlier life trauma had been associated with being ignored and unprotected. If this corrective emotional experience occurs when the old memory and old painful feelings are activated, this may constitute the kind of critical moment that Daniel Stern (2004) describes and is the second step in the three-step process of change that we describe.

The third step in the LRNG model is the transition from episodic to semantic memory and the "working through" process. By providing new experiences in therapy that update prior event memories through reconsolidation, the semantic structures derived from experiences will also change. Applying the new knowledge and experiencing the results in a variety of contexts can be conceptualized as creating multiple episodic experiences that will broaden the range of applicability of new knowledge encoded in semantic memory. As proposed in our integrated memory model, linkage to emotional responses is expected to translate into greater adaptive flexibility and success relative to the difficulties that led the patient to seek treatment.

Discussion

It is fascinating to consider how the present model of change resonates with concepts put forward at the inception of the modern era of psychotherapy with the publication of Breuer and Freud's (1895/1955) "Studies on Hysteria." These authors held that memories and their associated affects were the problem (the source of the symptoms or dysfunction), the analyst's job was to facilitate overcoming the patient's resistance to enable recall of the memory and affect, and the curative aspect was to experience and express the affect that had been pent up (assuming that catharsis was the mechanism of cure). If recall could be accompanied by the experience and expression of the affect associated with the trauma, the memory would go through a process of what Freud called "retranscription." This process of retranscription would change and update the memory and the symptoms would be resolved (Freud, 1896/1966). It is therefore remarkable to note that, to our knowledge, Freud's concept of "retranscription" was the first reference to what has now come to be known as memory reconsolidation.

Freud's early thinking has also contributed in a major way to the conceptualization of affect as described in our model. It is customary in PDT to view affect as always pressing for discharge or expression while being kept out of awareness by virtue of defensive processes (Brenner, 1973). According to this view, the essential therapeutic task is to uncover the affect or emotion that had been previously formulated and known in order to allow its conscious registration. Although such phenomena are well established in PDT, the current model places particular emphasis on a developmental process whereby emotion is transformed from a purely bodily state to one that is mentally represented, i.e., from implicit to explicit. In that regard, my colleagues and I have proposed the concept of "affective agnosia" to highlight how deficits in the ability to mentally represent emotional states at the conceptual level (Lane et al., 2015b), such as that often seen in the context of trauma, provide a complementary perspective to the concept of defense. Indeed the two are not mutually exclusive in that deficits may help to explain why certain conflicts are not resolved and defenses become entrenched (Summers, 2013). It is therefore notable that the term "agnosia" was coined by Freud in 1891 while practicing as a neurologist before he created the field of psychoanalysis (Freud, 1953). This concept is not one that Freud pursued once psychoanalysis was established (Levine, 2012) but its relevance in the current context provides an opportunity to extend Freud's legacy.

An important way that PDT differs from other major modalities is its unique and time-honored focus on the etiology of current dysfunction. Traditionally this focus has been associated with the assumption that *understanding* the (presumed) etiology of a problem, as well as its manifestations through the years up to the present, will be a major contributor to resolving it (Brenner, 1973). This stands in contrast to the focus by other major modalities on the factors that *maintain* current dysfunction. In some ways the concept of memory reconsolidation addresses this point directly. If one accepts the foundational premise of this model, namely that memories are not veridical records of the past (which as Freud asserted; Schimek, 1975) but instead accepts that memories of the past may have been updated through the years (which Freud also claimed; Freud, 1896/1966), one may view recollections of the past as the current version of memories that maintain the ongoing difficulties. This is not to discount the value of recall of past experiences as informative about earlier development. The current version of the recurrent pattern began at an early age and evolved over time. An adult's description of the early childhood environment, whether it is objectively accurate or not, can assist the clinician in identifying the specific nature of the current difficulties in relationships. What this amounts to is a developmental perspective on the factors that maintain the current difficulty. As such, this reframing of the concept of etiology in light of the phenomenon of memory reconsolidation allows for some convergence and potential overlap between psychodynamic theory and the theories underpinning other modalities.

The LRNG model emphasizes corrective emotional experiences as a necessary ingredient of the change process. In general, these are understood to be conscious emotional experiences that are counter to expectation and typically involve more positive emotions than anticipated. In the case of PDT these corrective experiences happen most importantly in the transference relationship with the therapist. As described by Daniel Stern (2004), progress in therapy may involve unusual critical moments that could not be planned or anticipated and are particularly memorable. In the context of PDT, it is also important to consider that the implicit process of relational knowing may involve interactions that induce more subtle feelings in the patient that may not be particularly memorable but over time may alter expectations and create hope that a new type of interpersonal experience may be possible. Indeed, Kächele & Thomä (2000) stated that "Psychoanalysis is more than the creation of a narrative; it is the active construction of a new way of experiencing self with other" (p. 218). Perhaps corrective emotional experiences that may or may not be noticed may be happening frequently and contribute an altered ability to relate to others in more trusting and less defensive ways. Perhaps the frequency of sessions and the intensity of the relationship with the therapist may provide a learning context for the transformation of recurrent patterns through reconsolidation that may differentiate PDT from other modalities and provide unique advantages.

Although the integrated memory model and the LRNG model focused on episodic memories, semantic memories, and their interaction, procedural memories were also described above in relation to transference, recurrent maladaptive patterns and the process of making behaviors more automatic through practice. In this regard, it is notable that the ability to change or update memories through reconsolidation is easiest for episodic memories, more difficult for semantic memories and harder still for procedural memories (Schacter, Wagner, & Buckner, 2000). Much less is known about the latter two compared to the former. This means that by virtue of corrective experiences and the updating of episodic and semantic memories patients will be better able to construe familiar problematic situations differently and will have the ability to respond emotionally in different and potentially more flexible ways. It will take considerable practice, however, to overcome the old automatic behavioral tendencies. In this context, conscious understanding of the recurrent patterns and their manifestations through insight can assist in interpersonal navigation and problem-solving when encountering new ambiguous circumstances.

To the extent that the process of change involves the three step LRNG process that applies to other modalities as well as PDT, questions arise about the necessity of certain time-honored traditions in PDT. For example, is it possible to bring about enduring change in PDT without working in the transference relationship with the PDT therapist? Or, if the interpersonal emotional field is the context in which change occurs, to what extent (and in what contexts) is it advisable to use the couch with the analyst out of view (Goldberger, 1995), potentially depriving the patient of emotional feedback in the form of facial expressions and body movements that often go beyond what words and vocal tone can convey? To the extent that the LRNG model is considered applicable to PDT, it provides a different vantage point for reconsideration of these questions.

One of the advantages of a specific theory of change is that it can help to explain what may have gone wrong in treatments that were not successful as well as provide guidance when progress is stagnant. Recall of past traumas or adverse experiences without competing emotional experiences will lead to a memory that is further reconsolidated and thus more likely to be retrieved during similar situations in the future. As the memory itself is strengthened, so too is the emotional response and the semantic structures that result in novel situations being interpreted in maladaptive ways. Recollection alone only serves to reinforce and further ingrain the patient's original version of the traumatic or adverse memories, and is insufficient to bring about clinical change. The LRNG model may be useful in thinking about how to alter the trajectory of the treatment.

In conclusion, the integrated memory model and the LRNG model of change provide a unifying framework across psychotherapy modalities that includes but is by no means limited to PDT. In some ways this basic mechanistic framework is analogous to the automobile; they all work in fundamentally the same way, and yet there are hundreds of different makes and models. Many factors determine which one a person might select. It makes a big difference what a person's starting point is and where she wants to go, and factors such as comfort, speed, and expense are important. It is also true that certain vehicles can do things that others can't. In the case of psychotherapy, problems vary in terms how deeply ingrained they are, the types of corrective emotional experiences that are needed to overcome previous learning and the number of repetitions needed to bring about the desired changes. For certain kinds of problems PDT works as well as other modalities; for certain others it may work better; and no doubt in many contexts other forms of therapy are to be preferred. An important goal for the future is to define what these contexts are.

Acknowledgment

I thank my co-authors Lee Ryan, Lynn Nadel, and Les Greenberg for their contributions to the model described here as originally published in *Behavioral and Brain Sciences* 2015; 38:1–19.

References

Aggleton, J.P., & Brown, M.W. (1999). Episodic memory, amnesia, and the hippocampal-anterior thalamic axis. *Behavioral and Brain Sciences*, 22, 425–489.

Alexander, F., & French, T.M. (1946). The corrective emotional experience. In *Psychoanalytic therapy: Principles and application*. New York: Ronald Press.

Bargh, J.A., & Morsella, E. (2008). The unconscious mind. *Perspectives on psychological science*, 3(1), 73–79.

Barrett, L.F. (2017). *How emotions are made: The secret life of the brain*. Boston: Houghton Mifflin Harcourt.

Barsalou, L.W. (1988). The content and organization of autobiographical memories. In: U. Neisser & E. Winograd (Eds.), *Remembering reconsidered: Ecological and traditional approaches to the study of memory* (pp. 193–243). New York: Cambridge University Press.

Bartlett, F.C. (1932). *Remembering: a study in experimental and social psychology*. New York: Cambridge University Press.

Bergman, E.T., & Roediger, H.L. (1999). Can Bartlett's repeated reproduction experiments be replicated? *Memory & Cognition*, 27, 937–47.

Bornstein, R.F. (2001). The impending death of psychoanalysis. *Psychoanalytic Psychology*, 18(1), 3–20.

Boston Change Process Study Group (2007). The foundational level of psychodynamic meaning—implicit process in relation to conflict, defense and the dynamic unconscious. *Int J Psychoanalysis*, 88, 843–860.

Bower, G.H. (1981). Mood and memory. *American Psychologist*, 36(2), 129.

Brenner, C. (1973). *An elementary textbook of psychoanalysis*. Madison, CT: International Universities Press.

Breuer, J., & Freud, S. (1955; Original work published 1895). Studies on hysteria. In: J. Strachey (Ed.), *Standard edition of the complete psychological works of Sigmund Freud*. London, UK: Hogarth Press.

Clore, G.L., & Ortony, A. (2000). Cognition in emotion: always, sometimes or never? In: R. Lane & L. Nadel (Eds.), *Cognitive neuroscience of emotion* (pp. 24–61). New York: Oxford University Press.

Clyman, R.B. (1991). The procedural organization of emotions: A contribution from cognitive science to the psychoanalytic theory of therapeutic action. *Journal of the American Psychoanalytic Association*, 39, 349–382.

Darwin, C. (1872). *The expression of the emotions in man and animals.* London, UK: John Murray.

de la Fuente, V., Freudenthal, R., & Romano, A. (2011). Reconsolidation or extinction: transcription factor switch in the determination of memory course after retrieval. *Journal of Neuroscience*, 31, 5562–5573.

Eagle, M.N. (2000). A Critical evaluation of current conceptions of transference and countertransference. *Psychoanalytic Psychology*, 17(1), 24–37.

Edelman, G.M. (1989). *The remembered present: A biological theory of consciousness.* New York: Basic Books.

Elsey, J.W., Van Ast, V.A., & Kindt, M. (2018). Human memory reconsolidation: A guiding framework and critical review of the evidence. *Psychological bulletin*, 144(8), 797–848. doi: 10.1037/bul0000152.

Freud, S. (1895/1950). Project for a scientific psychology (1950 [1895]). In *The standard edition of the complete psychological works of Sigmund Freud, Volume I (1886–1899): pre-psycho-analytic publications and unpublished drafts* (pp. 281–391).

Freud, S. (1910). The origin and development of psychoanalysis. *The American Journal of Psychology*, 21(2), 181–218.

Freud, S. (1966). Letter 52 from extracts from the Fliess papers. In: *The standard edition of the complete psychological works of Sigmund Freud, Volume I (1886–1899): pre-psycho-analytic publications and unpublished drafts* (pp. 233–239).

Freud, S. (1953). *On aphasia: A critical study* (Originally published 1891). New York: International Universities Press.

Friston, K. (2010). The free-energy principle: a unified brain theory? *Nature Reviews Neuroscience*, 11, 127–138.

Gazzaniga, M. (1998). *The mind's past.* Berkeley, CA: University of California Press.

Goldberger, M. (1995). The couch as defense and as potential for enactment. *The Psychoanalytic Quarterly*, 64, 23–42.

Greenberg, L.S. (2010). *Emotion-focused therapy: Theory and practice.* Washington, DC: DCAPA Press.

Hardt, O., Einarsson, E.O., & Nader, K. (2010). A bridge over troubled water: Reconsolidation as a link between cognitive and neuroscientific memory research traditions. *Annual Review of Psychology*, 61, 141–167.

Hoscheidt, S., Dongaonkar, B., Payne, J., & Nadel, L. (2013). Emotion, stress, and memory. In: D. Reisberg (Ed.), *Oxford handbook of cognitive psychology* (pp. 557–570). New York: Oxford University Press.

Hupbach, A., Gomez, R., Hardt, O., & Nadel, L. (2007). Reconsolidation of episodic memories: A subtle reminder triggers integration of new information. *Learning & Memory*, 14, 47–53.

Hupbach, A., Hardt, O., Gomez, R., & Nadel, L. (2008). The dynamics of memory: Context-dependent updating. *Learning & Memory*, 15, 574–579.

Inda, M.C., Muravieva, E.V., & Alberini, C.M. (2011). Memory retrieval and the passage of time: From reconsolidation and strengthening to extinction. *Journal of Neuroscience*, 31, 1635–1643.

Kächele, H. & Thomä, H.(2000). Lehrbuch der psychoanalytischen Therapie, Band 3 Forschung/Psychoanalytic Practice Vol 3 Research. Ulmer Textbank. Ulm (new edition in preparation).

Kihlstrom, J.F., Mulvaney, S., Tobias, B.A., & Tobis, I.P. (2000). The emotional unconscious. In: E. Eich, J.F. Kihlstrom, G.H. Bower, J.P. Forgas & P.M. Niedenthal (Eds.), *Cognition and emotion* (pp. 30–86). New York: Oxford University Press.

Lambie, J.A., & Marcel, A.J. (2002). Consciousness and the varieties of emotion experience: a theoretical framework. *Psychological Review*, 109(2), 219–259.

Landauer, T.K., & Dumais, S.T. (1997). A solution to Plato's problem: The latent semantic analysis theory of acquisition, induction, and representation of knowledge. *Psychological Review*, 104, 211–40.

Lane, R. (2000). Neural correlates of conscious emotional experience. In: R. Lane, & L. Nadel (Eds.), *Cognitive neuroscience of emotion* (pp. 345–370). New York: Oxford University Press.

Lane, R.D., & Garfield, D.A. (2005). Becoming aware of feelings: Integration of cognitive-developmental, neuroscientific, and psychoanalytic perspectives. *Neuropsychoanalysis*, 7, 5–30.

Lane, R.D. (2008). Neural substrates of implicit and explicit emotional processes: A unifying framework for psychosomatic medicine. *Psychosomatic Medicine*, 70, 214–231.

Lane, R.D., Ryan, L., Nadel, L., & Greenberg, L. (2015a). Memory reconsolidation, emotional arousal and the process of change in psychotherapy: New insights from brain science. *Behavioral and Brain Sciences*, 38, 1–19.

Lane, R.D., Weihs, K.L., Herring, A., Hishaw, A., & Smith, R. (2015b). Affective agnosia: Expansion of the alexithymia construct and a new opportunity to integrate and extend Freud's legacy. *Neuroscience & Biobehavioral Reviews*, 55, 594–611.

Lane, R.D. (2018). From reconstruction to construction: The power of corrective emotional experiences in memory reconsolidation and enduring change. *Journal of the American Psychoanalytic Association*, 66(3), 507–516.

Leichsenring, F., & Rabung, S. (2008). Effectiveness of long-term psychodynamic psychotherapy – A meta-analysis. *JAMA*, 300(13), 1551–1565.

LeDoux, J.E. (1996). *The emotional brain*. New York: Simon and Shuster.

Levenson, R.W. (1994). Human emotion: A functional view. In: P. Elkman & R.J. Davidson (Eds.), The nature of emotion – fundamental questions (pp. 123–126). New York: Oxford University Press.

Levine, H.B. (2012). The colourless canvas: Representation, therapeutic action and the creation of mind. *The International Journal of Psychoanalysis*, 93, 607–629.

Liberzon, I., & Sripada, C.S. (2008). The functional neuroanatomy of PTSD: A critical review. In: E.R. de Kloet, M.S. Oitzel, & E. Vermetten (Eds.), *Progress in* Brain Research (pp. 151–169). Amsterdam, Netherlands: Elsevier Science Publishing.

Maren, S. (2011). Seeking a spotless mind: Extinction, deconsolidation, and erasure of fear memory. *Neuron*, 70, 830–845.

McGaugh, J.L. (2003). Memory and emotion: The making of lasting memories. New York: Columbia University Press.

Milad, M.R., & Quirk, G.J. (2002). Neurons in medial prefrontal cortex signal memory for fear extinction. *Nature*, 420, 70–74.

Modell, A.H. (2010). The unconscious as a knowledge processing center. In: J. Petrucelli (Ed.), *Knowing, not-knowing and sort-of-knowing: Psychoanalysis and the experience of uncertainty* (pp. 45–61). London: Karnac.

Nadel, L., & Jacobs, W.J. (1998). Traumatic memory is special. *Current Directions in Psychological Science*, 7, 154–157.

Nadel L, Samsonovich A, Ryan L, Moscovitch M (2000). Multiple trace theory of human memory: Computational, neuroimaging, and neuropsychological results. *Hippocampus*, 10(4), 352–368.

Nadel, L., Campbell, J., & Ryan, L. (2007). Autobiographical memory retrieval and hippocampal activation as a function of repetition and the passage of time. *Neural Plasticity*, 2007, 90472.

Nader, K., Schafe, G.E., & Le Doux, J.E. (2000). Fear memories require protein synthesis in the amygdala for reconsolidation after retrieval. *Nature*, 406, 722–726.

Newman, K.M. (2013). A more usable Winnicott. *Psychoanalytic Inquiry*, 33, 59–63.

Quirin, M., Kazén, M., & Kuhl, J. (2009). When nonsense sounds happy or helpless: The implicit positive and negative affect test (IPANAT). *Journal of Personality and Social Psychology*, 97(3), 500.

Ryan, L., Cox, C., Hayes, S.M., & Nadel, L. (2008a). Hippocampal activation during episodic and semantic memory retrieval: Comparing category production and category cued recall. *Neuropsychologia*, 46, 2109–2121.

Ryan, L., Hoscheidt, S., & Nadel, L. (2008b). Perspectives on episodic and semantic memory retrieval. In: E. Dere, A. Easton, J. Huston, & L. Nadel (Eds.), *Handbook of episodic memory/handbook of behavioral neuroscience* (pp. 5–18). Amsterdam, Netherlands: Elsevier.

Ryan, L., Lin, C.Y., Ketcham, K., & Nadel, L. (2010). The role of medial temporal lobe in retrieving spatial and nonspatial relations from episodic and semantic memory. *Hippocampus*, 20, 11–18.

Safran, J.D., Muran, J.C., & Eubanks-Carter, C. (2011). Repairing alliance ruptures. *Psychotherapy*, 48(1), 80.

Schacter, D.L., & Tulving, E. (1994). What are the memory systems of 1994? In D.L. Schacter & E. Tulving (Eds.), *Memory systems 1994* (pp. 1–38). Cambridge, MA: MIT Press.

Schacter, D.L., Wagner, A.D., & Buckner, R.L (2000). Memory systems of 1999. In E. Tulving, & F.I. Craik (Eds.), *The Oxford handbook of memory* (pp. 627–643). New York: Oxford University Press.

Schimek, J.G. (1975). A critical re-examination of Freud's concept of unconscious mental representation. *International Review of Psycho-Analysis*, 2, 171–187.

Schwabe, L., Joëls, M., Roozendaal, B., Wolf, O.T., & Oitzl, M.S. (2012). Stress effects on memory: An update and integration. *Neuroscience & Biobehavioral Reviews*, 36(7), 1740–1749.

Shedler, J. (2010). The efficacy of psychodynamic therapy. *American Psychologist*, 65(2), 98–109.

Smith, R., & Lane, R.D. (2016). Unconscious emotion: A cognitive neuroscientific perspective. *Neuroscience and Biobehavioral Reviews*, 69, 216–238.

Spezzano, C. (1993). *Affect in psychoanalysis: A clinical synthesis*. Hillsdale, NJ: Analytic Press, Inc.

Stern, D.B. (1983). Unformulated experience: From familiar chaos to creative disorder. *Contemporary Psychoanalysis*, 19, 71–99.

Stern, D.N. (2004). *The present moment in psychotherapy and everyday life*. New York: W.W. Norton & Company.

Summers, F. (2013). *The psychoanalytic vision*. New York: Routledge.

Tulving, E. (2002). Episodic memory: From mind to brain. *Annual Review of Psychology*, 53, 1–25.

Tulving, E., & Markowitsch, H.J. (1998). Episodic and declarative memory: Role of the hippocampus. *Hippocampus*, 8, 198–204.

Wachtel, P.L. (2009). Knowing oneself from the inside out, knowing oneself from the outside in. The "inner" and "outer" worlds and their link through action. *Psychoanalytic Psychology*, 26(2), 158–170.

Wallerstein, R.S. (1990). The corrective emotional experience: is reconsideration due? *Psychoanalytic Inquiry*, 10(3), 288–324.

Wilson, M.A., & McNaughton, B.L. (1994). Reactivation of hippocampal ensemble memories during sleep. *Science*, 265, 676–679.

Winkielman, P., & Berridge, K. (2004). Unconscious emotion. *Current Directions in Psychological Science*, 13(3), 120–123.

Zajonc, R.B. (2000). Feeling and thinking: Closing the debate over the independence of affect. In: J.P. Forgas (Ed.), *Feeling and thinking: The role of affect in social cognition* (pp. 31–58). Cambridge, UK: Cambridge University Press.

Chapter 13

Emotions in psychodynamic process and outcome research

Manfred E. Beutel, Les Greenberg, and Richard D. Lane

The purpose of this manuscript is to explore the role of emotion in psycho-dynamic psychotherapy technique and outcome. While a focus on emotional change has been proposed as a hallmark of psychodynamic psychotherapy and an indicator of structural change, there has been little attention to specific technique for changing emotional processes and their relationships with outcome. We advance the hypothesis that integrating techniques from Emotion-Focused Therapy (EFT) will help psychodynamic psychotherapists in identifying, addressing and changing emotional processes and thus contribute to successful treatment outcomes, particularly in patients who have difficulties accessing their emotions (Beutel et al. 2018). Integrating experiential techniques into psychodynamic psychotherapy has the potential to support and intensify emotional activation and experiencing, and thereby improve outcome in patients who have limited access to their emotional experiences.

What are emotions?

Emotions entail cognitive, body-centered-expressive, and feeling-centered-motivational components. Inborn emotional components are generated fast and automatically, when evolutionary adaptive neurobiological and mental processes are activated. Basic emotions include interest, happiness, grief, anger, disgust, and fear. Each of the seven to nine inborn emotions acts like a flashlight alerting us to what needs cognition motivating us to use cognition in a specific way. Striving for emotion is an important motivation factor, and emotion regulation is a key aspect of human motivation (Greenberg 2004).

According to appraisal-theories, emotional responses result from cognitive appraisals to internal or external stimuli, which are considered relevant for important concerns of the organism. As opposed to basic and discrete emotions, dimensional theories differentiate emotions according to valence (good–bad; linked to the functioning of the orbitofrontal cortex, and activation (low–high), linked to the amygdala.

There is a general consensus among researchers on emotions that (Greenberg 2004):

- emotions signal what is important to us and if things develop in our interest (source of information),
- they help us survive by providing efficient, automatic responses in important situations,
- and they prepare us for action, in order to assert our wishes and needs, and they integrate experience, provide meaning, values and direction.

Emotional experience includes all verbal and nonverbal processes involved in the patient's generation, experience, regulation and the cognitive elaboration of a felt sense of a specific emotion. Becoming aware of emotions has been conceived as a developmental process along a continuum from implicit (emotional procedures) to explicit emotional experience (Lane & Garfield 2005).

As the burgeoning affective (neuro)sciences have shown, affective processes are crucial to understand psychopathology. The most frequent emotional ("internalizing") disorders have been characterized by neuroticism and emotional dysregulation. Thus, evolving transdiagnostic manuals for depression and anxiety have been focusing on maladaptive emotion processing (Busch et al. 2012; Leichsenring & Salzer 2014; Barlow et al. 2017).

As proposed by Lane et al. (2015), repetitive maladaptive reactions (affective reactions, cognitive appraisal, behavior) rest upon emotional memories and semantic structures (Lane et al. 2015). The basic change process in psychotherapy requires a sequence of reactivating and experiencing the avoided emotional memories fully and consciously ("hot, gut-level, visceral") and imbuing the related scene or interpersonal situation with new perspectives and meanings. The new experience is incorporated into new memory structures via reconsolidation and working through (rational, logical, head-level, "cold"). Thus, activation and processing of emotions is crucial for successful outcomes, even though different treatment approaches focus on specific entry points into the memory structure (e.g., memory episodes in psychodynamic psychotherapy, semantic structures in cognitive-behavioral, and emotional experience in emotion-focused therapy).

What is the role of emotions in the development of psychodynamic psychotherapy?

The conception of emotions in psychoanalysis has shifted throughout its history. To give a few prominent examples (Fisher et al. 2016):

- Breuer and Freud (1895/1955) postulated that an inability to express conflict tension at the time of trauma causes hysteria. Symptoms vanish, when previously repressed feelings come into consciousness and are relived. Insight is the important mechanism of change.
- Alexander and French (1946) proposed "corrective emotional experience" as a basic therapeutic principle exposing the patient to emotional conflicts under more favorable (therapeutic) than the previous (pathogenic) conditions.

- According to Bion (1984), the experience of painful emotions in the presence of the therapist, who has the ability to contain these emotions, enables the patient to gain more tolerance for his/her emotions.
- Recent psychodynamic short-term psychotherapies activate emotional responses: experiential brief dynamic therapy strives to reliving intensive or painful emotions in a safe and supportive relationship ("affect phobia," McCullough et al. 2003). Experiential Dynamic Therapy proposes that patient defenses (D) and anxiety (A) block the experience and expression of underlying adaptive feelings (F), leading to maladaptive relating/symptom formation. Thus, the therapist actively strives to (1) help patients become aware and let go of maladaptive defenses, (2) regulate anxiety and (3) helps the patient access and "viscerally" process underlying adaptive affects. There is strong evidence of efficacy across a variety of mental disorders (Lilliengren et al. 2017).

What is the impact of emotional experiencing on treatment outcome?

Based on a thorough review of the literature, Hilsenroth 2007 has identified the focus on emotions and emotional change as core criteria of psychoanalytic therapies and an indicator for significant (structural) change. Emotions are considered helpful to recognize what needs to be explored and interpreted in the patient's material. They are a reliable marker of the immediate, lively self-state. Yet, emotional experiencing of patients found comparably little attention in psychodynamic process or outcome research. There have been few studies on the relationship of specific technique and emotional change (Subic-Wrana et al. 2016).

Low emotional awareness predicted less improvement in psychodynamic short-term psychotherapy in panic disorder (Beutel et al. 2013). Pre-treatment social anxiety was a negative predictor of outcome (39% of variance). Only a few additional baseline characteristics predicted better treatment outcome (lower comorbidity and interpersonal problems) with a limited proportion of incremental variance (Wiltink et al. 2016).

In psychodynamic psychotherapy (PD) of personality disorders (Cluster C), an increase of emotional activation predicted better outcome (Ulvenes et al. 2012). The therapeutic alliance predicted mental functioning via emotional experiencing (Fisher et al. 2016). Overall, therapeutic improvement was associated with changes in neuronal networks underlying emotional processes (Abbass et al. 2014).

How can therapists promote emotional experience?

Psychodynamic treatment technique conceptualizes emotions as one mental content among others. Thus, there are no specific rules or strategies defined.

A tendency to speak about and not from emotional experience may interfere with "visceral" experiencing. However, difficulties to experience and express emotions are core characteristics of common (internalizing) mental disorders. For example, the preoccupation with anxiety symptoms wards off painful, conflicted emotions. Worrying, ruminating, catastrophizing are cognitive concerns, which entail little emotional processing. These strategies are often used by insecurely attached (preoccupied–avoidant) patients with limited emotional awareness. Emotional experience often begins implicitly (body sensations, action tendency), and patients may not attend inner sensations or feelings ("affect phobia").

From a psychodynamic framework, different ways of accessing emotional experience have been proposed:

- According to a more "classical approach," clarifying, confronting and interpreting emotions may include questions like "what did you feel then? … What happened next? … Were you also angry at him?" (Busch et al. 2012). "What would happen if you told your boss that you are angry at him? What would he do, what would you do …?" "You were upset. Could you try to describe this feeling more precisely?" (Leichsenring & Salzer 2014).
- A stronger focus on emotional experiencing may include statements such as "Do you feel how your voice softens and your eyes get wet … what is just happening inside of you …" Therapist softly and attuned to patient (tone of voice, posture): "there is so much pain/grief in you …" "do you feel how you become subdued and lower your head when your speak about … as if you are ashamed …" (Ulvenes et al. 2012).

In the meta-analysis of ten psychodynamic short-term psychotherapy studies (Diener et al. 2007), the effect size of therapist activities promoting emotional experiencing and expression was $r = 0.30$, comparable in size to the therapeutic alliance. In personality disorders (Cluster C) therapeutic focus on affect predicted better outcome in psychodynamic and worse in CBT treatment (Ulvenes et al. 2012). A moderate degree of psychodynamic (interpretations) and emotion-focused techniques predicted best treatment outcome (McCarthy et al. 2016). According to Town et al. (2012), support was more predictive of emotional experience of the patient than questions, self-disclosure and information. Lilliengren et al. (2017) and Town et al. (2011) reported that mobilizing unprocessed complex emotions (e.g., grief, rage, guilt) from stressful relational events predicted good outcome in generalized anxiety disorder (GAD). Experience of previously avoided affects increased by insight into defensive patterns and motivation to give them up (Aafjes-van Doorn & Barber 2017).

Psychodynamic online self-help for affect phobia

As we have shown previously, psychodynamic psychotherapy may be enhanced by online self-help. The goals of the psychodynamic program KEN

Online (Kraft Eigener Emotionen Nutzen; using the power of your emotions) are (Zwerenz et al. 2017):

- recognizing and relinquishing maladaptive defenses,
- exposure to conflicted feelings, and
- improvement in sense of self and relationships.

Eight modules over ten weeks provide texts and exercises to work through. The online self-help program is based on three theoretical concepts:

- the affect phobia model (McCullough & Andrews 2001),
- the triangle of conflict (Malan 1963),
- and emotional mindfulness (Kabat-Zinn 1994).

There is cumulating evidence for its effectiveness based on Swedish trials with patients with generalized anxiety disorder and depression (Johansson et al. 2013). A German trial for patients with mixed diagnoses as an aftercare to inpatient psychotherapy demonstrated that patients could learn to access and process their emotions. Building emotional competence helps them to reduce anxiety and depressive symptoms.

What we can learn from Emotion-Focused Psychotherapy (EFT)

Emotion-Focused Psychotherapy (EFT) considers emotions as constituents of self; activation of emotion schemata evokes emotional experiencing, based on past emotional learning (outside of consciousness). It integrates elements from client centered and Gestalt therapy. Good evidence for treatment of depression, couples, new approaches to anxiety. Emotional experiencing is defined as the patient's ability to approach emotions, activate them, remain in contact with and symbolize emotional experience. Full emotional processing leads to psychic change.

This view is supported by process–outcome research in EFT. Accordingly, a moderate degree of emotional activation, respectively depth of emotional processing predicted best outcome (Carryer & Greenberg 2010; Missirlian et al. 2005; metaanalysis by Pascual-Leone & Yeryomenko 2017: $r = 0.19$ to 0.25). Therapeutic alliance acted as a mediator.

How can we define emotional experiencing? The Experiencing Scale specifies different types of emotional involvement (Klein et al. 1986):

1   Objective and intellectual, giving no evidence of the personal significance of events they describe.
2   Personal but detached; no explicit reference to feelings, reactions, or internal states.

3   Reactions to external events begin to appear.
4   Marked shift inward with a focus on exploration of feelings and internal experiences. At Level 4 clients are in direct contact with their fluid experience and speak "from" it as opposed to "about" it.
5   Questions about experience and the self are raised and explored from an internal perspective.
6   Newly realized feelings and experiences are integrated and explored to produce personally meaningful constructions and resolve issues.
7   Shifts and new understandings in one particular area of experience are broadened to a wider range of experiences giving clarity and meaning (Pascual-Leone & Yeryomenko 2017).

As we have delineated recently (Beutel et al. 2018), common grounds of emotion theory between psychodynamic and emotion-focused therapy include the following assumptions:

- emotional schemes result from past interactions with significant others, which are only partly conscious,
- emotional experience and the therapeutic bond are considered important for outcome,
- defense is motivated by the avoidance of negative, sometimes overwhelming or traumatic affect.

Psychodynamic psychotherapy proposes that (Subic-Wrana et al. 2016):

- insight into the nature and origin of largely unconscious maladaptive emotional patterns interrupts these patterns eliciting avoided emotions,
- interpretation (e.g., defense, transference) links emotional experience, cognitive understanding and corrective experience.

According to EFT, however,

- maladaptive emotional responses are activated and experienced viscerally; these are modified by processing and generating meaning,
- the therapist's task is to facilitate experiencing by engaging the patient emotionally and circumventing resistance,
- thereby the patient recovers subjective ownership of the "painful" emotion, which has been lost due to defensive processes (Greenberg & Pascual-Leone 2006).

Different types of emotional experience ("phenomenology") are specified which require different kinds of therapeutic interventions:

- primary adaptive emotions are responsive to circumstances, shifting, fresh and new (e.g., grieving, self-assertive anger), and they provide access for information and change,

- primary maladaptive emotions have a disorganizing quality, stuck in past reaction patterns (e.g., hopeless despair, lingering anger), and they are accessed therapeutically to transform them,
- as a response to primary emotions, secondary emotions obscure emotional experiencing, and they feel inhibited, confused, a whining quality (e.g., reproachful anger instead of fear). Exploration leads to more primary information,
- instrumental emotion include strategic affect (e.g., blaming, crocodile's tears): awareness of the aim (Greenberg 2004).

EFT has defined a wide range of therapeutic techniques to facilitate emotional experience. These include (Elliott et al. 2004; Greenberg 2004):

- a crucial aspect is the therapeutic presence (being completely in the moment, empathically responsive) enabling empathic attunement to the patient,
- evocative empathic response involves extending the patient narrative with vivid examples and metaphors,
- guiding attention requires and supports the patient to attend and "stay with" feelings "inside,"
- focusing implies pursuing felt sense, bodily here-and now experiences, and symbolizing them,
- identifying and articulating needs helps patients to foster the awareness of needs as core agent of change,
- emotional activation is promoted by techniques adopted from Gestalt therapy. E.g., in the empty chair technique, the patient is instructed to vividly confronting self-interruption, anxiety, and self-criticism. So-called two chair techniques help patients face avoided emotions in interpersonal conflicts as imagined in the significant other in the opposite chair,
- an important strategy to promote emotion regulation is to encourage self-soothing.

Future directions

The focus on emotions and emotional change are core characteristics of psychodynamic psychotherapies. Yet, emotional experiencing has been neglected in psychoanalytic treatment technique and research. Given that the most frequent mental disorders and internalizing disorders entail difficulties experiencing and regulating emotions, transdiagnostic manuals focus increasingly on emotional experience.

Emotional experiencing and activation predict symptom improvement across humanistic, experiential and psychodynamic therapies and have increasingly found attention in cognitive behavioral therapy (Aafjes-van Doorn & Barber, 2017).

We should therefore pursue the current trend clearly specifying which overarching mechanisms we address therapeutically. It is worthwhile to explore, when, how, and how much affective experiencing can be effective and facilitated by which means by the therapist in psychodynamic psychotherapy (in the context of a good therapeutic relationship). In guiding the patient to attend his/her emotional experience it is important to maintain therapeutic neutrality and a questioning stance (process-guiding, not content-guiding). We surmise better access to treatment-refractory patients with ego-structural deficits of emotional awareness (implicit expression, limited ability to symbolize their feelings). Transdiagnostic improvement of emotional competence by psychodynamic online self-help ("affect phobia") may be used in a preventive or blended care approach.

We recently proposed Emotion Focused Psychodynamic Psychotherapy (EFPP) as a generic treatment approach for anxiety disorders, which are characterized and maintained by emotional avoidance (Beutel et al. 2018). Beyond simply adding EFT techniques to psychodynamic psychotherapy, the combined approach helps reactivate and experience avoided emotional memories fully and consciously, as our first experiences in treating single cases have illustrated. Related scenes or interpersonal situations are imbued with new perspectives and meanings and reconsolidated (transference, working through). Emotional poignancy (or liveliness) is the important indicator for emotional processing throughout treatment. Anxiety needs to be evoked in treatment in order to be worked through and resolved. In short-term treatments the therapist needs to assume a more active role (time-limitation, focus). Reactions of the patient need to be reflected under transference aspects (ambivalent-dependent relationship patterns in anxiety disorder patients).

References

Abbass, A.A., Nowoweiski, S.J., Bernier, D., Tarzwell, R., & Beutel, M.E. (2014). Review of psychodynamic psychotherapy neuroimaging studies. *Psychotherapy and Psychosomatics*, 83(3), 142–147.

Aafjes-van Doorn, K., & Barber, J.P. (2017). Systematic review of in-session affect experience in cognitive behavioral therapy for depression. *Cogn Ther Res*, 41, 807–828.

Alexander, F., & French, T.M. (1946). The principle of corrective emotional experience. In: Alexander, F., French, T.M. (Eds.), *Psychoanalytic therapy: Principles and application* (pp. 66–70). New York: Ronald Press.

Barlow, D.H., Farchione, T.J., Bullis, J.R., Gallagher, M.W., Murray-Latin, H., Sauer-Zavala, S., Bentley, K.H., Thompson-Hollands, J., Conklin, L.R., Boswell, J.F., Ametaj, A., Carl, J.R., Boettcher, H.A.T., & Cassiello-Robbins, C. (2017). The unified protocol for transdiagnostic treatment of emotional disorders compared with diagnosis-specific protocols for anxiety disorders a randomized clinical trial. *JAMA Psychiatry*, 74(9), 875–884.

Beutel, M., Greenberg, L., Lane, R.D., & Subic Wrana, C. (2018). Treating anxiety disorders by emotion-focused psychodynamic psychotherapy (EFPP)—An integrative, transdiagnostic approach. *Clin Psychol Psychother*, 1–13.

Beutel, M.E., Scheurich, V., Knebel, A., Michal, M., Wiltink, J., Graf-Morgenstern, M., ... Subic-Wrana, C. (2013). Implementing panic focused psychodynamic psychotherapy into clinical practice. *The Canadian Journal of Psychiatry*, 58(6), 326–334.

Bion, W. (1984). *Learning from experience*. London: Karnac.

Breuer, J., & Freud, S. (1895/1955). Studies on hysteria. In: J. Strachey (Ed.), *Standard edition of the complete psychological works of Sigmund Freud*. London: Hogarth Press. (Original work published in 1895.)

Busch, F.N., Milrod, B.L., Singer, M.B., & Aronson, A.C. (2012). *Manual of panic focused psychodynamic psychotherapy: Extended range*. New York NY: Routledge.

Carryer, J.R., & Greenberg, L.S. (2010). Optimal levels of emotional arousal in experiential therapy of depression. *Journal of Consulting and Clinical Psychology*, 78(2), 190–199.

Diener, M.J., Hilsenroth, M.J., & Weinberger, J. (2007). Therapist affect focus and patient outcomes in psychodynamic psychotherapy: A meta-analysis. *American Journal of Psychiatry*, 164(6), 936–941.

Elliott, R., Watson, J.C., Goldman, R.N., & Greenberg, L.S. (2004). *Learning emotion-focused therapy: The process-experiential approach to change*. Washington, DC: American Psychological Association.

Greenberg, L.S. (2004). Emotion-focused therapy. *Clinical Psychology & Psychotherapy*, 11(1), 3–16.

Greenberg, L.S., & Pascual-Leone, A. (2006). Emotion in psychotherapy: A practice-friendly research review. *Journal of Clinical Psychology*, 62(5), 611–630.

Hilsenroth, M.J. (2007). A programmatic study of short-term psychodynamic psychotherapy: Assessment, process, outcome, and training. *Psychotherapy Research*, 17(1), 31–45.

Johansson, R., Björklund, M., Hornborg, C., Karlsson, S., Hesser, H., Ljótsson, B., et al. (2013). Affect-focused psychodynamic psychotherapy for depression and anxiety through the Internet: a randomized controlled trial. *PeerJ*, 1, e102.

Kabat-Zinn, J. (1994). *Wherever you go, there you are: Mindfulness meditation in everyday life*. New York: Hachette Books.

Klein, M.H., Mathieu-Coughlan, P.L., & Kiesler, D.J. (1986). The experiencing scales. In L.S. Greenberg, & W.M. Pinsof (Eds.), *The psychotherapeutic process: A research handbook* (pp. 21–71). New York, NY: The Guilford Press.

Lane, R.D., & Garfield, D.A.S. (2005). Becoming aware of feelings: Integration of cognitive-developmental, neuroscientific, and psychoanalytic perspectives. *Neuropsychoanalysis*, 7(1), 5–30.

Lane, R.D., Ryan, L., Nadel, L., & Greenberg, L. (2015). Memory reconsolidation, emotional arousal, and the process of change in psychotherapy: New insights from brain science. *Behavioral and Brain Sciences*, 38, e1.

Leichsenring, F., & Salzer, S. (2014). A unified protocol for the transdiagnostic psychodynamic treatment of anxiety disorders: An evidence-based approach. *Psychotherapy*, 51(2), 224–245.

Lilliengren, P., Johansson, R., Town, J.M., Kisely, S., & Abbass, A. (2017). Intensive short-term dynamic psychotherapy for generalized anxiety disorder: A pilot effectiveness and process-outcome study. *Clinical Psychology & Psychotherapy*, 24(6), 1313–1321.

Malan, D.H. (1963). *A study of brief psychotherapy*. New York: Plenum.

McCullogh, L., & Andrews, S. (2001). Assimilative integration: Short-term dynamic psychotherapy for treating affect phobias. *Clin Psychol*, 8(1), 82–97.

McCarthy, K.S., Keefe, J.R., & Barber, J.P. (2016). Goldilocks on the couch: Moderate levels of psychodynamic and process-experiential technique predict outcome in psychodynamic therapy. *Psychotherapy Research*, 26(3), 307–317.

Missirlian, T.M., Toukmanian, S.G., Warwar, S.H., & Greenberg, L.S. (2005). Emotional arousal, client perceptual processing, and the working alliance in experiential psychotherapy for depression. *J Consult Clin Psychol.*, 73(5), 861–871.

Pascual-Leone, A., & Yeryomenko, N. (2017). The client "experiencing" scale as a predictor of treatment outcomes: A meta analysis on psychotherapy process. *Psychotherapy Research*, 27(6), 653–665.

Subic-Wrana, C., Greenberg, L.S., Lane, R.D., Michal, M., Wiltink, J., & Beutel, M.E. (2016). Affective change in psychodynamic psychotherapy: Theoretical models and clinical approaches to changing emotions. *Zeitschrift für Psychosomatische Medizin und Psychotherapie*, 62(3), 207–223.

Town, J.M., Hardy, G.E., McCulluough, L., & Stride, C. (2012). Patient affect experiencing following therapist interventions in short-term dynamic psychotherapy. *Psychotherapy Research*, 22(2), 208–219.

Ulvenes, P.G., Berggraf, L., Hoffart, A., Stiles, T.C., Svartberg, M., McCullough, L., & Wampold, B.E. (2012). Different processes for different therapies: Therapist actions, therapeutic bond, and outcome. *Psychotherapy*, 49, 291–302.

Wiltink, J., Hoyer, J., Beutel, M.E., Ruckes, C., Herpertz S., Joraschky, P., Koranyi, S., Michal, M., Nolting, B., Poehlmann, K., Salzer, S., Strauss, B., Leibing, E., & Leichsenring, F. (2016). Do patient characteristics predict outcome of psychodynamic psychotherapy for social anxiety disorder? *PLOS ONE*, 11(1).

Zwerenz, R., Becker, J., Johansson, R., Frederick, R.J., & Andersson, G. (2017). Transdiagnostic, psychodynamic web-based self-help intervention following inpatient psychotherapy: Results of a feasibility study and randomized controlled trial. *JMIR Ment Health*, 4(4), e41.

Chapter 14

Discussion from a clinical perspective

Clara Raznoszczyk Schejtman

It is a great pleasure and a responsibility to discuss these impressive contributions. Not only for their theoretical and methodological quality but also for the amount of research data involved. More so since it entails the effort to delve deeper in the notion of affective change in the therapeutic approach.

Briefly, I will endeavor to convey some three main ideas inspired in Dr Beutel's and Dr Clarkin's chapters: (1) Clinical Psychoanalysis, outcome research and pluralism, (2) the role of affect in development, psychopathology and clinical work and (3) the present and future dialogue amongst researchers and clinicians and training new generations.

Clinical psychoanalysis, outcome research and pluralism

> Is research in psychotherapy outcome and evidence-based proposals an answer for the present Zeitgeist?

> Are there universal foundations of psychoanalytical knowledge or are they sensitive to change and to be customized over times and cultures?

> Is pluralism a new paradigm for updating psychoanalysis?

Written outpour in psychoanalysis is huge, highly intellectual and diverse all over the world but the bridges between these products and current research has not been so fluid. Evidence-based manualized therapies that are psychoanalytically oriented are a necessary path to recognition in mental health policies. In Latin America, especially in Buenos Aires and Montevideo, there has been a strong tradition of psychoanalytical education, due to the early translation of Freudian writings into Spanish and to its hegemony in the free public Universities. Even in public hospitals and private health insurance psychoanalytically oriented therapies are the selected method. Psychoanalysts produce changes in the classical tradition and enabled more flexible settings (once or twice a week) and a pluralistic approach in our psychoanalytic associations.

Inspired by Joseph Sandler's ideas, Beatriz de Leon de Bernardi (2017) has presented lately a consistent qualitative research on pluralism. Sandler faced difficulties while trying to build a definitions index of central psychoanalytic concepts and he concluded that this difficulty was related to a tendency in the analysts to build and use in their practice private implicit theories. He referred to it as the "elasticity" of concepts, which have a spectrum of meaning-movement related to a clinical context. Although acknowledging this plurality has been a liberating advance within the analytic community, it had also the potential of inhibiting attempts of integrating concepts (Bohleber et al., 2013).

Most of the analysts maintain that the exploration within the session with the patient is their research method and that the analyst's tools are their own analysis, supervision, and interactive seminars. Several of them are still reluctant to consider empirical research as a suitable methodology to expand psychoanalytical knowledge. Strong controversies had been displayed in this issue, such as the ones held between John Bowlby and the British Psychoanalytic Society, or between Robert Wallerstein and Andre Green, amongst others. Fortunately, debates kept going but some ghosts and persecutory feelings amongst groups diminished and more psychoanalytic societies include today different theoretical frameworks in their trainings and research programs.

De Leon (2017) worked with candidates at the Uruguay Psychoanalytic Association analyzing their supervision reports and their public presentations, together with their written Master's dissertation and a long personal interview about their psychoanalytic education.

In her sample, candidates were satisfied with their pluralistic training and expressed that the integration of concepts did not work consciously while conducting the session. She also found that there was a gap between what was presented in the public presentations and what was going on in the consulting rooms. De Leon (2017) concludes that so-called trans-theoretical bridging concepts are integrated in a tacit way and this tendency is linked to the collective traditions each scientific society builds. At the same time, these traditions promote feelings of membership and cohesiveness that may press the members not to raise certain ideas and concepts that could be critical to the main stream of a society.

She also found that the analysts in the sample attributed different meanings to psychoanalytic concepts, including the fundamental ones.

Is this polysemy in dealing with the concepts a consequence of pluralism? Is this an advantage or a disadvantage for the discipline?

Recently Bob Emde in an interview with Galatzer Levy (2017) suggested an interplay between evidence-based practice and practice-based evidence. He proposes to consider the idea: What works under what circumstances, how, and for whom, in what community, stressing that the community involvement has an additional input to better practices.

Evaluating outcome of psychotherapies is a current demand in order to plan mental health offers and manualization is a useful tool for research. Manualization does not mean simplification. As Clarkin, Maxwell, and Sowislo (in this volume) state about TFP (Transference Focused Psychotherapy) and we can extend to EFPP (Emotional Focused Psychodynamic Psychotherapy) presented by Beutel, Greenberg, and Lane (in this volume): these therapeutic models embrace the heterogeneity across patients, they are not a "cook-book" approach to intervention.

From different methodological data recollection such as those gathered by De Leon through candidates reports and those gathered from Clarkin et al. and Beutel et al. in their therapeutic proposal, the affective rapport with the patient is reported as a main tool to successful psychotherapy. This brings us to our next point.

The role of affect in development, psychopathology and psychotherapy

Clarkin and Beutel have presented us their psychotherapeutic approaches and they highlight the role of affect in the therapeutic achievement. Clarkin et al. (2018) propose that TFP is mostly directed to patients with difficulties with self-identity and interpersonal dysfunction, and acknowledges that affect arousal in a safe setting provides the opportunity to modify extreme cognitions and to relate affects in the emotionally "hot" and immediate experience with others. The hypothesized mechanism of change in TFP is increased affect regulation achieved through the growing ability of the patient to reflect psychologically and put momentary affect arousal, especially in social interactions, into a more benign integration of emotion, thought and behavior.

Beutel et al. proposed that clinical practice and theoretical research have linked personality disorders to repetitive maladaptive reactions or vicious circles of affective arousal, emotion-centered autobiographic memory and semantic structures. Their EFPP model stresses the role of emotional display in the basic change processes in psychotherapy, updating painful emotional memories, which have been guiding maladaptive responses and engaging in new experiences that are incorporated via reconsolidation and reinforcing the new memory.

I want to introduce some ideas about the developmental perspective that links affect regulation-dysregulation in infancy with the building of a sense of identity and internal symbolic representations of self and others and the potential psychopathology that maladaptive affects can produce.

Early affect development is one of the foundational basis of Freudian theory. In "Culture and its Discontent" (Freud, 1930), Freud points out that an infant at the breast does not as yet distinguish his ego from the external world as the source of sensations flowing upon him. He gradually learns to do so, in response to the fact that some sources of excitation, which he will later recognize as his own bodily organs, can provide him with sensations at any moment, whereas other sources evade him from time to time. This first relationship between ego and object is closely related to the presence of a human being that is capable to diminish the displeasure through feeding and reducing the baby's anxiety. The pleasure-displeasure series is the first psychic differentiation.

A pure pleasure ego then is built characterized by a primitive perception of a threatening hated world "outside." The development of the *Bindung* between affects and representations consolidates the ego and the recognition of an "outside" external world opposite to an inside one, though these boundaries are not fixed. Freud stresses that this structural situation is the starting point of pathological disturbances (Freud, 1930).

Several approaches from psychoanalysis and findings produced in infant observation research are in line with these Freudian assumptions. Human babies are born as the most helpless of the species and their dependency on the adult is the strongest and the longest. They are not even aware of their most basic needs and feelings. The five level of emotional awareness theory attempt to integrate neurobiological and psychological findings on emotion processing which is compatible with psychoanalytic developmental and clinical theories (Lane & Schwartz, 1987). At level 1 there is a predominance of consciously unaware stimulus-reflex patterns; affect-related tension is experienced as a physical sensation, whereas level 2 refers to an action response to affective arousal, which is experienced as positively or negatively valence state of tension or as action tendencies.

This radical unawareness of the infant's own affective states and the primary experience of overwhelming affect could be associated with helplessness and has potentially traumatic effects in different periods of life. The action of the adult caregiver has a foundational influence in solving the basic needs and at the same time transforming the original human helplessness.

Debates on the starting of psychic life come from different authors. Laplanche and Pontalis (1973) suggested that affect is the qualitative expression of drives quantitative energy and its shifts. Solms (2017) suggests that conscious states are inherently affective and that emotions are "peremptory forms of motor discharge" (p. 21), which place them at the ID level. According to Freud, Solms sustains that the distinctive feature of affective consciousness would be linked to pleasure-unpleasure series, motorically expressed as approaching/withdrawal behaviors.

Sensory regulation is a first step to affective regulation. The first experiences are basically discharge of tension, non-verbal, unrepresentable and do not have yet a psychic status (Levine et al., 2013). The adult's awareness that affective and motor expressions of the infant are messages to be interpreted in the pleasure-unpleasure series is the way to transform the bodily self into subjective structure. Moreover, the adult capacity to transform infants' negative effect has a crucial role in its discrimination between self and object (me and not me) and between inside and outside world. Myron Hofer (1995) suggests that parents provide hidden regulators of the deep structures of the brain stream which mediate the achievement of sleep-wake cycles and other bodily functions. We can assume that these hidden regulators may be linked to parents' unconscious that has a bearing on their parental function. The intense bodily relationship between the helpless and needy infant and the primary caregiver was a central issue in psychoanalysis from the foundational discoveries of Freud that linked mental psychopathology to early experiences. Pathology has made us acquainted with a great number of states in which the boundary lines between the ego and the external world become uncertain or in which they are actually drawn incorrectly. There are cases in which parts of a person's own body, even portions of his or her own mental life—perceptions, thoughts and feelings—appear alien and as not belonging to his or her ego; there are other cases in which the subjects ascribe to the external world, representations that are originate in their own ego.

From the field of infant research, important contributions have been made to know more about the enigmatic first time of life. Sroufe (1996) suggests that states of pleasure and discomfort are precursor emotions that precede the development of the more discrete states of joy, fear, anger, and others more sophisticated such as shame, nostalgia, jealousy, and pride. Sharing interactive affective experience can thus shape the general intensity and valence of emotional activation in children and an amplification of pleasurable emotions that increases intense engaged affect. Positive dyadic affective engagement builds new joint senses of the world between infant and adult. At the same time the reparation of negative affect is a crucial function of the parental transforming capacity (Tronick, 1989, 2008).

Siegel (1999) suggests that in depressed dyads the shared amplification of positive emotional states is missing or poor and the capacity to emotionally regulate and to enjoy these intense states may be underdeveloped. Feeling comfortable with intense arousal and engagement with others may have its origins in both constitutional and experiential features of the individual. It is often at moments in which emotion becomes most intense that we seem to crave the greatest need to be understood and that defines our subjective emotional vulnerability. "Feeling felt" is a good medicine towards helplessness.

Parents hold the amplification of affective input but also the shift to infant's self-regulation. Vulnerability is present not only in moments of intense pleasurable emotions that may overwhelm the immature infant, but also at separation moments when a sensitive attachment figure that feel in resonance with the infant may lower the possibilities of isolation and withdrawal. Acknowledging the inevitable moments of the infant's unintended disconnection can allow us to repair the normal ruptures in alignment and enables us to learn to tolerate increasing levels of emotional intensity, lowering the effects of extreme vulnerability. The extreme sensitivity of infants towards internal and external stimuli brings out to develop a protective shield or a protective envelop. The adult is part of the infant's protective system and his capacity to transform and repair affects may diminish the potentiality of overwhelming threatening early affects. The parent's psychic structure and unconscious conflicts have a strong impact in this crucial parental function.

Environmental failure in building connection and in repairing negative effects may produce emotional pain, deep anxiety of loss and can carry developmental, physical, emotional and mental damage and a defensive closeness towards the outside world. We can consider these circumstances as maladaptive affect regulation and we can infer that these are in the basis of severe personality disorders as it was described by Beutel et al. and Clarkin et al. in this volume.

In our longitudinal research program at University of Buenos Aires and the IPA, based on a videotaped healthy mother-infant sample we found that successful dyadic regulation brings to the achievement of the capacity to modulate affects and more complex states of mind and to a more smooth transition from dyadic affect regulation to infant's self-regulation. Frequent affective dysregulation and negative affect may produce developmental drawbacks and defensive closure and the protective shield may become rigid, leading to withdrawal and in some cases to partial withdrawal in normal development (Schejtman et al., 2012). Another finding of our team is the subtle differentiation between the building of self-regulation resources by using toys and a more defensive self-regulation that can lead to withdrawal. Self-regulation resources scaffold infants' states of high positive arousal and are a message to the adult to deal with over-engagement. The adult maintains a distal connection while the infant is exploring his own regulatory resources. This process can be related to Winnicott's conceptualization of the foundational paradox about the early capacity of "being alone in the presence of other." Interactive regulation and infant self-regulation are two sides of one dyadic affective regulatory process in which the infant and the mother provide mutual regulatory input that supports self-regulation in the infant (Tronick, 1989, 1998, 2008). We suggested that an infant's self-regulation may be linked to autoerotism. Maternal libidinal input works with the infant's autoerotic self-regulation to scaffold the infant's state of high positive arousal. Autoerotic self-regulation is a healthy narcissistic resource to deal with temporary excessive internal and external stimuli and with short maternal absence (Vardy & Schejtman, 2008).

Self-regulation in the presence of a caring mother that can attune with the affective display of the infant and let the baby be engaged in a libidinal self-exploration may be considered a challenge in the increasing organized complexity of developmental changes.

Through a detailed observation of videotaped material, we differentiate two kinds of infant responses. The first is self-regulatory resources to repair negative affect. The second is a more defensive self-regulatory message of infant withdrawal in response to maternal over-engagement. Distinguishing between the achievement at six months of age of self-regulation as opposed to defensive withdrawal is of high clinical value and was one of the strong contributions of research to clinical work in early infancy (Schejtman et al., 2012, 2014).

The ego capacity to cope with increasing amounts of external and internal stimuli in the infant can be linked to the building of a healthy narcissism as an emotional immunological system. A strong adherence to small familiar sensorial signs is essential to cope with the enormous strangeness that the variations of stimuli from the inner and outer world produce (Solan, 2015). This system may contribute to interpersonal emotional communication and to build relationships with others despite their otherness and inevitable conflicts. Laplanche (1992) suggested that a complex heterogeneous relationship exists between the affective and physical action of the adult towards the infant's body and the inner impact of that action on the movement of the infant's drives. There is no direct effect between the parents' unconscious and the child's structure; but the impact of the adult's actions and representations produce in the child a libidinal movement generated from inside its psyche. The intersubjective parent–infant movement leads to a specific intrapsychic structure in the child and to a particular mode of discharge of drives. Locating intersubjective interactive failures and/or intrapsychic conflicts in the child or in the parents is a new challenge for our clinical practice.

Recently Miller (2013) in a research conducted in Uruguay found that children with higher levels of emotional dysregulation showed emotional and behavioral disturbances, aggression, manifestations of anxiety, depression, and attentional disorders. Another significant point about the parental capacity to deal with the affective display and its regulation in infancy is the parental reflective function. Parental capacity for recognizing an infant's or child's mental states, feelings, thoughts, and connecting them in meaningful ways has an impact in the development of a sense of himself as both connected to and separated from the parent (Fonagy, Gergely et al., 2002; Slade et al., 2003).

Connection and separation are central in development. Separations involves suffering and mourning both for the child and the parent, even if they are necessary for development. The concept of alterity in the intimate relationship conveys the capacity of feeling together and separated at the same time. When normal separation is felt as abandonment, the original helplessness may appear with its potentially traumatic effects and its consequences in a maladaptive affective regulation.

In a healthy sample of dyads of preschool children, we found that mothers who were less reflective regarding their attitudes towards their child's anger and dysregulated manifestations showed greater intrusiveness and critical verbalization in a videotaped playing interaction with their children (Schejtman, 2017). Parent recognition of a link between the infant's mental states and their behavior will contribute to develop a mental model of the affective experience, and thus contribute to the developing capacities for affective self-regulation. Likewise, the mother's capacity to appreciate the dynamics of her own affective experience is regulating as well. Our proposal is to diagnose early presence of partial withdrawal, rigid defenses and maternal over engagement in normal development. Diagnosing means capturing the unique qualities of each baby and family, focusing in healthy resources. Short-term dyadic early interventions may diminish developmental drawbacks of emotional, cognitive and social potentialities of the child.

Clarkin and Beutel sustain that affective display is essential for a positive result in psychotherapy, both in TFP and in EFPP. In TFP the objective is to produce a new benign regulation that can be assimilate to the patient's structure while in EFPP the assumption is that the only way to produce a change is to elicit most primary affects.

Some questions that these proposals raise:

- Is affective arousal in psychotherapy a new opportunity of affective interactive amplification like the one between infant and adult?
- May this affective amplification also elicit early overwhelming negative affects?
- Is emotional activation the key path to therapeutic change regardless the theoretical approach?
- What could be considered a consistent change regarding the theoretical conception of each therapeutic approach?

As John Clarkin et al. (2018) state about borderline patients and probably for other severely disturbed patients, the main difficulty is the lack of accurate perception between self and other, difficulties in building intimacy and dysregulated expressions in everyday life. Both TFP and EFPP propose that emotional arousal activation in the therapy has a strong impact in the process of change. The difference may consist that in EFPP the analyst uses activation techniques to elicit emotional arousal.

But how to relate this active position of the analyst with neutrality and abstinence?

How the relationship between transference-counter transference-resistances would be displayed in the session?

Could the therapist initiative enhance resistance or reactivate early defensive shields in the patient?

Is necessary a diagnosis of psychic vulnerability in order to choose which psychotherapeutic method is the suitable for each patient?

Privileging affective interchange between patient and therapist, rather than verbal interpretations and intellectual reflection, is an emotional challenge for the therapist and requires permanent self-reflection, self-analysis and intensive training to cope with this emotional amplification. Coming to the training and education of analysts, I get to my third point.

Present and future of mutual enrichment between researchers and clinicians: training new generations

Manfred E. Beutel et al. foresee in the future of psychoanalytical practice transdiagnostic approaches. Emde in Galatzer Levy (2017) reminds us Serge

Lebovici's idea of psychoanalysis as a *trans* discipline, as integrative but multidisciplinary in outlook.

Interdisciplinary and transdisciplinary approaches may enhance psychoanalytical treatment efficacy and may enhance our presence and contributions to mental health policies, infancy rights, violence inside and outside families and other.

But what should we focus on in the training of new generations of psychotherapists training? Is research a new pathway to training professionals and must be included in the institutes programs? How to put together the deep elaboration each theoretical approach is offering with a pluralistic perspective, not only in the mental health field but also in connecting disciplines? How to train analysts with affective implication in their practices?

Dialogues and collaboration are taking place in different projects. In Brazil, Rogerio Lerner and his colleagues have managed to include psychoanalysts in the building of an evaluation system for early detection of autistic signs IRDI. A new multidisciplinary seminar on complex cases in infancy is being held in the Argentine Psychoanalytic Association. New bridges between psychoanalysis and research are part of the research and teaching programs at the University of Buenos Aires.

Workshops with clinicians and researchers, like the Research Training Program of the IPA and different models of working parties, are popular in our societies and international congresses. Marianne Leuzinger Bohleber is working with refugees and migrants in Germany with emotional involvement towards the most vulnerable. Susana Vinocur Fischbein and I were working on social violence in Latin America. Mark Solms is disseminating Neuropsychoanalysis. The IPA is publishing the "Open Door Review," summarizing decades of systematic psychotherapy research.

Research outcome is a useful tool to clinicians that are not necessarily engaged in research and that are practicing different psychotherapeutic approaches. Meaningful dialogues between researchers and clinicians may help to bridge data with deep theoretical conceptualization that guide the clinical work.

I wish a present and future of cross fertilization between research, clinical practice and its implications in renewing theories and outreach activities directed to our communities. Emotional involvement, pluralism and critical scientific attitudes in the therapist's education may improve our practices oriented to deal with vulnerability and subjective suffering.

References

Bohleber, W., Fonagy, P., Jiménez, J.P., Scarfone, D., Varvin, S., & Zysman, S. (2013). Towards a better use of psychoanalytic concepts: A model illustrated using the concept of enactment. *International Journal of Psychoanalysis*, 94, 501–530.

Clarkin, J., Cain, N., & Lenzenweger, M. (2018). Advances in transference-focused psychotherapy derived from the study of borderline personality disorder: Clinical insights with a focus on mechanism. *Current Opinion in Psychology*, 21, 80–85. doi: 10.1016/j.copsyc.2017.09.008.

De Leon de Bernardi, B. (2017). *Efectos del pluralismo teórico en la formación y la práctica psicoanalítica*. Disertación doctoral, Universidad de Buenos Aires, 2017.

Fonagy, P., Gergely, G., Jurist, E., & Target, M. (2002). *Affect regulation, mentalization: Developmental clinical and theoretical perspective*. New York: Others Press.

Freud, S. (1930). Culture and its discontents. In: *Standard edition of complete works*. New York: Hogarth Press.

Galatzer Levy, R. (2017). An interview with Robert Emde. *The American Psychoanalyst*, 51 (4), 5–6, 19–20.

Hofer, M.A. (1995). Hidden regulators: implications for a new understanding of attachment, separation and loss. In: S. Goldberg, R. Muir & J. Kerr (Eds.), *Attachment theory: Social development and clinical perspectives* (pp. 203–230). Hillsdale, NJ: The Analytic Press, Inc.

Lane, R.D., & Schwartz, G.E. (1987). Levels of emotional awareness: A cognitive-developmental theory and its application to psychopathology. *Am J Psychiatry*, 144, 133–143.

Laplanche, J. (1992). *La Révolution copernicienne inachevée. Travaux 1967–1992*. Paris: Aubier.

Laplanche, J., & Pontalis, J.-B. (1973). *The language of psycho-analysis*. New York: Hogarth Press.

Levine, H.B., Reed, G.S., & Scarfone, D. (2013). *Unrepresented states and the construction of meaning*. London: Karnac Books.

Miller, D. (2013). *Las huellas del afecto*. Grupo Magro Editores, Universidad Católica Uruguay.

Schejtman, C.R. (2017). *Función materna. Relación entre variables intrapsíquicas y variables interactivas observacionales*. Tesis de doctorado Facultad de Psicología, Universidad de Buenos Aires.

Schejtman, C.R., Huerin, V., Vernengo, M.P., Esteve, M.J., Silver, R., Vardy, I., Laplacette, J.A., & Duhalde, C. (2014). Regulación afectiva, procesos de simbolización y subjetividad materna en el juego madre-niño. *Revista de Psicoanálisis de la Asociación Psicoanalítica de Madrid*, (71), 3–24. Madrid, España. ISSN 1135-3171.

Schejtman, C.R., Huerin, V., & Duhalde, C. (2012). A longitudinal study of dyadic and self affective regulation and its link with maternal reflective functioning along the first 5 years of life. *The Signal, WAIMH (Asociación Mundial de Salud mental infantil)*, 20(2), abril–junio 2012. www.waimh.org/files/signal//signal_2_2012.pdf.

Siegel, D. (1999). *The developing mind: Toward a neurobiology of interpersonal experience*, New York: Guilford Press.

Slade, A., Aber, J., Berger, B., Bresgi, I., & Kaplan, M. (2003). *PDI-R2. Parent development interview revised*. New Haven, CT: Yale Child Study Center, Yale University.

Solan, R. (2015). *The enigma of childhood*. London: Karnac.

Solms, M. (2017). "The unconscious" in psychoanalysis and neuroscience: An integrated approach to the cognitive unconscious. In: M. Leuzinger-Bohleber, S. Arnold, & M. Solms (Eds.), *The unconscious. A bridge between psychoanalysis and cognitive neurosciences* (pp. 16–35). London/New York: Routledge.

Sroufe, L.A. (1996). *Emotional development. The organization of emotional life in the early years.* New York: Cambridge University Press.

Tronick, E.Z. (1989). Emotions and emotional communication in infants. *American Psychologist, 44,* 112–119.

Tronick, E.Z. (1998). Dyadically expanded states of conscious and the process of therapeutic change. *Infant Mental Health Journal, 19,* 290–299.

Tronick, E.Z. (2008). Conexión intersubjetiva, estados de conciencia y significación. In C.R. Schejtman (Ed.). *Primera Infancia. Psicoanálisis e Investigación* (pp. 155–168), Buenos Aires: Akadia Editorial.

Vardy, I., & Schejtman, C.R. (2008). Afectos y regulación afectiva. Un desafío bifronte en la primera infancia. In: C.R. Schejtman (Ed.). *Primera Infancia. Psicoanálisis e Investigación* (pp. 53–70). Buenos Aires: Akadia Editorial.

Part III

Critical thinking and research in psychoanalytic education

A clinician's view of research, critical thinking, and culture in psychoanalytic education

Linda S. Goodman

Introduction

As a clinician, I'm taken with the subtitle of this volume: Researchers and Clinicians in Dialogue. I imagine some believe the survival of psychoanalysis depends on this: Researchers and Clinicians in Dialogue. What is the prospect for that to happen? How do we understand what might promote or hinder this? My chapter takes this up and begins with an institute classroom experience. I'll then offer some local and national context for the prospect of such dialogue. My point will be to locate our current prospects for survival within a broader cultural context. I believe beyond stimulating interest and engagement with research, and promoting tolerance of psychoanalytic pluralism, we'll enhance the meaningfulness of our educational initiatives for our candidates and for ourselves and our prospects for a vibrant future, first, by strengthening and energizing integrative initiatives. Second, I imagine the benefits of these initiatives will optimally occur as we are able to affirm psychoanalytic values to guide us through times of uncertainty and discontinuity. I imagine by navigating in light of psychoanalytic values we'll retain our identity and foster our integrity as we venture on. That's a sketch of what's ahead.

For now, I'd like to relate a classroom experience:

A psychoanalytic classroom vignette

A paper made a low arc and landed on the seminar table. Tossed casually, and into the proximity of fellow candidates, I noticed some looked up. It was indeed an expressive gesture. What to make of it?—Dismissive? Frustrated? Contemptuous-rejecting? Or, something else? The introductory course aimed to advance an initiative for integrating psychoanalytic concepts, clinical material and an example of relevant research. The topic of the class session was interpretation. It aimed to demonstrate the value of clinical nuance. As clinicians, most of our candidates already knew intuitively that characteristics of the individual patient, as well as timing, tact and dosage, make a significant difference in how the work goes, and now this paper demonstrated something further: namely, that systematic research showed a moderating variable about the patient can also make a difference. In this case, the moderating variable was poor versus more mature object relations. And here was some evidence that the positive effect of transference interpretation on outcome is more likely in patients with poor object relations versus in patients with more mature object relations (see Hoglend et al, 2007). Another way of knowing had been introduced. And it offered, perhaps, a surprising finding, not what one would imagine our analytic fathers and mothers would have taught. Had I just witnessed an understandable "foreign body" reaction—as *both* systematic research was introduced, and as conventional wisdom was questioned? I sensed there was a great deal more to understand.

I looked up at the candidate and recalled that earlier in the class a description of the candidate's analysand had been offered. The analysand's style had come across as a non-stop and voluminous out-pouring. The candidate was frank to disclose feeling overwhelmed by the too-muchness of the material and the sense of helplessness in the face of it. Reflecting back, I imagined the tossed paper could be announcing "and now the instructor gives me moderating variables to deal with? I don't think so." Was I seeing what one might call a "crass resistance" to my "poor timing"? And/or, could the gesture have been an attempt to regulate anxiety? Given the candidate's sense of overwhelm, that paper wasn't helpful—"so toss it."

Yet there was more: speaking toward the end of the class, the candidate observed that this paper isn't even about psychoanalysis, it's about psychodynamic psychotherapy. Now, the candidate was raising the question of its relevance. More evidence of resistance? Or, was it also a reasonable question in the service of critical thinking? Perhaps both and more. I expressed appreciation for the critical thinking and reformulated the observation as a question about relevance. That (actually) it's not a settled question whether research findings on psychodynamic psychotherapy are relevant to psychoanalysis. Frequency of sessions (what some call "dosage") might make a telling difference. I didn't press on further. It was time to stop and it seemed the candidate already had a plateful. I wondered if the candidate might be feeling some relief to think there was no need to bother with presumably irrelevant research findings.

After class, I recall feeling more challenged than I had expected by what had happened. When I reflected back on the entirety of it, I came to feel grateful for this glimpse into the tangled intertwining of clinical education (including elements of transference and countertransference), critical thinking and research. The experience provided a rare glimpse of something not often seen overtly, but most probably something, that is commonly there. I came to see my experience as not only a valuable challenge for me, but also for my colleagues and generally for the field of psychoanalysis. There is so much here and I will return later to give further context for the vignette.

Backstory

First, I'd like to introduce myself. I'm a clinician—a clinical psychologist trained at a research-oriented university and a psychoanalyst from the New Center for Psychoanalysis (NCP). I've chaired, or co-chaired, our NCP Research Committee for many years and along with other chairs and co-chairs [specifically Drs Morris Eagle and Joshua Pretsky who join me here today], we've collaborated with a fine group of bright and congenial NCP colleagues in taking up research relevant to psychoanalysis. We are basically an interest group. From time to time we have invited scholars and research speakers for formal presentations in conjunction with support from the NCP Program Committee and Robert Stoller Foundation. And finally, from time to time, we provided encouragement, and some supportive consultation as we could, for a few research projects. Our efforts have been modest, and we were not the first pioneers in our community. Our Research Committee met as a congenial interest group for many years. We regularly invited others to join us. As you might guess, there weren't many rsvp's.

However, as some of you probably know, a growing number of analysts and psychodynamic clinicians have been convinced the time had come to confront our resistances, "step up our game," and implement a more energized educational mission of encouraging greater open-ness and curiosity about knowledge from bordering fields. Perhaps it was four years ago, our colleague and then co-chair Allan Compton strongly suggested we propose a modest pilot project to integrate some relevant research in a few selected courses in which instructors were open to this idea. The idea was reviewed (thoughtfully, if not perhaps warily) by NCP Curriculum Committee and approved. The pilot was to make a modest maiden voyage.

Ironically, our experimental pilot project on its "maiden voyage" met up with major transformations in the organizational culture of APsaA. National gate-keeping functions in education and training were giving way to ideas of "local option" and "institute choice." It seemed the small NCP pilot craft had "caught a wave" and was an idea whose time had come. Morris Eagle and I were invited to Co-chair the Research Education Section of APsaA's newly minted Department of Psychoanalytic Education. We, perhaps naively, accepted.

As I alluded to earlier, cultural context matters and I return to it now: At both the micro level in our clinical practices and at the macro level, cultural shifts and emerging realities also influence the course of psychoanalytic history. Without going into detail, here are some obvious factors: emerging and elaborating psychoanalytic pluralism, reductions in numbers of analytic patients, cost control pressures from third party payers as well as changing expectations from patients. I imagine you could add others. In addition, the slowly developing corpus of psychoanalytic process and outcome research wasn't given the recognition it deserved. This is in part due to its small audience.

Research findings were regularly ignored in Institute classes and at psychoanalytic meetings. All of these factors and more have contributed to a sense that the health of psychoanalysis is in serious hazard.

Alerts, warnings and proposed remedies

During this time, some of our leaders have issued various alerts and warnings. Otto Kernberg has pressed this case in a crescendoing series of papers. First delivered 20 years ago, his paper "A Concerned Critique of Psychoanalytic Education" (Kernberg 2000) advised:

> The systematic neglect of research training and of developing a research attitude is a major problem of contemporary psychoanalytic education, reflecting a dangerous lack of concern for the scientific standing of psychoanalysis in the world that surrounds us.
>
> (p. 109)

Kernberg continues:

> It needs to be stressed that psychoanalytic research includes a broad spectrum of investigation, ranging from clinical research in the psychoanalytic situation to scholarly critique of psychoanalytic concepts; from hermeneutic research regarding the clinical application of conceptual models, to empirical research within and outside the psychoanalytic situation.
>
> (p. 109)

And he carries on that these investigations are crucial because they "foster progress in psychoanalytic knowledge and its acceptance in the intellectual world" (p. 109).

Six years later Kernberg (2006) followed with "The Pressing Need to Increase Research in and on Psychoanalysis" wherein the psychoanalytic community was called out—for keeping a safe distance from research findings that paradoxically psychoanalytic theoreticians and clinicians had inspired or catalyzed. Kernberg urged that it was time for a broad spectrum of research to be undertaken from individual candidate's work to collaborative institutional projects and to establish or reestablish links with universities (p. 923).

More recently Kernberg's tone became more imperative (2012). In "Suicide Prevention for Psychoanalytic Institutes and Societies," he envisioned that any attempt to alter a failing psychoanalytic society was likely to "generate intense anxiety, frequently expressed as a desperate clinging to "standards" "which is actually an attempt to maintain a comfortable status quo." He advocates developing "rescue teams" that require intensive individual and organizational training and yet he anticipates that any efforts to teach survival skills in the context of threatening realities are likely to generate "worries about the victim's 'identity' and existential doubt about whether one is still what he or she does" (p 707). In other words, he anticipates very considerable resistance in response to attempts to promote change. Observing the well-known caution that a drowning victim may resist rescue efforts and drown their rescuer as well as themselves, the rescuer must be prepared to deal with desperate and blind resistance at times.

What is Kernberg's rescue plan? Here, condensed, are his six points:

1 Establishing a life line with local universities to counteract professional and scientific isolation.
2 Developing psychoanalytically oriented psychotherapy programs. In doing so, Kernberg anticipated reactions that such programs could threaten the identity of analysts and stimulate reactions that an institute's mission is to focus exclusively on training psychoanalysts.
3 Injecting a "research orientation" into your organizational life—letting go of monofocal perspectives in favor of tolerance of multiple and even contradictory theories and a tolerance and openness to multiple perspectives, as well as findings from neighboring fields.
4 Present a realistic public image of your scientific achievements and concerns as well as your clinical and professional contributions.
5 Innovate in psychoanalytic education—though he warned this will be the most difficult aspect as his first suggestion was to abolish the training analyst system as it existed in 2012. He recommended instead an alternative certification process based on a realistic assessment of psychoanalytic competence. In addition, he advised the selection of faculty on the basis of excellence in teaching as well as intellectual interests and areas of specialized knowledge, and participation in the scientific activities of institute, etc.
6 Finally, he urged rescuers to familiarize themselves with typical expressions of opposition to change—even sophisticated, subtle descriptions implying qualitative distinction between psychoanalysis and psychodynamic psychotherapy if the distinction is based on the assumption that they are in opposition to one another. In fact, he alluded to a growing body of evidence that both empirical research and conceptual developments show they are complementary rather than in opposition.

While valuable, it seems to me Kernberg's rescue guidelines for institutes and training programs would benefit from emphasizing a still larger historical and cultural context. Pluralism of different schools in psychoanalysis do, in fact, give rise to anxiety among some analytic clinicians as seen in the following comments expressed on the APsaA listserve. I don't expect this anxiety would, in the short term, be salved by greater attention simply to research findings, nor by adjustments in who gets to be faculty or training and supervising analysts. Here's a portion of one listserve posting after a recent APsaA national meeting (All quotes are given with permission):

Personally, I believe that beneath what we call politics is anxiety about reviewing the efficacy of psychoanalysis as taught and practiced in today's world. OR, are we each doing work tailored to the individual but hesitant to talk about it. Is there a pull as some(one) suggest to preserving the status quo?

In my mind we have huge questions but not enough opportunities for discussion. Is this because of anxiety, arrogance, certitude, or what? I honestly do not know.

On another posting, the writer traces influences that brought new ideas and perspectives infusing further talent and creativity into the field. The writer continues describing that which,

gave rise to pluralism which albeit creative is putting forth conflicting propositions and calls for conflicting educational prescriptions. We now have the overflow of interesting ideas but insufficient structures to arrive at multifold integration of them. […] Many interesting voices clamor for deserving attention, but often talk past each other. Books and articles are written but how successfully do they get woven into the discourse? It seems unlikely that attending worthwhile panels could bring this about sufficiently. Many of us do such integrations on our own, but for psychoanalysis to be successful we need to do it together, don't we?

I join the last writer in placing high value on efforts to integrate our psychoanalytic thinking and pluralism. It is not enough to tolerate pluralism, however politely or ecumenically we sit together. Beyond becoming research consumers, I believe we also need to work toward and support efforts toward *an integrative perspective*. However, in my view, only an integrative perspective that includes research findings will permit a meaningfully innovative and evolving future.

Analytic identity and the psychoanalyst's ego ideal

Focusing on the current cultural context in psychoanalysis, it's fair to ask will those who lead beyond the traditional and the status quo be wisely received or cast out? Given our pluralism, it seemed the field was nearly past the conversation-stopping pronouncement: "that's not analysis." Kernberg's point about needing to familiarize ourselves with typical expressions of opposition to change is true but incomplete. It's not just desperate clinging to the past to avoid, say, the anxiety of change. We need to understand and discern between resistance when change also threatens the violation of valued standards versus resistance to fend off valid challenge by raising disqualifying questions about the challenger's analytic identity. I imagine sometimes this will be a tough and anxiety provoking call. This might be especially so when change also threatens a shame-inducing violation of a psychoanalyst's internalized ego ideal.

Jonathan Lear (2008) discussed the role of shame vis a vis the internalized "other." He wrote movingly about it in his book *Radical Hope: Ethics in the Face of Cultural Devastation*. He described how the Crow Indian nation's loss of the buffalo brought in its wake a near cultural collapse. This was the case because it triggered the loss of the hunter/warrior role model—an ideal of authority and leadership. While changes in psychoanalysis hardly match the cataclysmic challenges faced by the Crow nation, perhaps there is value in considering some cultural resonances. Lear wrote of the Crow Chief:

> who continued to experience shame at the prospect of certain acts [that] might show he was stuck in a past world psychologically unable to face the radically new circumstances that confronted him ... after all, how is one to change one's second nature?
>
> (p. 87)

Lear referenced Bernard Williams discussing Sophocles' Ajax and the role of shame vis a vis the internalized other:

> What countenance can I show my father Telemon?
> How will he bear the sight of me
> If I come before him naked, without any glory,
> When he himself had a great crown of men's praise?
> It is not something to be born.
>
> (pp 87–88)

Lear (2008) described how in fact the survival of the Crow nation involved a remarkable transformation of the internalized ideals one aspires to—(to avoid shame) in short, to a transformed ego ideal. Led by the Chief's dream and the elders interpretation of it, an ancillary Crow icon of the Chickadee was elevated to help the tribe survive the cultural devastation that was upon them. The dream advised:

> become a Chickadee! He is least in strength but strongest of mind among his kind. He is willing to work for wisdom. The Chickadee-person is a good listener. Nothing escapes his ears, which he has sharpened by constant use. Whenever others are talking together about their successes and their failures, there you will find the Chickadee person listening to their words.
>
> (p. 80)

Lear (importing Aristotelean ethics) terms Chickadee virtue a new form of courage that is integral to a transformed ego ideal.

Allan Compton (2008) in reviewing Lear's book described the Chief as an exemplar of a state of mind that Lear calls "radical hope," and wrote that Lear's intent was to demonstrate the possibility of achieving that state of mind. Compton inferred:

> The person who demonstrates radical hope and courage is a leader who can find a way to adapt to calamities without losing the essence of what made him himself or her herself. Given a situation of cultural devastation, it is conceivable that a person could respond neither with despair nor with denial. To respond optimally requires an underlying 'radical courage,' in order to be able to deal with the unimaginable.
>
> (p. 493)

While I don't believe psychoanalysis is in comparable cultural ruin, the kinds of changes encouraged by Kernberg and others may well be experienced by some as the need to transform a psychoanalytic ego ideal.

Compton (2008), in his concluding remarks, observed how Lear's inspiring book:

> makes us realize how much the values appropriate to the treatment situation may have impoverished other aspects of psychoanalytic culture, such as our public presentation to each other and to the rest of the world. To pursue the "goods" that Aristotle outlined with the overriding good of excellence guiding us, leaders must have courage and must encourage hope. They must act neither in a timorous, retiring way nor in an impulsive, needlessly disruptive way, but from a standpoint in between, and with wisdom. Further, they must be able to act (not just think) wisely in situations that vary from mildly upsetting to totally catastrophic.... For psychoanalysts, in view of the gradual but steady decline of our profession within American culture, these are particularly urgent recommendations. Positive values have become (or have usually been) foreign to open discussion by psychoanalysts, though there are certainly exceptions....
>
> (p. 501)

Integrative thoughts and positive values

It might be understandable, at this point, to question what all this has to do with a clinician's view of research, critical thinking and culture in psychoanalytic education?

Positive values of truthfulness and patient welfare are ones that psychoanalytic treatment and research broadly share. These values—truthfulness and patient welfare—merit a rich and ongoing dialogue. And this would be the case not only for traditional psychoanalytic practice but also for analytic clinicians meeting bordering fields of knowledge and expanded domains of action. What will allow clinicians to move ahead without losing essential analytic values, without sacrificing one's analytic identity and guidance by an essentially analytic ego ideal?

It seems we will be best served when our educational mission reaches beyond research consumption and theoretical integration. As we affirm analytic values which include truthfulness and patient welfare and confirm psychoanalytic identities, both in our thinking and professional activities, it seems possible resistances to altering currently engrained educational practice might give way to greater imagination and creativity. Doing so may foster a more productive dialogue between clinicians and researchers, and consequently further the educational mission with an integration of research findings, critical thinking, and clinical wisdom. I'm closing with what I hope you will find an inspiring thought as well as a meaningful prospect.

References

Compton, A. (2008). Radical Hope: Ethics in the Face of Cultural Devastation Jonathan Lear. Cambridge, MA: Harvard University Press, 2008. *American Imago*, 65(3): 489–502.

Hoglend, P., Amlo, S., Marble, A., Bogward, K-P., Sorbye, O., Sjaastad, M.C., & Heyerdaahl, O. (2006) Analysis of the Patient-Therapist Relationship in Dynamic Psychotherapy: An Experimental Study of Transference Interpretations. *American Journal of Psychiatry*, 164(10), 1739-1746.

Kernberg, O.F. (2000). A Concerned Critique of Psychoanalytic Education, *International Journal of Psychoanalysis*, 81(1): 97–120.

Kernberg, O.F. (2006). The Pressing Need to Increase Research in and on Psychoanalysis. *International Journal of Psychoanalysis*, 87(4): 919–926.

Kernberg, O.F. (2012). Suicide Prevention for Psychoanalytic Institutes and Societies. *Journal of the American Psychoanalytic Association*, 60(4): 707–719.

Lear, J. (2008). *Radical Hope: Ethics in the Face of Cultural Devastation*. Cambridge, MA: Harvard University Press.

Chapter 16

Teaching empirical research in psychodynamic psychotherapy

How to make research *really* matter

Joshua Pretsky

Teaching psychodynamic psychotherapy and psychoanalytic students about empirical research methods and findings is imperative in developing their clinical capacities and in cultivating their critical thinking. They should not only be informed about research findings but also persuaded that the empirical literature is of compelling relevance to how they think about and approach their patients clinically each day in their offices. I aim to spark their interest and provide them tools to continue a relationship with the research literature as lifelong learners.

I've come to this conclusion based on a number of formative professional experiences that I will share. I will then describe the settings in which I teach, each with its own unique context, student characteristics and emphases, and then provide a list of teaching topics that I have found most effective over the years.

My passion for teaching empirical research to psychoanalytic and psychodynamic therapy students grew out of a number of formative professional experiences during my psychoanalytic journey. The main influence was, and has been, my own experience as a practicing psychotherapist. Compelled by the clinical challenges and needs faced in my office, I evolved away from the traditional analytic technique of my training toward a more flexible, actively engaged and experientially-focused approach. This shift, I feel, has been reflective of changes in the profession overall caused by the evolution of psychoanalytic theory, the decline in psychoanalyses, and the "contemporary crisis of psychoanalysis."

A few important mentors helped shape my path. During analytic training at the New Center for Psychoanalysis (NCP) in Los Angeles I was fortunate to have as my primary supervisor Gerald Aronson, an empirically minded and highly compassionate person who taught me that analytic technique served therapeutic outcome and was not a means unto itself. A brilliant polymath, he made room during our meetings for open inquiry, challenges to analytic theory and an experimental approach to clinical technique. He encouraged and fostered my critical thinking and helped attenuate a self-generated pressure to conform to the views of my educational authorities. Earlier, during psychiatry residency at Columbia University in New York City, Lisa Mellman invited me to join her research project converting the Wallerstein Scales of Psychological Capacities to a self-report form. This gave me first-hand experience in scale development, statistics and the intellectual rigor needed for research. At Columbia I also met with Beatrice Beebe, who taught me about the use of video coding systems and time-series regression analysis in the study of mother-infant dyads. Each in their own way, these mentors imparted the value of science in psychoanalysis.

My own ten-year training analysis was another major influence. My training analyst was and is a warm, astute, vibrant and wise man. He was much more open and comfortable with himself than I was with myself at the time and he helped me greatly. Yet, the use of the couch and the relatively abstinent stance of pure-form analysis created a certain interpersonal distance that my defenses exploited. Somewhere around year three he did not utter a single word for an entire week. I appreciate now, and appreciated then, his attempt to try something radical in order to shake me up. But, that move only drew me further into my defended self. When the planned termination came years later he had me sit back up in the chair opposite him for about three weeks. We both observed how much more emotionally open and accessible I was in that arrangement. I wonder how much deeper and shorter my analysis might have been had I sat up for most of it. This experience left me thinking about the overall effectiveness of psychoanalysis and how, in some cases, analytically desirable results might be achieved more efficiently with a more active, focused and emotionally engaged stance.

The next significant influence was not being passed for certification by the American Psychoanalytic Association three years after graduation from analytic training. The brief explanatory letter stated that I failed to address as resistance to analysis the patient's decision to go to graduate school and cut back on treatment from four times to one or two times per week, even though this decision occurred after a number of years of three to four day a week analysis and measurable clinical improvement. This explanation was not accompanied by any objective justification or evidence. I was left with the impression that official psychoanalysis privileged strict analytic technique above clinical improvement. I was also greatly troubled by the implication that the patient's decision was further evidence of pathology rather than a sign of psychological growth that emerged from the therapeutic work of the already extensive analysis. Like many others before me, I came away from that experience rather dismayed and critical of the process, having seen directly the biases and validity problems inherent in it.

The next major influence was my own research on analytic practice patterns by psychoanalytic graduates. The major finding of our study was that graduate analysts had, on average, less than one case of analysis in their practice (Pretsky, Aizaga, & Cherry 2009). This finding led me to consider the training goals of psychoanalytic training and the continued emphasis of institutes on their psychoanalytic over their psychodynamic therapy training programs.

Last but not least, a significant influence has been, and continues to be, the overall support for research and research education from the leadership of my analytic home, NCP. NCP has maintained a research committee since its inception; it has sponsored lectures on research topics by visiting scholars; it embarked on a new research teaching pilot program a few years ago; at the time of this publication two of its members (Drs. Goodman and Eagle) head the American Psychoanalytic Association Department of Education research education section; and NCP was a co-sponsor of the 2018 Joseph Sandler psychoanalytic research conference. I am grateful for the open-minded, embracing stance toward research found in this organization, recognizing this is not necessarily the case at other institutes.

All of these influences evoked a passion for teaching psychotherapy research. However, I have come to appreciate the challenges faced in trying to engage students on this topic; one that they may experience as esoteric, irrelevant, confusing, or boring. Some opposition emerges from a particular student's opinions and experiences and some is generic; more to do with the problems of the research literature itself (i.e., experience distant, opaque, mechanistic, statistics-laden, at times full of jargon and poorly written). How then can one make empirical research really matter to students? Clinical immediacy is the lode star. The teacher must convey this information in ways that captures the students' imagination, persuades them of its relevance to their clinical work and leaves them more interested in, and more equipped to engage with the literature throughout their career. Along the way, the teacher must increase the student's ability and freedom to think critically about the teachings they encounter in their training. As an effective translator the teacher must stay current on the literature and be able to explain basic research design and statistical concepts simply and clearly, linking them to clinical examples.

In terms of settings, I teach senior psychiatry residents at the University of California, Los Angeles. These students are well versed in research methods, the value of empirical research, and how to interpret study findings. Some of these students are medical or basic science researchers themselves. They are a homogeneous group which values the scientific method and statistical analysis. However, they are quite inexperienced as psychotherapists. They need help conceptualizing how this information might apply to their own clinical experience.

With this group I focus on research in the areas of attachment, the therapy relationship, alliance rupture and repair, and defense work to help shape their therapeutic stance and clinical identity. I also firmly establish psychodynamic psychotherapy as an evidence-based treatment and discuss how it compares favorably to the other types of therapy that they are required to learn (mainly CBT).

At NCP I teach psychoanalytic psychotherapy students. These students have varying levels of psychodynamic psychotherapy experience but are generally experienced clinicians who are well-versed in other modalities, such as DBT and supportive, problem focused therapy. More of them tend to work in clinic settings rather than in private practice. Many of those in clinic settings are often asked to deliver manualized treatments and to engage in onerous data tracking at their workplace. They find it either meaningless or anti-therapeutic as it's perceived not to reflect what is really going on for the patient. Their antipathy also relates to the administrative paperwork these approaches impose on them. They crave more meaning and deeper interactions with patients in their work. Other of these psychotherapy students are experienced private practice therapists also looking to deepen their work. In this population, research fluency is variable and, despite their frustrations with evidence-based approaches in their own experience, they are excited to hear that psychodynamic psychotherapy is proven to be effective. They also enjoy seeing how psychoanalytic concepts are operationalized for research purposes through the use of psychoanalytically meaningful ways of codifying process and outcome.

With this group I emphasize technique, asking them to consider the relational, affective and experiential aspects of a psychodynamic approach as it lines up with the robust findings on common factors and outcome. I also focus on the use of the self of the therapist in understanding countertransference reactions, in managing the working alliance, in being authentic and in considering the use of judicious self-disclosure.

Finally, along with Morris Eagle, I co-teach an introduction to empirical research and critical thinking to first-year analytic students at NCP. This is part of the new educational pilot program where research findings are brought into a number of courses across the four year curriculum. These students are generally experienced, seasoned clinicians, with the exception of those who come from non-mental health fields such as the humanities, social sciences and the law. All psychoanalytic students come seeking greater depth and meaning to their work. They have varied research exposure and training backgrounds and tend to be either uninformed, neutral, skeptical, or contemptuous of empirical research as it pertains to psychoanalysis. However, they typically appreciate the logic and reasoning of the scientific method and can be persuaded by a well-made case that the psychological scales and measures, study designs and findings of empirical research capture the complexity and depth of psychoanalytic thinking and are, therefore, meaningful and applicable.

With this group, I encourage the students to adopt an active critical thinking attitude as they embark on their training. In this setting I emphasize an exploration of the biases and distortions of clinical data commonly found in psychoanalytic case reports that weaken the validity of their theoretical assertions. We discuss criteria that make for an empirically sound case report and the role and purpose of individual case and population-based studies. I also emphasize the importance of therapeutic outcome and encourage students to question the "but it's not analysis" orientation so embedded in psychoanalytic culture. We cover some of the problems of teaching by appeals to authority often found in psychoanalytic education and discuss the ways in which empirical research can help guide the field. Finally, the epistemological debate between constructivist and objectivist positions is addressed as it tends to be an engaging topic for these students and further animates their curiosity.

With this in mind, I offer the following eight teaching domains with references that I have found most effective in developing a research curriculum across a range of settings:

1 Psychodynamic psychotherapy is an evidence-based treatment

Students at psychoanalytic institutes have invested significant time and money in their training. Showing them that psychodynamic psychotherapy is evidence-based relative to other evidence-based therapies (Shedler, 2010; Gerber et al., 2011; Thoma et al., 2012) bolsters their conviction and enthusiasm for what they are pursuing. In defining "evidence-based," this area covers some basic research concepts such as reliability; validity (i.e., construct, content, ecological and experimental); statistical vs. clinical significance; effect size; efficacy vs. effectiveness; and meta-analysis. This is also an opportunity to look critically at the biases against psychodynamic psychotherapy that students encounter in their graduate programs or work settings (Abbass et al., 2017) and some problems with how "evidence-based" is defined and proven in medicine (Shedler, 2015).

2 Empirical research speaks to the clinical setting

This topic is mostly devoted to issues related to scale development and how to operationalize psychoanalytic concepts while maintaining their conceptual validity and richness. I like to demonstrate this using scales that can measure psychoanalytically meaningful outcomes such as the Shedler Westen Assessment Procedure (Shedler & Westen, 2007), the Inventory of Interpersonal Problems (Salzer et al., 2010) and the Reflective Functioning Scale (Katznelson, 2014). We also examine measures of process such as the Psychotherapy Q-Sort (Ablon & Jones, 2005). The students always appreciate and enjoy reviewing these measures in detail, looking at some of the individual items to see how and where the clinical phenomena are captured.

3 Empirical research addresses clinical technique

Research on various specific techniques, such as transference interpretation (Høglend et al., 2008; Levy & Scala, 2012; Høglend, 2014), therapeutic alliance management (Safran, Muran & Eubanks-Carter, 2011; Hersoug et al.,

2013; Cameron, Rodgers & Dagnan, 2018), frequency and total number of sessions, and different analytic approaches (Waldron et al., 2013; Gazzillo et al., 2014) are presented. This is an opportunity to explore the value of process-outcome studies. One interesting example shows how outcome in CBT may be related more to psychodynamic strategies than to strict adherence to CBT protocol (Ablon, Levy & Smith-Hansen, 2011). The possible convergence of technique in the next wave of psychotherapy—based on these findings and those in affective neuroscience—and the use of unified protocols is considered (Allen, McHugh & Barlow, 2008). This topic prompts a look at the importance of adapting technique to clinical needs based on specific patient characteristics such as quality of object relations (Høglend, 2006; Blatt & Shahar, 2004). It eases the pressure to conform to strict analytic technique (i.e., transference interpretation as a gold standard intervention) and eases the shame associated with the invariable deviation from it.

4 A "systematic-empirical" approach encompasses different kinds of research: case study vs. population study

The robust debate (Hoffman, 2009, 2012; Eagle & Wolitzky, 2011; Aron, 2012; Safran, 2012; Fonagy, 2013) between constructivist and objectivist positions, sparked by Irwin Z. Hoffman's plenary address to the American Psychoanalytic Association in 2007 is the basis for this topic. Here I discuss the role and utility of idiographic and nomothetic approaches and how they complement each other to the benefit of the field (Blatt, Corveleyn, & Luyten, 2006). I invite a critical examination of the threats to validity in both types of studies and discuss the way in which the presentation of clinical data in classical analytic papers weakens their inferential power. Bias and distortion is examined more carefully, as well as how the scientific method attempts to redress them (Meehl, 1997).

5 Neuroscience is relevant to psychodynamic theory and technique

The emerging engagement of psychoanalysis with neuroscience is an exciting topic and there are a broad range of issues to choose from (Westen & Gabbard, 2002; Solms & Panksep, 2012; Van der Kolk, 2006; Schore, 2007; Porges, 2011; Geller & Porges, 2014; Lane et al., 2015). The key is demonstrating how neuroscience findings and neuroscientific theories are directly relevant to clinical technique. This often takes shape around attachment, affect, memory and interpersonal regulation, leading to discussions of analytic technique, including the use of the couch and the role of corrective emotional experiences. The significance and role of nonverbal communication and a careful examination of the trauma model are addressed.

6 Equivalence of outcome between different psychotherapy modalities (the dodo bird effect) and the role of common factors has real implications, but may challenge our allegiances

The finding that all bona fide psychotherapies are more or less equally effective (Steinert et al., 2017; Wampold et al., 1997; Budd & Hughes, 2009) leads to a consideration of which factors most influence outcome in psychotherapy. We discuss the finding that common factors account for a larger portion of the variance in outcome than do differences between individual treatment models (Laska, Gurman & Wampold, 2014; Wampold & Imel, 2015). I emphasize the relational aspects of these factors, such as alliance, collaboration and goal consensus, and therapist factors such as flexibility, empathy and transparency. I emphasize how these findings fundamentally support a psychoanalytic perspective on the importance of relationship in treatment (Norcross, 2002). We also look at other therapist variables (Lingiardi, Muzi, Tanzilli & Carone, 2018) such as attachment style and reflective function capacities (Bateman et al., 2018). At times these findings threaten a student's investment in the perceived superiority of psychoanalysis. In addressing this, I emphasize how a common factors model is not a one size fits all approach (Laska & Wampold, 2014) and that there are conceptual challenges to this model as well (de Felice et al. 2019).

7 Expertise research and deliberate practice findings are refreshing and offer the therapist a career-long path to improvement

It is a well-established finding that some therapists have better results than others. The area of research that studies the differences between highly effective therapists and others is a fruitful approach to training and skill acquisition (Tracey, Wampold, Lichtenberg & Goodyear, 2014; Miller, Hubble & Chow, 2018). The finding that there is no stable correlation between experience and expertise opens the door to a critical look at training models and what brings about expertise. The role of and nature of supervision, the use of session video recording, programs for measurement of clinical outcome and obtaining patient feedback are considered (Rousmaniere, Goodyear, Miller & Wampold, 2017). We discuss to what extent these elements are found in psychoanalytic training programs and why.

8 Research resources are available for ongoing learning

One of my main goals is to help students become future consumers of research. Here we consider ways in which clinicians and researchers can collaborate to address clinically valuable questions (Tasca et al., 2015; Tasca,

Grenon, Fortin-Langelier, & Chyurlia, 2014). Because there isn't time to teach research fluency, I offer instead resources that already synthesize and summarize research findings for them. In my view, the best resources for this are the PPRNet blog from the University of Ottawa and the IPA Open Door Review.

To conclude, teaching empirical research to psychoanalytic and psychodynamic therapy students is challenging, interesting and necessary for the future of our field and for students' clinical capacities and critical thinking. Knowledge generated by the scientific method, however limited, flawed, or subjectively constructed, remains our best approach to getting at the truth. A research orientation and exposure to empirical methods must be integrated into training to support an open, critical thinking stance and to free up the creativity of students (Kernberg, 2016). Research findings also have consequences for curricular frameworks (Gerber & Knopf, 2015). Training in psychoanalytic institutes should emphasize technique as it is known to relate to positive, psychoanalytically meaningful treatment outcomes. That means revising the curriculum from a theory focused, chronological and historical approach that always starts with Freud, to one that leads with, and focuses on, the most contemporary, empirically supported techniques and those psychoanalytic theories that underpin them.

References

Abbass, A., Luyten, P., Steinert, C., & Leichsenring, F. (2017). Bias toward psychodynamic therapy: Framing the problem and working toward a solution. *Journal of Psychiatric Practice, 23*(5), 361–365.

Ablon, S.J., & Jones, E.E. (2005). On analytic process. *Journal of the American Psychoanalytic Association, 53*(2), 541–568.

Ablon, J.S., Levy, R.A., & Smith-Hansen, L. (2011). The contributions of the psychotherapy process Q-set to psychotherapy research. *Research in Psychotherapy: Psychopathology, Process and Outcome,* 14–48.

Allen, L.B., McHugh, R.K., & Barlow, D.H. (2008). Emotional disorders: A unified protocol. In D.H. Barlow (Ed.), *Clinical handbook of psychological disorders: A step-by-step treatment manual* (pp. 216–249). New York, NY: The Guilford Press.

Aron, L. (2012). Rethinking "doublethinking": Psychoanalysis and scientific research—an introduction to a series. *Psychoanalytic Dialogues, 22*(6), 704–709.

Bateman, A., Campbell, C., Luyten, P., & Fonagy, P. (2018). A mentalization-based approach to common factors in the treatment of borderline personality disorder. *Current Opinion in Psychology, 21*, 44–49.

Blatt, S.J., Corveleyn, J., & Luyten, P. (2006). Minding the gap between positivism and hermeneutics in psychoanalytic research. *Journal of the American Psychoanalytic Association, 54*(2), 571–610.

Blatt, S.J., & Shahar, G. (2004). Psychoanalysis–With whom, for what, and how? Comparisons with psychotherapy. *Journal of the American Psychoanalytic Association, 52*(2), 393–447.

Budd, R., & Hughes, I. (2009). The Dodo Bird Verdict—controversial, inevitable and important: A commentary on 30 years of meta-analyses. *Clinical Psychology & Psychotherapy: An International Journal of Theory & Practice*, *16*(6), 510–522.

Cameron, S.K., Rodgers, J., & Dagnan, D. (2018). The relationship between the therapeutic alliance and clinical outcomes in cognitive behaviour therapy for adults with depression: A meta-analytic review. *Clinical Psychology & Psychotherapy*, *25*(3), 446–456.

de Felice, G., Giuliani, A., Halfon, S., Andreassi, S., Paoloni, G., & Orsucci, F.F. (2019). The misleading Dodo Bird verdict. How much of the outcome variance is explained by common and specific factors?. *New Ideas in Psychology*, *54*, 50–55.

Eagle, M.N., & Wolitzky, D.L. (2011). Systematic empirical research versus clinical case studies: A valid antagonism?. *Journal of the American Psychoanalytic Association*, *59*(4), 791–818.

Fonagy, P. (2013). There is room for even more doublethink: The perilous status of psychoanalytic research. *Psychoanalytic Dialogues*, *23*(1), 116–122.

Gazzillo, F., Waldron, S., Genova, F., Angeloni, F., Ristucci, C., & Lingiardi, V. (2014). An empirical investigation of analytic process: Contrasting a good and poor outcome case. *Psychotherapy*, *51*(2), 270.

Geller, S.M., & Porges, S.W. (2014). Therapeutic presence: Neurophysiological mechanisms mediating feeling safe in therapeutic relationships. *Journal of Psychotherapy Integration*, *24*(3), 178.

Gerber, A.J., Kocsis, J.H., Milrod, B.L., Roose, S.P., Barber, J.P., Thase, M.E., … & Leon, A.C. (2011). A quality-based review of randomized controlled trials of psychodynamic psychotherapy. *American Journal of Psychiatry*, *168*(1), 19–28.

Gerber, A., & Knopf, L. (2015). An empirically-based psychoanalytic curriculum. *Psychoanalytic Inquiry*, *35*(sup1), 115–123.

Hersoug, A.G., Høglend, P., Gabbard, G.O., & Lorentzen, S. (2013). The combined predictive effect of patient characteristics and alliance on long-term dynamic and interpersonal functioning after dynamic psychotherapy. *Clinical Psychology & Psychotherapy*, *20*(4), 297–307.

Hoffman, I.Z. (2009). Doublethinking our way to "scientific" legitimacy: The desiccation of human experience. *Journal of the American Psychoanalytic Association*, *57*(5), 1043–1069.

Hoffman, I.Z. (2012). Response to Safran: The development of critical psychoanalytic sensibility. *Psychoanalytic Dialogues*, *22*(6), 721–731.

Hoffman, I.Z. (2012). Response to Eagle and Wolitzky. *Journal of the American Psychoanalytic Association*, *60*(1), 105–120.

Høglend, P. (2014). Exploration of the patient–therapist relationship in psychotherapy. *American Journal of Psychiatry*, *171*(10), 1056–1066.

Høglend, P., Amlo, S., Marble, A., Bøgwald, K.P., Sorbye, O., Sjaastad, M.C., Heyerdahl, O. (2006). Analysis of the patient–therapist relationship in dynamic psychotherapy: An experimental study of transference interpretations. *American Journal of Psychiatry*, *163*(10), 1739–46.

Høglend, P., Bøgwald, K.P., Amlo, S., Marble, A., Ulberg, R., Sjaastad, M.C., … & Johansson, P. (2008). Transference interpretations in dynamic psychotherapy: Do they really yield sustained effects?. *American Journal of Psychiatry*, *165*(6), 763–771.

Katznelson, H. (2014). Reflective functioning: A review. *Clinical Psychology Review, 34*(2014), 107–117.

Kernberg, O.F. (2016). *Psychoanalytic education at the crossroads: Reformation, change and the future of psychoanalytic training.* New York: Routledge.

Lane, R.D., Ryan, L., Nadel, L., & Greenberg, L. (2015). Memory reconsolidation, emotional arousal, and the process of change in psychotherapy: New insights from brain science. *Behavioral and Brain Sciences, 38.*

Laska, K.M., Gurman, A.S., & Wampold, B.E. (2014). Expanding the lens of evidence-based practice in psychotherapy: A common factors perspective. *Psychotherapy, 51*(4), 467.

Laska, K.M., & Wampold, B.E. (2014). Ten things to remember about common factor theory. *Psychotherapy, 51*(4), 519–524.

Levy, K.N., & Scala, J. (2012). Transference, transference interpretations, and transference-focused psychotherapies. *Psychotherapy, 49*(3), 391.

Lingiardi, V., Muzi, L., Tanzilli, A., & Carone, N. (2018). Do therapists' subjective variables impact on psychodynamic psychotherapy outcomes? A systematic literature review. *Clinical Psychology & Psychotherapy, 25*(1), 85–101.

Meehl, P.E. (1997). Credentialed persons, credentialed knowledge. *Clinical Psychology: Science and Practice, 4*(2), 91–98.

Miller, S.D., Hubble, M.A., & Chow, D. (2018). The question of expertise in psychotherapy. *Journal of Expertise, 1,* 121–129.

Norcross, J.C. (2002). Empirically supported therapy relationships. *Psychotherapy Relationships that Work: Therapist Contributions and Responsiveness to Patients,* 3–16.

Pretsky, J.E., Aizaga, K., & Cherry, S. (2009). Analytic practice patterns among psychoanalytic institute graduates: A bicoastal comparison. *Journal of the American Psychoanalytic Association, 57*(2), 450.

Porges, S.W. (2011). *The polyvagal theory: neurophysiological foundations of emotions, attachment, communication, and self-regulation (Norton Series on Interpersonal Neurobiology).* New York: W.W. Norton & Company.

Rousmaniere, T., Goodyear, R.K., Miller, S.D., & Wampold, B.E. (Eds.). (2017). *The cycle of excellence: Using deliberate practice to improve supervision and training.* Hoboken, NJ: John Wiley & Sons.

Safran, J.D. (2012). Doublethinking or dialectical thinking: A critical appreciation of Hoffman's "doublethinking" critique. *Psychoanalytic Dialogues, 22*(6), 710–720.

Safran, J.D., Muran, J.C., & Eubanks-Carter, C. (2011). Repairing alliance ruptures. *Psychotherapy, 48*(1), 80.

Salzer, S., Leibing, E., Jakobsen, T., Rudolf, G., Brockmann, J., Eckert, J., … & Keller, W. (2010). Patterns of interpersonal problems and their improvement in depressive and anxious patients treated with psychoanalytic therapy. *Bulletin of the Menninger Clinic, 74*(4), 283–300.

Schore, A.N. (2007). Psychoanalytic research: Progress and process. Developmental affective neuroscience and clinical practice. *Psychologist-Psychoanalyst, 27*(3), 6–15.

Shedler, J. (2010). The efficacy of psychodynamic psychotherapy. *American psychologist, 65*(2), 98.

Shedler, J. (2015). Where is the evidence for "evidence-based" therapy?. *The Journal of Psychological Therapies in Primary Care, 4*(1), 47–59.

Shedler, J., & Westen, D. (2007). The Shedler–Westen assessment procedure (SWAP): Making personality diagnosis clinically meaningful. *Journal of Personality Assessment, 89*(1), 41–55.

Solms, M., & Panksepp, J. (2012). The "Id" knows more than the "Ego" admits: Neuropsychoanalytic and primal consciousness perspectives on the interface between affective and cognitive neuroscience. *Brain Sciences, 2*(2), 147–175.

Steinert, C., Munder, T., Rabung, S., Hoyer, J., & Leichsenring, F. (2017). Psycho-dynamic therapy: As efficacious as other empirically supported treatments? A meta-analysis testing equivalence of outcomes. *American Journal of Psychiatry, 174*(10), 943–953.

Thoma, N.C., Mckay, D., Gerber, A.J., Milrod, B.L., Edwards, A.R., & Kocsis, J.H. (2012). A quality-based review of randomized controlled trials of cognitive-behavioral therapy for depression: An assessment and metaregression. *American Journal of Psychiatry, 169*(1), 22–30. doi:10.1176/appi.ajp.2011.11030433.

Tasca, G. et al. (2015). What clinicians want: Findings from a psychotherapy practice research network survey. *Psychotherapy, 52*(1), 1–11.

Tasca, G., Grenon, R., Fortin-Langelier, B., & Chyurlia, L. (2014). Addressing chal-lenges and barriers to translating psychotherapy research into clinical practice: The development of a Psychotherapy Practice Research Network in Canada, *Canadian Psychology, 55*(33), 197–203.

Van der Kolk, B.A. (2006). Clinical implications of neuroscience research in PTSD. *Annals of the New York Academy of Sciences, 1071*(1), 277–293.

Waldron, S., Gazzillo, F., Genova, F., & Lingiardi, V. (2013). Relational and classical elements in psychoanalyses: An empirical study with case illustrations. *Psychoanalytic Psychology, 30*(4), 567.

Wampold, B.E., & Imel, Z.E. (2015). *The great psychotherapy debate: The evidence for what makes psychotherapy work.* New York: Routledge.

Wampold, B.E., Mondin, G.W., Moody, M., Stich, F., Benson, K., & Ahn, H.N. (1997). A meta-analysis of outcome studies comparing bona fide psychotherapies: Empirically," all must have prizes." *Psychological Bulletin, 122*(3), 203.

Westen, D., & Gabbard, G.O. (2002). Developments in cognitive neuroscience: II. Implications for theories of transference. *Journal of the American Psychoanalytic Associ-ation, 50*(1), 99–134.

Chapter 17

The role of critical thinking and research in psychoanalytic education

Morris N. Eagle

The debate regarding the enhancement of critical thinking and the integration of research findings, including those from related disciplines, into psychoanalytic training and education is not new. Many current critiques of psychoanalytic education and training practices echo previous disaffections. As far back as 1952, Glover wrote:

> It is scarcely to be expected that a student who has spent some years under the artificial and sometimes hothouse conditions of a training analysis and whose professional career depends on overcoming 'resistance' to the satisfaction of his training analyst, can be in a favorable position to defend his scientific integrity against his analyst's theory and practice....

Glover continues:

> An analyst, let us say, of established prestige and seniority, produces a paper advancing some new point of view or alleged discovery in the theoretical or clinical field. Given sufficient enthusiasm and persuasiveness, or even just plain dogmatism on the part of the author, the chances are that without any check, this view or alleged discovery will gain currency, will be quoted and re-quoted until it attains the status of an accepted conclusion. Some few observers who have been stimulated by the new idea may test it in their clinical practice. If they can corroborate it they will no doubt report the fact; but if they do not, or if they feel disposed to reject it this scientific "negative" is much less likely to be expressed, at any rate in public, and so, failing effective examination, the view is ultimately canonized with the sanctioning phrase "so and so has shown". In other words, an ipse dixit acquires the validity of an attested conclusion on hearsay evidence only.
>
> (p. 403)

It is humbling—and discouraging—to recognize that we continue to have the same debate, with few significant changes in psychoanalytic educational practices and habits of mind.

The impression one gets from much of the psychoanalytic literature is that whereas critical thinking as expressed, for example, in basing one's inferences on evidence, is a necessary and integral aspect of research and science, it is not central to the clinical situation, where the critical means of knowing and understanding are based largely on intuition and accessing one's countertransference reactions to the patient. Consider the following assertions regarding the use of countertransference (now understood as the totality of the analyst's feelings and thoughts) as a means of understanding the patient: "The thoughts and feelings which emerge [in the analyst] will be, precisely, those which did not emerge in the patient, the repressed and the unconscious" (Racker, 1968, p. 17).

Or:

There is a pragmatic value in assuming that even those thoughts and emotional experiences that clearly arise within the analyst from the analyst's own personal life and have seemingly little to do with the specific patient at hand—for example, when the analyst's personal life events intrude upon the hour to such an extent so as to encroach upon or even override his or her capacities to analyze effectively—can be presumed to have a patient-related component that contributes to their appearance in a given hour in a particular way.

(Levine, 1997, p. 48)

In addition, rather than appealing to evidence, including clinical evidence, to support one's clinical inferences, it is not uncommon to find instead references to authoritative figures (see Spence, 1990). If evidence is presented at all, it is often limited to illustrative self-selected clinical vignettes.

I am not arguing that one's countertransference reactions may not provide useful information about the patient as well as therapist–patient interaction. Indeed, it may. It may, however, provide more useful information about oneself than about the patient. Whether, however, one is justified in asserting that recognition of the usefulness of the analyst's countertransference constitutes the "common ground" that cuts across different psychoanalytic theories (Gabbard, 1995) or that one's countertransference reactions will be precisely what is repressed in the patient is another matter. Perhaps most important in the present context, an uncritical over reliance on countertransference as a means of learning about the patient may distract one from recognizing the need for corroborating evidence.

It seems clear that, as Kernberg (2000; 2006; 2012) has cogently argued over many years, if psychoanalysis is to survive, there need to be changes in the nature of training and education. Let me turn more directly to the question of the role of research in psychoanalytic education and training. First, one needs to clarify what one means by research. Too often, a negative attitude toward research is fed by the implicit assumption to the effect that research equals experimental design and quantitative data. Although a good deal of systematic research is, indeed, based on experimental design and quantitative data, broadly understood, research also includes naturalistic studies, N of 1 designs, cross-over designs, qualitative studies, mixed designs, use of quasi-experimental design for clinical data, and disciplined case studies.

With regard to this last point, it has been argued (e.g., Hoffman, 2009) that case studies merit the same epistemological status as large scale quantitative studies employing experimental designs. I have some sympathy for this point of view, with the important caveat that large scale quantitative projects and case studies serve different epistemological purposes and aims (see Eagle and Wolitzky, 2011). However, the fact is that despite the defense of case studies as a legitimate means of gaining knowledge, one finds few disciplined case studies in the psychoanalytic literature. Instead, as noted, one generally finds theoretical formulations and assertions accompanied by presumably illustrative self-selected clinical vignettes intended to support a particular theoretical and/or clinical point of view.

In 1991, the American Psychoanalytic Association Committee headed by Klumpner and Frank reviewed the 60 most frequently referenced "psychoanalytic articles" that had been published in three prominent journals between 1969 and 1982 and scrutinized the top 15. They reported that

> [n]ot a single one of these 15 papers included any significant amount of ordinary clinical data. Our sample contained no case studies. What evidence was given in support of the conclusions could only be described as sketchy. We found no verbatim examples and only one dream fragment.... Our most frequent description of the 15 papers were, "no clinical data," "no evidence," "overgeneralized" or "assumptions not testable."
>
> (as cited in Portuges, 1994, p. 12)

There have been attempts to identify and recommend standards for the case study method that would enhance its comprehensiveness, clinical usefulness, reliability and validity (e.g., Edelson, 1985; Eagle & Wolitzky, 2011). However, these attempts have had little impact on papers published in psychoanalytic journals. In short, little has changed since the Klumpner and Frank (1991) report.

In arguing for the importance of integrating research and research findings into psychoanalytic education, I am not suggesting a hagiographic and uncritical attitude toward research. That would be as unwise as the other extreme of total neglect of research findings. As Kazdin (2006), a prominent researcher himself, has written, much experimental research lacks robust ecological validity, that is, relevance to phenomena in the real world. Also, as has been aired as a public issue, many research findings in a range of disciplines are not successfully replicated. In short, research is a fallible human activity. However, although seemingly paradoxical, it is primarily critical thinking, a research attitude, and the use of research methods that has uncovered and identified the factors and problems that have distorted and corrupted research findings and that point to necessary correctives. In short, although subject to human fallibility, the internalization of scientific habits of mind and the use of scientific methods constitute the most reliable means of dealing with our fallibility.

To repeat, endorsing the importance of an expanded role for research in psychoanalytic education does not mean that research findings should be unquestioned and treated as gospel. They are as subject to critical evaluation as is clinical inference. The difference, however, is that whereas research training attempts to develop values and habits of mind characterized by critical thinking and accountability to evidence—even if, as we have seen, such thinking and values can be corrupted—psychoanalytic training and education as it is currently constituted tends to develop habits of mind too much characterized by appeal to authority, loyalty to this or that psychoanalytic "school" and somewhat idiosyncratic and questionable means of gaining knowledge and understanding.

I am aware that psychoanalytic candidates are not likely to become researchers—and that is as it should be. However, they do need to be educated to become intelligent research consumers who can make critical and open-minded judgments regarding the value and ecological validity of research findings. I want to add that, in my view, this is not best achieved by introducing separate courses on formal research design and statistical methods. I have been teaching in and/or directing doctoral programs in clinical psychology for many years and the pattern that I have repeatedly observed is that what is learned in these courses is simply not retained once the courses are completed. And remember, this pattern is common for Ph.D. students who are presumably being trained to do research. Thus, rather than offer separate courses on research methods, the inclusion of research findings and issues as an integral component of ongoing psychoanalytic courses is far more likely to contribute to the development of critical thinking and interest in research.

In contrast to the past, we now have a cadre of talented psychoanalytic researchers, working mainly in the area of process and outcome psychotherapy research, whose findings, however, are largely unrepresented in psychoanalytic education. And when research findings are referred to at all, they tend to be selectively cited in order to make a public relations case for the effectiveness of psychodynamic or psychoanalytic psychotherapy. I recall an experience during the time that I was President of the Division of Psychoanalysis (Division 39) of the American Psychological Association. Although there was generally little interest in research among most of the members and officers of Division 39, a sudden apparent interest in research emerged in reaction to a spate of published criticisms launched against the lack of evidence for the effectiveness of psychoanalytic treatment. A number of Division 39 officers proposed the formation of a committee whose task was to amass all the evidence available demonstrating the effectiveness of psycho-dynamic and psychoanalytic treatment. For the most part, the attitude toward research of individuals making this proposal generally ranged from indifference to hostility; it had been turned to only for its demonstration and public relations value. There is something unseemly about, on the one hand, taking the position that psychotherapy research is irrelevant to psychoanalysis and to psychoanalytic education and, at the same time, turning to it for its public relations value.

There are, indeed, features of some research methods that limit the applicability and relevance of research findings to the clinical situation and to clinical phenomena. Many research studies, including psychotherapy research studies, report the statistical significance of differences between conditions on particular measures. For example, the outcome of a particular therapeutic approach may be compared with the outcome of a control condition or, the outcomes of two different therapeutic approaches may be compared with each other. Although other more sophisticated designs are employed, this design of testing the statistical differences between means has been a mainstay in much research.

Clinicians, including psychoanalytic candidates, have correctly observed that general research findings, such as reports of mean differences in outcomes, are often not very helpful in understanding and working with individual cases. For one thing, statistically significant findings do not necessarily translate to clinical significance. Often, effect sizes in therapeutic outcome are so small that, although statistically significant, they have virtually no practical clinical significance. Also, significant differences between two conditions does not mean that *every* member in Condition A behaves in one same way and that *every* member of Condition B behaves in another different way. The fact is that some members in Condition A will behave in a *similar way* to some members of Condition B. Thus, as a clinician reading such studies, you have no reliable way of knowing where to place your individual patient. Hence, whereas research findings of this sort are potentially useful in adding to the store of the clinician's background information, they are often not especially useful in guiding clinical work with individual patients.

One of the ways of at least partly ameliorating this problem is obtaining individual difference measures and reporting not just main effects (i.e., differences between conditions A and B), but also *interaction effects*, that is, interactions between individual difference variables and outcomes. Let me illustrate by describing a longitudinal study by Dodge and his colleagues (e.g., Dodge, 2006; Weiss, Dodge, Bates, & Pettit, 1992). They reported that compared to young adults who were not physically punished as children (Group A), young adults who were physically punished as children (Group B) showed more hostility and aggression. This is a mildly interesting, but not unexpected main effect finding. The more interesting and informative finding was that the differences in young adult aggressive behavior between Groups A and B were mainly due to those members of Group B who had developed a "hostile attributional style." In other words, there was a significant interaction effect. That is, the development of a hostile attributional style *interacting* with early physical punishment tends to lead to greater young adult aggressive behavior.

This is a far more interesting finding than simply knowing mean differences between groups. For one thing, based only on main effects, one might promulgate the incomplete, over-simplified, and therefore somewhat misleading conclusion, that physical punishment in childhood leads to aggressive behavior in young adulthood. Second, the interaction findings generate further important questions to be investigated, including the question of the factors involved in explaining why only a subgroup of those subject to physical punishment in childhood develop a hostile attributional style. Third, these interaction findings suggest processes that mediate between early physical punishment and later aggressive behavior. Fourth, one would want to know how many individuals in the non-physically punished in childhood group developed a hostile attributional style and whether they, too, developed aggressive behavior. And finally, the inclusion of individual difference interaction effects is one step in rendering research findings somewhat more relevant to the clinician insofar as they are descriptive of smaller subgroups of individuals. It is important to note, particularly in the present context, that unless the Dodge study had included an individual differences variable, in this case, the development of a hostile attributional style, we would not know that it mediates the relationship between early physical punishment and aggressive behavior in young adulthood.

The lesson here is that productive research is likely to include both experimental design, that is comparisons between experimental and control conditions, as well as relevant measures of individual differences. This issue is the focus of a classic 1957 paper entitled "The two disciplines of scientific psychology", the American Psychological Association Presidential address given by Cronbach. The paper addresses the issues underlying the tensions between two different research approaches, which, interestingly enough, parallel the issues that generate tension between clinician and researcher. Although Cronbach's paper was published in 1957, it has much to tell us today.

The two disciplines to which Cronbach refers are "experimental psychology" and "correlational psychology" (p. 671). Cronbach writes that in the discipline of experimental psychology, "the experimental method [is one in which] the scientist changes conditions in order to observe their consequences ..." and where "the experimenter is interested only in the variation that he himself creates" (p. 671). Contrastingly, in the correlational psychology approach, the researcher "finds his interest in the already existing variation between individuals ..." (p. 671). Whereas the experimenter wants to "discover the general laws of mind or behavior", the correlational psychologist is "concerned with individual minds" (p. 673). Cronbach continues: "Just as individual differences are a source of embarrassment to the experimenter, so treatment variation attenuates the results of the correlator" (p. 674). The combination of main effects and interaction effects essentially constitutes the employment of both the experimental and correlational research methods.

Insofar as the experimental researcher is mainly interested "in the variation he himself creates", that is, in the question of differences in outcome in two different groups, ordinary psychotherapy outcome research, which is concerned with comparing outcomes between two different conditions, employs an experimental method. In this approach, there is no interest in "existing variation" within either group. Indeed, in order to test the statistical significance of differences between the means of the two groups on a particular outcome, one needs to assume that the variance in each group (i.e., the individual differences within each group) is approximately the same and that the individuals in the two groups do not systematically differ on any relevant variables (e.g., age; socioeconomic status; level or type of pathology, gender, etc.) other than in the conditions manipulated in the experiment (e.g., being a patient in therapy approach A versus in therapy approach B). In short, in the experimental approach, individual differences are treated as variables to be controlled rather than systematically investigated.

In a purely correlational study, the focus would be on individual differences *within* a given condition. For example, one might want to investigate the relationship between individual differences in age, level or type of pathology, defensive style, attachment pattern—all "existing variations" between individuals—and outcome in regard to a particular therapeutic approach. Thus, whereas in the experimental approach, individual differences are treated as "noise" or error variance, in the correlational approach the individual differences that already exist constitute the primary data that are correlated with outcome. For example, one might find that patients with personality features X have better outcome in approach A, whereas patients with personality features Y have better outcomes in therapy approach B. Cronbach (1957) writes that "In general, unless one treatment is clearly best for everyone, treatments should be differentiated in such a way as to maximize their interaction with aptitude variables" (p. 681). Cronbach makes this comment in the context of discussing educational interventions—hence, the reference to "aptitude variables". However, his comment is entirely applicable to the therapeutic context, where one would refer not to "aptitude variables", but to personality or diagnostic variables.

Consider recent studies by Hoglend et al. (2006, 2007, 2008) which reported no significant differences in therapeutic outcome as a function of presence or absence of transference interpretations. That is, there were no main outcome effects with regard to presence or absence of transference interpretations. However, there were interaction effects such that the effects of transference interpretations on outcome interacted with the patient's level of object relational functioning. Contrary to clinical wisdom, patients with low levels of object relationships benefited from transference interpretations, whereas patients with high levels of object relations did not.

However, this is not the end, but only the beginning of a story in which successive research projects in a research program address questions and issues raised by the previous research projects. For example, a clinician might note that the Hoglend studies do not tell us anything about the influence of the content or timing of transference interpretations on outcome (see Hobson & Kapur, 2010), and whether these factors interact with specific individual difference variables, questions of considerable clinical significance. The clinician would be quite correct in raising these issues. However, a research program sensitive to ecological validity would be equally interested in addressing these questions. Thus, there is a convergence here between clinical and research interests. The point is that the more the research program zeroes in on questions generated by successive research studies, the greater and more specific their relevance to clinical work. Put more broadly, one can say that the greater the number of individual difference variables studied in an ongoing research program, the less the difference between ideographic and nomothetic approaches and the less gap between researcher and clinician.

An example of an approach that serves to narrow the gap between clinician and researcher is a recent study by Silberschatz (2017), who argues against what he refers to as the "homogeneity assumption" made in much psychotherapy research, that is, the assumption that all patients within a given diagnostic category are homogeneous and that all interventions within a given therapeutic modality are homogeneous. The results of the Silberschatz study show that the compatibility of therapist interventions with *specific* patient characteristics and problems (i.e., the nature of their core pathogenic beliefs) was robustly related to therapeutic outcome.

Influenced by the development of personalized medicine, and similar to the Silberschatz study, a recent program of research that also narrows the gap between clinician and researcher, has attempted to identify the particular treatment approach to depression that is likely to lead to a better outcome for a given patient (Cohen & Rubeis, 2018). In one such research approach, each patient receives a Personalized Advantage Index (PAI) score based on a number of pre-treatment variables (e.g., marital status, life events, comorbid personality disorder). An important finding is that the patient's PAI score identifies the treatment approach (e.g., cognitive behavior therapy [CBT] versus interpersonal therapy), which, based on past research, is predicted to produce better outcome for a given patient. An important finding is that when patients were randomly assigned to a treatment approach that, based on their PAI score, is judged to be optimal, they show better outcome than when assigned to a treatment approach that, based on their PAI score, is judged to be non-optimal (Huibers, Cohen, Lemmens, Arntz, Peters et al., 2015).

It seems to me that clinicians need to be aware of such findings, which suggest that one size does not fit all, that is, that a particular therapeutic modality, including a psychoanalytic or psychodynamic modality, will not necessarily constitute the optimal treatment for all patients. One cannot assume that the approach in which one was trained is necessarily the optimal treatment for any given patient. Further, in order to make a judgment regarding what is likely to be an optimal treatment for a given patient, one needs to be aware of the above kind of findings and have at least some working knowledge of available treatment modalities. As far as I am aware, psychoanalytic institutes offer little or no information regarding non-psychoanalytic treatment approaches. Given the above findings, this state of affairs does not seem defensible.

It is important to note that just as one cannot assume homogeneity among patients, one cannot also assume homogeneity among therapists within a given therapeutic modality, manuals notwithstanding. As I have noted elsewhere (Eagle, 2018), a number of studies have shown that differences between therapists' effects on outcome are consistently greater than differences between treatment effects (e.g., Luborsky et al., 1985; Wampold, 2001). Indeed, in one study, "the therapists whose clients showed the fastest rate of improvement had an average rate of change 10 times greater than the mean for that sample" (Okiishi et al., 2003, p. 373). Consider also Kim et al.'s (2006) report of the results of a re-analysis of data from the NIMH Treatment of Depression Collaborative Research Program. They report that about 8% of the variance in outcomes was attributable to therapists, whereas 0% was attributable to type of treatment. There is a growing body of research demonstrating striking differences in therapeutic outcome among different therapists that cut across different therapeutic modalities that need to be included in psychoanalytic training and education.

Psychotherapy is not a disembodied process. It is carried out by individual therapists who differ on many dimensions. Thus, in comparing treatments, the ecologically valid unit of study is not simply different therapeutic approaches, but different therapeutic interventions carried out in particular ways by different therapists with varying personality characteristics and abilities working with different patients also with varying personality characteristics, etc.

As Dr. Goodman (this volume) notes in her chapter, one should expect resistance to radical change, a resistance that is based, at least in large part, on fear of losing one's psychoanalytic identity and ego ideal as well as fear of compromising one's psychoanalytic values. These concerns cannot be dismissed or minimized and must be dealt with in a constructive way. I must admit that I do not have any easy way of dealing with this problem beyond the practical step of an ongoing dialogue between clinician and researcher, one in which the clinician's legitimate concerns with clinical relevance and more broadly, with ecological validity are recognized and taken into account by the researcher.

However, in my view, what is ultimately required is a revamping of psychoanalytic education in which research findings, critical thinking, clinical insights and formulations, as well as insights from other disciplines are integrated into every course and every aspect of training; and in which the general aim is increasing awareness of and connection with other perspectives rather than nurture a fantasy of splendid isolation. There is no point minimizing the degree to which such revamping entails nothing less than challenging psychoanalytic culture and certain habits of mind. The specific challenges facing the possibility of change include the realities that many psychoanalytic candidates are simply not interested in research and view research as irrelevant and even antithetical to their primary goal of learning how to carry out treatment; that the candidates' negatively tinged attitudes toward research is mirrored by the majority of faculty at many psychoanalytic institutes; and that candidates are far more shaped and influenced by their training analyst and supervisors than by any course work.

Perhaps confrontation with the fears identified by Dr. Goodman can provide an opportunity for us to re-think the nature of our psychoanalytic identity and psychoanalytic values. Failure to confront the need for change is likely to result in a thoroughly marginalized status for psychoanalysis, whereas confronting the need for change provides an opportunity for continued integration and growth.

References

Cohen, Z.D., & DeRubeis, R.J. (2018). Treatment selection in depression. *Annual Review of Clinical Psychology, 14*, 209–236.

Cronbach, l. (1957). The two disciplines of scientific psychology. *American Psychologist, 12*(11), 671–684.

Eagle, M.N. (2018). *Core concepts in contemporary psychoanalysis: Clinical, research evidence and conceptual critiques.* New York: Routledge.

Eagle, M.N., & Wolitzky, D.L. (2011). Systematic empirical research versus clinical case studies: A valid antagonism? *Journal of the American Psychoanalytic Association, 59*(4), 791–818.

Edelson, M. (1985). *Hypothesis and evidence in psychoanalysis.* Chicago: University of Chicago Press.

Gabbard, G. (1995). Countertransference: The emerging common ground. *International Journal of Psychoanalysis, 76*, 475–485.

Glover, E. (1952). Research methods in psychoanalysis. *International Journal of Psychoanalysis, 33*, 403–409.

Hobson, R.P., & Kapur, R. (2010). Working in the transference: Clinical and research perspectives. *Psychology and Psychotherapy: Theory, Research and Practice, 78*(3).

Hoffman, I.Z. (2009). Doublethinking our way to "Scientific" legitimacy: The desiccation of human experience. *Journal of the American Psychoanalytic Association, 57*, 1043–1069.

Hoglend, P., Amlo, S., Marble, A. Bogwald, K.-P., Sorbye, O. Jaastad, M.C., & Heyerdaahl, G. (2006). Analysis of the patient-therapist relationship in dynamic psychotherapy: An experimental study of transference interpretations. *American Journal of Psychiatry, 164*(10), 97–120.

Hoglend, P., Bogwald, K.P., Amlo, S., Marble, A., Ulberg, R., Sjassted, M.C., & Johansson, P. (2008). Transference interpretations in dynamic psychotherapy: Do they really yield sustained effects? *American Journal of Psychiatry*, *65*, (6), 763–771.

Hoglend, P., Johansson, P., Marble, A., & Bogwald, K.P., & Amlo, S. (2007). Mediators of the effects of transference interpretations in brief dynamic psychotherapy. *Psychotherapy Research*, *17*, 2, 162–174.

Huibers, M.J.H., Cohen, Z.D., Lemmens, LHJm … DeRubeis, R.J. (2015). Predicting optimal outcomes in cognitive therapy or interpersonal psychotherapy for depressed individuals using the Personalized Advantage Index approach. *PLOS/One* https://doi.org/10.1371/journal.pone.0140771

Kazdin, A. (2006). Arbitrary metrics: Implications for identifying evidence-based treatment. *American Psychologist*, *61*, 42–49.

Kernberg, O.F. (2000). A concerned critique of psychoanalytic education. *International Journal of Psychoanalysis*, *81*(1), 97–120.

Kernberg, O.F. (2006). The pressing need to increase research in and on psychoanalysis. *International Journal of Psychoanalysis*, *87*(4), 919–926.

Kernberg, O.F. (2012). Suicide prevention for psychoanalytic institutes and societies. *Journal of the American Psychoanalytic Association*, *60*, 707–719.

Kim, D.M., Wamplod, B.E., & Bolt, D.M. (2006). Therapist effects in psychotherapy: A random-effects modeling of the National Institute of Mental Health treatment of depression collaborative research program data. *Psychotherapy Research*, *16*(2), 161–172.

Klumpner, G.H., & Frank, A. (1991). On methods of reporting clinical material. *Journal of the American Psychoanalytic Association*, *39*, 537–551

Levine, W.B. (1997). The capacity for countertransference. *Psychoanalytic Inquiry*, *17*(1), 44–68.

Okiishi, J., Lambert, M.J., Nielsen, S.L., & Ogles, B.J. (2003). Waiting for supershrink: An empirical analysis of therapist effects. *Clinical Psychology & Psychotherapy*, *10*(5), 361–373.

Portuges, S. (1994). Knowledge knots: Problems of psychoanalytic research in clinical psychoanalysis. Paper presented at annual meeting of American Psychological Association. Washington, DC.

Racker, H. (1968). *Transference and countertransference*. Madison, CT: International Universities Press.

Silberschatz, G. (2017). Improving the yield of psychotherapy research. *Psychotherapy Research*, *27*(1), 1–13.

Spence, D.P. (1990). *The rhetorical voice of psychoanalysis: Displacement of evidence by theory*. Cambridge, MA: Harvard University Press.

Weiss, B., Dodge, K.A., Bates, J.E., & Pettit, G.S. (1992). Some consequences of early harsh discipline: Child aggression and a maladaptive information processing style. *Child Development*, *63*(6), 1321–1335.

Index

Page numbers in **bold** denote tables, those in *italics* denote figures.

effectiveness of; RCTs (randomized controlled trials)
outcome, terminology of 15, 41

PAI (Personalized Advantage Index) 256
pain, chronic 112
panic disorder 107; *see also* anxiety disorders
panic instinct 27
Panksepp, J. 33n3
Passett, Peter 9
PAT (psychoanalytic long-term therapy): LAC Study 138, 141–2, 143, 148, 151, *151*, 152–3, *153*, 154–5, 156, 157, 158, **159**, 166
patients: exclusion from outcome research 49; factors contributing to change 89–90; values and preferences 53
PDT (psychodynamic psychotherapy) 211; allegiance factor in 129; as an evidence-based treatment 242; anxiety disorders **102–3**, 107–10, 118, 119, 129; avoidant personality disorder **105**, 117; BPD (borderline personality disorder) **104–5**, 114–16, 118; Cluster C personality disorders **105**, 116–17, 118; definition of PDT 100–1; depressive disorders **102**, **103**, 106–7, 110, 118, 129; eating disorders **103–4**, 112–13, 119, 129; equivalency testing 130; internet-guided self-help 107; mixed personality disorders **105**, 117–18, 118–19, 129; pathological grief 107, 118; PDT models 101; PTSD (posttraumatic stress disorder) 110–11, 118, 129; qualities of studies included in research 128–9; RCT studies 99–120; role of emotions in 207–8; somatoform disorders **103**, 111–12, 118; substance-related disorders **104**, 113–14, 118, 129; teaching of empirical research in 238–45; Wolfe's clinical discussion of 128–34; *see also* LRNG (Lane, Ryan, Nadel, and Greenburg) model of change
Penn State Worry Questionnaire 108
personality disorders 17, **105**, 117–18, 118–19, 129; AVDP (avoidant personality disorder) **105**, 117; Cluster

C personality disorders **105**, 116–17, 118, 208, 209; impact of emotional experiencing on treatment outcomes 208; and maladaptive affect regulation 218, 221; *see also* BPD (borderline personality disorder)
personality organization, and BPD 177–8
personality theory 68
Personalized Advantage Index (PAI) 256
personalized medicine 40, 256
person-centred approach 16
Peterson, Bradley 1
physical punishment, impact of on children 253–4
Physiological Institute 3
Piper, W.E. 107
Plänkers, T. 7
play instinct 28
Plötzl, Otto 4
pluralism 216–18, 231, 233, 234
Pontalis, J.-B. 219
population studies, and empirical research 243
Porcellana, M. 110
Porcerelli, J. 77
Portuges, S. 251
postmodernism 10
posttraumatic stress disorder *see* PTSD (posttraumatic stress disorder)
PPRNet blog, University of Ottawa 245
predictions, automatization of 28–9, 29–30
Pretsky, Joshua 19–20, 231, 238–48
process research *see* psychotherapy process research
process-outcome research 58
prolonged exposure therapy 50
psychic life, starting of 219
psychoanalysis: as an independent discipline 3; attacks on in evidence-based medicine era 11–12; effectiveness of 26, 30–2, 53, 58, 90–1, 136–7, 174; healthful effects of 132–3; historical overview 2–12; loss of importance of in medicine 10–11; marginalization of 10; origins of 2–5; scientific basis of 26–32; and scientific research 57–8; traumatic history of Nazi period 5; values in 236–7; *see also* PDT (psychodynamic psychotherapy)

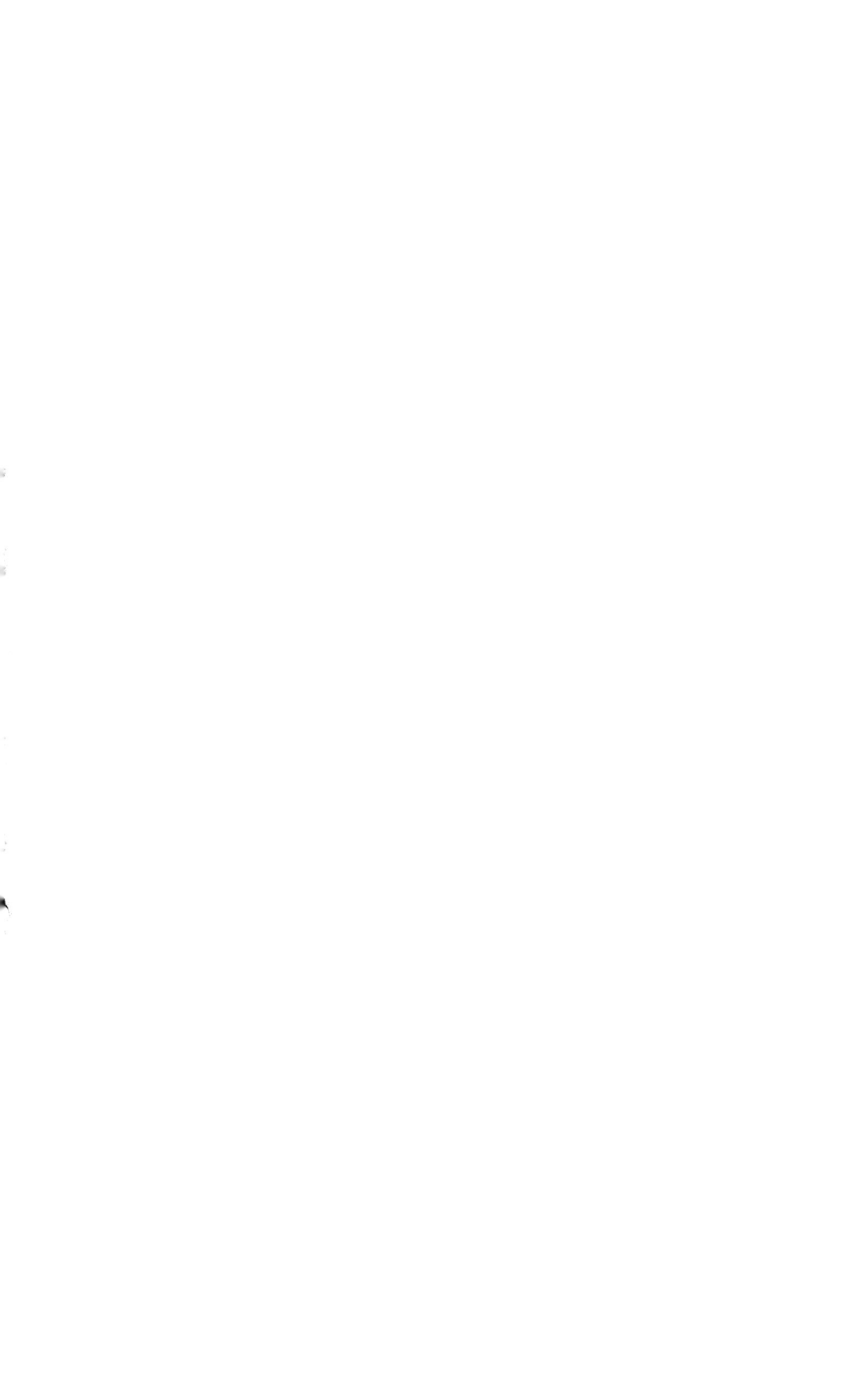

For Product Safety Concerns and Information please contact our EU
representative GPSR@taylorandfrancis.com
Taylor & Francis Verlag GmbH, Kaufingerstraße 24, 80331 München, Germany

www.ingramcontent.com/pod-product-compliance
Lightning Source LLC
Chambersburg PA
CBHW060346220326
41598CB00023B/2820